Trance and Healing in Southeast Asia Today

Trance and Healing
in
Southeast Asia Today

Ruth-Inge Heinze

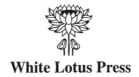

White Lotus Press

© 1997 by Ruth-Inge Heinze. All rights reserved.
Published 1988, First edition
Second revised and expanded edition, 1997

White Lotus Co., Ltd
G.P.O. Box 1141
Bangkok 10501
Thailand

Tel. (662) 332-4915, 741-6288-9
Fax (662) 311-4575, 741-6287
Internet: ande@loxinfo.co.th

Printed in Thailand
Typeset by COMSET Limited Partnership

Library of Congress Cataloging-in-Publication Data

Ruth-Inge Heinze
Trance and healing in Southeast Asia today

Bibliography: p.
Includes index.

    1. Shamanism-Asia, Southeastern. 2. Shamans-Asia, Southeastern. 3. Mediums-Asia, Southeastern. 4. Healers — Asia, Southeastern. 5. Healing-Asia, Southeastern. 6. Spirit possession-Asia, Southeastern. 7. Asia, Southeastern — Religious life and customs.
I. Title, II. Ruth-Inge Heinze
BL2370.S5H42 1988 306!.6 87-37256

ISBN 974-8496-59-7 pbk.   White Lotus Co., Ltd.; Bangkok
ISBN 1-879155-64-8 pbk.   White Lotus Co., Ltd.; Cheney

Contents

List of Illustrations		ix
Acknowledgements		xiii
Introduction		xv
1.	The Split Between Science and Religion	xv
2.	Research Tools and Questions	xvi
3.	Fieldwork	xviii
	Notes to Introduction	xxiii

Part 1
Theoretical Considerations

Chapter 1	Who Is a Shaman?	3
1.1.	Definition	3
1.2.	Historical Development of Shamanism	8
1.3.	Is Shamanism an Elementary Form of the Religious Life?	11
Chapter 2	The Social Setting	15
2.1.	Thailand	15
2.2.	Malaysia	17
2.3.	Singapore	20
2.4.	The Complexity of Interlocking Social Systems	22
Chapter 3	Elements of Shamanism	33
3.1.	The Shaman	33
3.1.1.	Field data	33
3.1.2.	Belief Systems	33
3.1.3.	Age	34
3.1.4.	Gender	34
3.1.5.	Occupation	35
3.1.6.	Socio-economic Status	35

Contents

3.1.7.	Character	35
3.1.8.	Differences Between Thailand, Malaysia, and Singapore:	37
3.1.8.1.	Thailand	37
3.1.8.2.	Malaysia	40
3.1.8.3.	Singapore	40
3.1.8.3.1.	Taoist priests	40
3.1.8.3.2.	Shamans, mediums and healers	41
3.1.9.	How Does One Become a Shaman?	42
3.1.9.1.	Hereditary	42
3.1.9.2.	Revelations or visions	42
3.1.9.3.	Decision	42
3.1.10.	Preparation	43
3.1.10.1.	Solely advised by spiritual entities	43
3.1.10.2.	Formal training	43
3.1.11.	Initiation and Change of Life Style	43
3.1.12.	Reasons to Continue	45
3.1.12.1.	Altruistic	45
3.1.12.2.	Gain in status	45
3.1.12.3.	Other reasons	46
3.1.12.4.	Exploited by others	46
3.2.	Entourage (see also, introduction, footnote 7)	46
3.2.1.	Characteristics	46
3.2.2.	Functions	48
3.3.	Clients	49
3.3.1.	Characteristics	49
3.3.2.	How Do Clients Meet Shamans, Mediums, and Healers?	50
3.3.3.	When Are Shamans, Mediums, and Healers Consulted?	50
3.4.	Shamanic Performances	52
3.4.1.	Operational Base	52
3.4.2.	Paraphernalia	53
3.4.3.	Varieties of Trances	58
3.4.4.	When Trances Are Used	71
3.5.	Nature of Spiritual Beings	72
3.6.	Interethnic Overlap	89

Chapter 4 Socio-Psychological Considerations
4.1.	Introduction	93

4.2.	Belief in and Knowledge of Modern Medicine	102
4.3.	Belief in and Knowledge of Traditional Medicine	103
4.4.	Belief in and Knowledge of the Divine Source	107
4.5.	Are Shamans, Mediums, and Healers Beyond Criticism?	109
4.6.	What Are the Implications for Other Social Systems?	111

Part 2
Shamanic Practices: A Case History Approach

Case 1	A 39-year-old Housewife Becomes Possessed By a Deified General From the Three Kingdoms (Singapore Chinese)	125
Case 2	An Altar in Search of a Shaman and a Shaman in Search of an Altar (Singapore Indian)	129
Case 3	How Contacts to Mediums Develop (Singapore Chinese)	132
Case 4	How I Became a Medium (Singapore Chinese)	135
Case 5	How I Became A Medium (Singapore Chinese)	136
Case 6	Testimony of a Father about the Possession and Exorcism of His Son (Singapore Chinese)	140
Case 7	The Nine Imperial Gods in Singapore (Singapore Chinese)	146
Case 8	Automatic Writing In Singapore (Singapore Chinese)	164
Case 9	Glossolalia in Singapore (Singapore Chinese and Malay)	178
Case 10	Kuda Kepang: Horse Possession (Singapore Malay)	182
Case 11	A Male Muslim Bomoh in Singapore (Malay)	186
Case 12	A Female Muslim Bomoh in Singapore (Malay)	188
Case 13	Main Puteri Performed by a Muslim Shaman in Kelantan (Malay)	189
Case 14	One Female and Six Male Muslim Bomohs in Pattani, Thailand (Thai-Malay)	192
Case 15	A Brahmin Shaman in Bangkok (Thai)	198
Case 16	The Wife of Brahmā: Phrom Mali (Central Thai)	201
Case 17	The Divine Sages: Pu Sawan (Central Thai)	203
Case 18	Calling Phra Narai (Central Thai)	215
Case 19	Spirit Dances in Chiang Mai (Northern Thai)	217
Case 20	One Lineage of Spirit Mediums in Chiang Mai (Northern Thai)	221
Case 21	A Meo Shamaness (Northern Thai Hill Tribe)	225
Summary		226

Contents

Appendix 1	Chinese Terms Used in the Text	231
Appendix 2	Malay Terms Used in the Text	237
Appendix 3	Indian Terms Used in the Text	243
Appendix 4	Thai Terms Used in the Text	247
Appendix 5	Chinese Festivals	251
Appendix 6	Malay-Muslim Fextivals	255
Appendix 7	Hindu, Mainly Tamil, Festivals	257
Appendix 8	Thai Festivals	259
Notes		261
Glossary		271
Bibliography		303
Index		331

List of Illustrations

Figures

1	Kavadi carrier (Thaipusam), Singapore	25
2	Kavadi carrier (Thaipusam), Singapore	25
3	Overcome by ecstasy, Thandayuthapani Temple, Singapore	25
4	Preparations for fire walking (Timiti), Sri Mariamman Temple, Singapore	25
5	Preparations for fire walking (Timiti), Sri Mariamman Temple, Singapore	26
6	The God (Rāma) speaks, Snake Temple, Sembawang Shipyard, Singapore	26
7	Chinese medium in trance on a spike chair, after having consumed large portions of alcohol and opium, near Ord Bridge, Singapore	26
8	Chinese medium in trance on a spike chair, Ganges Road, Singapore	27
9	Chinese medium in trance, near Upper Thomson Road, Singapore	27
10	Chinese medium cooking food for a temple festival, near Upper Thomson Road, Singapore	28
11	Entourage, assisting clients, near Upper Thomson Road, Singapore	28
12	Altar of a house temple, near Upper Thomson Road, Singapore	29
13	Small shrine under a tree, ball-bearing factory, Jurong, Singapore	29
14	New shrine, ball-bearing factory, Jurong, Singapore	30
15	Using the mu bei in front of the factory shrine, Jurong, Singapore	30
16	Chinese medium blessing clients, near Upper Serangoon Road, Singapore	31
17	Chinese mediums exorcising a school, Singapore	31
18	Spike ball used by a Chinese medium, Pegu Road, Singapore	32

List of Illustrations

19	A Sea Goddess speaks through a Chinese medium while a Taoist priest recites from the Taoist Canon, Changi, Singapore	81
20	The Living Buddha speaks through a Chinese medium, Penang ..	81
21	Chinese medium, clad as Kuan Yin, at the Festival of the Nine Imperial Gods, Singapore	82
22	The Nine Imperial Gods are sent back to their heavenly abodes at the end of their festival, Singapore	82
23	Altar with the eight trigrams. The black flag indicates the presence of a medium, Chinese temple near Ord Bridge, Singapore	83
24	Dragon whips and Four General skewers, Chinese temple near Ord Bridge, Singapore	84
25	Typical Chinese altar, Singapore	85
26	Taoist priest dancing the pattern of the Big Dipper, Taiwan	85
27	Temple dedicated to receiving messages from the Highest God, Red Swastika Society, Singapore	86
28	Sand Box for Automatic Writing, Red Swastika Society, Singapore	86
29	Automatic Writing, Keng Yeo Taoist Association, Jurong, Singapore	87
30	Kuda Kepang, Rasa Singapura, Singapore	87
31	Falling out of trance during the Kuda Kepang, Rasa Singapura, Singapore	88
32	Kuda Kepang trainers, Changi, Singapore	88
33	Malay bomoh, preparing for a main puteri, Kelantan, Malaysia ..	113
34	Bomoh in trance, during a main puteri, Kelantan, Malaysia	114
35	Female bomoh, Pattani, southern Thailand	114
36	Sixty-year-old bomoh, Pattani, southern Thailand	114
37	Bomoh after a tiger possession, Pattani, southern Thailand	115
38	Monks performing a first-hair-cutting ceremony, Bangkok, Thailand	115
39	Abbot of Wat Tham Krabod, Saraburi, Thailand	116
40	Entrance to Phrom Mali's compound, Petchkasem Road, Bangkok, Thailand	116
41	Altar in Phrom Mali's practicing hall, Petchkasem Road, Bangkok, Thailand	117
42	Monk blessing medicine, Pu Sawan, Petchkasem Road, Bangkok, Thailand	117

List of Illustrations

43 Monk pouring blessed water after an exorcism, Pu Sawan, Petchkasem Road, Bangkok, Thailand 118
44 Calling Phra Narai (photo of the Thai king as a monk on the back wall), private residence, Bangkok, Thailand 118
45 Spirit dance, Wat Chet Yot, Chiang Mai, northern Thailand 119
46 Spirit medium, Sansei, outside Chiang Mai, northern Thailand ... 119
47 Hill tribe altar, near Chiang Mai, northern Thailand 120
48 Chinese-Kadazan mediums, Sabah, Borneo 120

Tables

Table 1 Alternate States of Consciousness (ASC) Characteristics and Uses 62
Table 2 Alternate States of Consciousness (ASC) Working Model 64

Acknowledgements

I wish to thank the Council for International Exchange of Scholars for providing me with Fulbright-Hays Research Grant #1069-83079 which made the research for this book possible. I also want to express my gratitude for the hospitality and intellectual companionship so generously offered by Dr. Sandhu and his staff at the Institute for Southeast Asian Studies during my stay in Singapore from June 1978 to June 1979. My thanks are extended to the colleagues from the Departments of Sociology, Philosophy, and Malay Studies at Singapore University (now National University) as well as to the colleagues from the Department of English at Prince Songhkla University, Pattani; the Department of Religious Studies at Mahidol University, Bangkok; and the Department of Anthropology, Chiang Mai University, Thailand. Professor Amin Sweeney, Department of South and Southeast Asia Studies, University of California, Berkeley, advised me on the use of Malay terms. I consulted Professor Wolfram Eberhard, Department of Sociology, University of California, Berkeley, on the pantheon of Chinese gods and he deciphered Chinese inscriptions and pamphlets for me. Professor George A. De Vos, Department of Anthropology, University of California, Berkeley, contributed useful comments on psychodynamic processes related to trances and healing. (Professors Sandhu and Eberhard have died since I wrote this book, and Professor De Vos has retired, my gratitude for their assistance has remained undiminished.)

I am deeply indebted to the shamans, mediums, and healers I worked with in Southeast Asia over the last thirty-six years. They did not only permit me to observe and participate in their activities, they also accepted me into their homes and treated me like a friend. The insights I gained through these close relationships allowed a better understanding of their role in three rapidly modernizing Southeast Asian countries. The knowledge shared with individuals coming from different ethnic groups and belonging to different socio-economic and religious systems led to unique experiences. I began to recognize "elementary forms of the religious life," as they still emerge in our time.

Acknowledgements

During this research, I also learned to access my own self-healing powers. Working with shamans, mediums, and healers of Southeast Asia has, indeed, changed my life in more than one aspect.

Ruth-Inge Heinze, Ph.D.

January 1996

Center for Southeast Asia Studies
University of California, Berkeley

Introduction

1. The Split Between Science and Religion

Three Southeast Asian nations—Thailand, Malaysia, and Singapore—provide the background for my research on trance and healing. To work in rapidly modernizing, multi-ethnic, and multi-religious countries, I had to prepare myself for complex networks of interconnected socio-economic and religious-cultural systems. The main difficulty, however, seemed to be the belief that shamans, mediums, and healers tap spiritual powers. Scholars hesitate to touch systems that depend on the faith of their followers because research results can be questioned by non-believers.

There is a marked difference between belief and faith. Alan Watts offered us a clear distinction when he said,

> ... in general practice, belief has come to mean a state of mind which is almost the opposite of faith. Belief ... is the insistence that the truth is what one would "lief" or wish to be. The believer will open his mind to the truth on condition that it fits in with his preconceived ideas and wishes. Faith, on the other hand, is an unreserved opening of the mind to the truth, whatever it may turn out to be. Belief clings, but faith lets go .... Most of us believe in order to feel secure, in order to make our individual lives seem valuable and meaningful. Belief has thus become an attempt to hang on to life, to grasp and keep it for one's own. But you cannot understand life and its mysteries as long as you try to grasp it (1951:240).

Why have issues of faith become unacceptable to science? The controversy is "rooted in the wrong understanding of faith as a type of knowledge which has a low degree of evidence but is supported by religious authority" (Tillich 1965:33). When one "dimension of meaning is not able to interfere with another dimension," the conflict is "actually not between faith and science but between a faith and a science which are not aware of their own valid dimensions" (Tillich 1965:82). Faith and science deal obviously with different dimensions.

Introduction

The split between science and religion occurred in Italy, in the 14th century, during the transitional period between medieval and modern times (Webster 1990:977). Scientists developed techniques of investigation which did not allow topics like spirituality to be included into their research design. Representatives of world religions, on the other hand, became defensive and tried to counteract the rationalization of the spiritual realm.

Where do I stand?

During the thirty-six years of research in Southeast, South, and East Asia, I have been asked over and over again whether I "believe" in the existence of spirits. Western scholars are more inclined to respect the power of the Holy Spirit but hesitate when spiritual powers are given different names in other cultures. My answer always will be,

> With our present scientific tools we can neither prove nor disprove the existence of spirits of whatever nature they may be and, since we have not yet established a multi-dimensional paradigm that allows the inclusion of other dimensions, we have to admit our limitations. We can, however, investigate what led up to such beliefs and we can evaluate results observed in the context of faith.

We have to be ready for refining and adjusting our tools. Most of all, we have to recognize the limits of reductionism and work on a new terminology and methodology to arrive at tangible results. We have, in fact, to develop new paradigms.

2. Research Tools and Questions

What tools do we have to study trances and healing?

The logical step would be to ask theologians. Depending on the codified faith (dogma) and the beliefs they are representing, theologians may declare mystics, shamans, mediums, and healers either to be divinely inspired or to be heretics, because they are possessed by "pagan" spirits. For the Christian Church, it is acceptable that the Holy Ghost descended on the first community. This belief, for example, survives in the practices of people who speak "in tongues" (for *glossolalia*, see Part 2, Case 9). Other miraculous events require the sanction of a religious authority who has limited tolerance for individual expressions. The manifestation of Our Lady of Lourdes had to be verified by the Catholic Church and, in our century, the Bishop of Arizona (USA), for example, issued a decree that the Church is not in favor of appearances of Our Lady.

Introduction

Scientifically, we have not been able to explain what happens when faith causes a shift of attention. I have observed numerous cases where transcendence effected physical conditions. The strength of faith, for example, is tested in fire walking that is still performed in South and Southeast Asia, mainly by Tamil Indians but also by Chinese. In Spring of 1979 I saw over eight hundred Tamil cross the fire pit at the Sri Mariamman Temple in Singapore during *Timiti* (see, Figs.1 and 2, Chapter 1.1., and Babb 1974a). Less than 10 per cent of the fire walkers got burned, that means, over 720 individuals passed the test of faith.

When we want to conduct a pragmatic test of truth, we have to be coherent and consistent. When coherence and consistency turn out to be paradoxes, we become painfully aware that science does not sufficiently explain all observable behavior. Pressured by the need to expand scientific boundaries, we have, on one hand, to be ready to make empirical adjustments to our hypothetical model and, on the other hand, we should never claim to represent any topic in all its aspects. When we are not able to control all variables, we have to admit that our reports are not complete. We can, however, balance the unevenness of our findings by using more than one point of reference (I will discuss the technique of "triangulation" later, see also, footnotes 8 and 9).

In this book, I want to give you the opportunity

1. to observe faith as a vital part of the belief systems in Southeast Asia and
2. to recognize the needs that created these religious-cultural systems,

so that you can

3. move toward understanding those who mediate between different levels of consciousness to fulfill the needs of their community.

The belief in spirits and that they can "possess" human beings is based on cultural theories which produced culture-specific belief systems (for the nature of spiritual entities, see Chapter 3.5.). Spirit possession, for example, can be feared and may require exorcism, but it can also be sought and used for beneficial purposes. In certain cultures, "possession" is not necessarily considered to be a mental illness (see Chapter 3.4.4).

While investigating these phenomena, I will also be offering answers to four additional questions:

Introduction

4. Is the demand for spiritual guidance and help increasing or declining?
5. Is the syncretism we find in modern belief systems strictly a theoretical issue that is of no importance to the participants in a ritual? And
6. Is shamanism an "elementary form of the religious life" (Durkheim 1931, 1917)?

Furthermore, when rituals continue to be recreated wherever and whenever physiological, psychological, intellectual, social, or spiritual needs arise,

7. do these needs lead to the emergence of new need-fulfillers?

If this be the case, we should not be surprised when elements of different religions appear in rituals of modern multi-ethnic and multi-religious societies. They fulfill similar basic needs.

3. Fieldwork

More research in the field of Southeast Asian folk religions and healing is needed. The persistence of shamans, mediums, and healers who work in rapidly modernizing countries has, in the past, either been ignored or played down. Academic studies of shamanism, trances and healing have been so far predominantly carried out by psychiatrists (Silverman 1967) and historians of religion (Eliade 1974). They introduced their professional biases to the topic.

Psychiatrists would draw character profiles of shamans, mediums, and healers, mainly based on their experiences with mental patients or prisoners. They would treat folk practices as "anecdotal" and "unproven" and consider the use of trances "abnormal." They have not yet recognized that lunatics and shamans differ in the way they process their trances. Lunatics are unable to grasp what they have experienced, while shamans tap into spiritual power and, like mystics, come "to know God" (Prabhavananda 1953). The rare occurrence of transcendental experiences does not seem to justify the use of the term "abnormal." Furthermore, misjudging the deep absorption of meditators, the psychiatrists' diagnosis was "regression" which proves that psychiatrists are unaware of the expansion of consciousness occurring right in front of their eyes. Psychiatrists have not yet the tools to measure different states of consciousness. (Biofeedback equipment, for example, still needs refinement.) Stereotyping any alternate state of consciousness[1] as abnormal precludes the possibility that these states could be used beneficially.

Introduction

We have reason to doubt that clinical terms, used in Western pathology, are appropriate for defining Eastern mystics, shamans, mediums, and healers. Trance experiences, occurring in the context of culture, are, for example, encouraged by Balinese, Chinese, Hindu, while they are vilified and pathologized by representatives of organized Western religions and Western science as well.

Looking for assistance from other disciplines, I found that, during the last decades, anthropologists and sociologists have begun to approach the study of shamanism, alternate states of consciousness[1] and traditional healing with a less biased mind.[2] Historians of religion, like Eliade (1974), had laid the ground for arriving at workable statements about shamans, mediums, and healers. Using historical data, we can, indeed, attempt to understand the role practitioners played in their societies. I examined the social systems in which they and their clients operated and I looked at their relationships to other systems. I, therefore, added socio-psychological tools and attempted to strike the middle way between natural and supernatural explanations. In sum, I used an interdisciplinary approach.

Where information had been collected already by anthropologists and sociologists, it lacked frequently adequate documentation. Fortunately, pioneering work had been done, for example, by Cuisinier (1936), Elliot (1955), Gimlette (1915), Laderman (1991), Peters (1980, 1981), Spiro (1957), Tambiah (1968, 1970, 1984), Wee (1976, 1977, 1980), and Winstedt (1920, 1924, 1925), to name a few. Their efforts were promising and clarified some of the issues. However, a general framework and more longitudinal studies are needed. Most of all, old methodologies have to be revised and scholars have to agree on procedures, before data can be compared cross-culturally.

To fulfill the need for scientific studies of trance and healing, the fieldwork for this book was conducted in three modern Southeast Asian countries: Thailand, Malaysia, and Singapore; among four major ethnic groups: Thai, Chinese, Malay, and Tamil Indian; in the framework of five world religions: Buddhism (*Theravāda*, *Mahāyāna*, or *Tantrayana/Vajrayana*), Taoism (folk religious practices, not the original philosophical way of life), Hinduism (mainly Tamil, from southern India), Islam, and Christianity, often coexisting with indigenous forms of shamanism, mediumship, and healing. (Animism, perceiving everything as being interconnected and attributing a soul even to stones, mountains, trees, etc., appears to be the matrix from which later belief systems and, in the last consequence, religions grew; see also Glossary).

Probing the trances in Southeast Asia, I discovered that they fulfill a large range of community needs. To come into the presence of spiritual powers, for example, is still an essential element of Southeast Asian healing rituals.

Introduction

Furthermore, the alternate states of consciousness[1] I observed in Southeast Asia differed considerably in nature and depth (see Chapter 3.4.3–4, and the Glossary).

During my fieldwork, it became evident that it takes a strong and healthy mind to go into trance on demand, regularly, and in culturally acceptable patterns (see, e.g., Hartog 1972a and b). His findings were confirmed by Kleinman who said that "Shamanistic healing clearly demands personal strengths and sensitivities incompatible with major psychopathology, especially chronic psychosis" (1980:214).

It would go beyond the scope of this book to discuss what is considered "normal" and what is considered "abnormal." Expert opinions differ (see, e.g., Devereux 1956:23–48) and the criteria for "normalcy" vary from one ethnic group to another. Furthermore, terminologies used by representatives of "modern" medicine differed considerably from the terminologies used by "traditional" practitioners.

How did I prepare myself for this task? I received my basic training at the Department of Ethnology (Free University of Berlin, West Germany) and the Department of Anthropology (University of California, Berkeley). At UC Berkeley, I participated, among others, in an American Identity study and conducted interviews on beliefs and attitudes in multi-ethnic and multi-religious America. Specializing in "Religion and Society," I found I should be able to read basic religious scriptures in the original. Greek and Latin I had studied already in Berlin (Germany), but for Southeast Asian religions the study of Sanskrit, Pāli, and Thai became necessary.

Reading the Vedas, Upanisads, Puranas,[3] and the Buddhist Canon in the original, however, did not tell me how the philosophies presented in these scriptures were applied in daily life. The scriptures also did not tell me why and how the respective religions survived for thousands of years.

Collecting data for my dissertation on "The Role of the Sangha[4] in Modern Thailand" in 1971–1972, I had observed already many Thai practices that did not seem to fit into the framework of the Buddhism I had read about. The apparently divergent practices showed the tendency of seeking a personal, direct experience of locally accessible spiritual powers, mainly with the help of shamans, mediums, or healers. Such attempts were prompted by very pragmatic considerations. I wanted to explore the underlying needs that could not be satisfied otherwise. Fulbright-Hays Research Grant #1069-83079, finally, gave me the financial independence to pursue this goal in Singapore, Malaysia, and Thailand for one year, 1978–1979.

Introduction

After nineteen years of work in the fields of sociology, anthropology, psychology, and comparative religion, after having traveled and worked in most Asian countries and, after having tested several social science models and psychological research techniques, I tried, in 1978, to embark on the research for this book with as unbiased a mind as possible.

No hypothesis was drawn up beforehand to avoid the fallacy of distorting data to fit them on a Procrustean bed or putting on blinders that would prevent the discovery of unforeseen factors. I was ready to accept the element of indeterminacy.[5]

The fieldwork was conducted in four stages:

First Stage: During the first months, commuting between Singapore, Malaysia, and Thailand, data were collected during participant observation. After having been introduced by a devotee,[6] I would ask for permission to be present when shamans, mediums, and healers worked with their clients. I told them that I wanted to "write a book" about the deities and spirits they evoked. Sitting among clients who were waiting in line, nobody objected to my presence neither before, during nor after the sessions. Discussions developed on the basis of mutual interests. During the first phase, I, therefore, did not ask any direct questions and left it open what I wanted to know. I carefully avoided anything which could be offensive and showed interest and respect for whatever they were doing.

The strategy worked. After three months, my informants made the first step in sending a delegation. They wanted to know why I had not ask any questions. My answer was, "What should I have asked?" A door had opened. There was no separation any more between informants who wanted to be understood and me, who wanted to start on the right foot and understand them on their own terms. My patience was rewarded. They had been given time to get used to my presence and they had been assured that I was without prejudice and genuinely respectful of their customs. Temple committees took the initiative and assigned members to tell me the story of the temple and, after I had demonstrated some previous knowledge about their mythology and legends, I was even consulted in disputes about certain details.

Shamans, mediums, and healers agreed to take psychological tests[7] and began to speak about their dreams and visions. Through a stroke of luck, I even was present at the birth of a legend when a shaman manifested some precious stones. So, over time, case data could be collected and followed by "free-flowing interviews."[8] The data from the first stage were, therefore, mainly, descriptive.

Introduction

Second Stage: During the second stage, I sat down and looked at the collected material to draw up preliminary hypotheses, establish models, and formulate conclusions.

Third Stage: During the third stage, back in the field, hypotheses and models were tested. This is the stage where researcher and informants crosscheck the data to filter out each other's biases. In any country, even the most unbiased researcher cannot completely escape subjectivity as much as informants cannot be completely objective about themselves. We have to be aware of the "Rashomon effect."[9] So I looked for somebody of the culture I was studying to comment on my data and tried to find the middle ground between self-report, participant observation, and comments of a third person.

During the **Fourth Stage**, I used socio-psychological approaches for the formulation of my conclusions (see Chapter 4).

Part 1 of this book is predominantly theoretical. The discussion of actual field data can be found in Part 2 where twenty-one cases from the author's fieldwork have been selected to demonstrate the wide range of variations in appearance and style found among practitioners belonging to four different ethnic groups and working in the framework of five world religions.

When discussing the role of shamans, mediums, and healers in three Southeast Asian countries today, I will, therefore, point to differences in paraphernalia and ritual where necessary, but I will also present elements common to all. Talking about practitioners, whether they may be Chinese *tang-ki*, Thai *ma khi* and *khon song*, Thai-Malay and Malay *bomohs*, or Tamil Indian *swamis*, I will use the term "shaman" for all (1) who employ alternate states of consciousness during their consultations, divinations, and healing, (2) who answer needs of their community which are otherwise not fulfilled, and (3) who are the mediators between the sacred and the secular.

For readers coming from different disciplines, a glossary, a bibliography, appendices, and an index have been added.

This book does not claim to cover all aspects of trance and healing in modern Southeast Asia. It has been written to survey the present situation and to lay the foundation for future monographs.

Introduction

Notes to Introduction

[1] In contrast to Tart's "altered states of consciousness" (1969), I prefer the term "alternate" because it indicates that there are several distinct states of consciousness which do not coincide but alternate when and wherever they appear.

[2] See Bourguignon (1965, 1966), Davidson (1965), Dickes (1965), Eister (1974), Eliade (1946, 1974), Kiev (1974), Laderman (1991), Lessa (1972), Prince (1966), Spiro (1967), Tart (1969, 1986), Wavell (1966) and others.

[3] Diacritical marks have been left out for all languages and dialects; they are identified only where necessary.

Furthermore, in the absence of an international agreement for transcription of foreign names, no attempt has been made to standardize the spelling of names. They may, therefore, be spelled differently, sometimes just phonetically, sometimes according to the author quoted.

Also, the plural of some foreign words has been anglicized in simply adding an "s" to the singular form of the word because the regular plural of some foreign words may not be easily recognizable as such to those not familiar with the respective language.

[4] In this case, the three Buddhist communities: (1) the group of spiritually advanced individuals (*arahats*), (2) monks, nuns, and novices, and (3) the Buddhist laity; basically all ordained and non-ordained individuals who follow Buddhist customs.

[5] Used by Victor Turner in a public lecture on the University of California, Berkeley Campus, on December 6, 1979.

[6] In Chapter 3.2, I will talk in more detail about the progressively growing group of followers: client - devotee - entourage. When a new shaman, medium or healer emerges, s/he will first be consulted by family members who spread the word to neighbors and acquaintances. Some of the clients become devotees and show their gratitude for what they have received by coming frequently just to stay close to the place where spiritual powers manifest. They enjoy the *liminal* state of the *communitas* Turner (1966) was talking about. Out of the group of devotees, the deity or the shaman, medium or healer may select helpers to assist with the rituals. The group of helpers then develops into a self-organizing entourage (see also Chapter 3, II).

[7] For example, the Thematic Apperception Test (TAT), during which individuals are asked to tell a story to each of twelve pictures with ambiguous scenes.

Introduction

⁸ Free-flowing interviews are unstructured. Though the points to cover may have been established beforehand, questions are asked only when the interviewee brings up the topic. These non-directional interviews reduce the possibility that informants tell what they think the interviewer might want to hear. It increases also the chance of discovering new aspects.

⁹ In the Japanese film *Rashomon*, a wife is raped and her Samurai husband murdered by a robber. When each of the three talk about the event, their accounts differ considerably in interpretation. Even the ghost of the dead husband does not seem to tell the entire "truth."

The reader is also referred to Devereux who mentioned that "a failure to differentiate between actually observed behavior and the statements of an informant can also lead to erroneous interferences (1967:200). He pointed to "the alarming possibility that field ethnography (and indeed all social science) . . . may be a species of autobiography" (1967:viii). Anthropologists who have studied at first hand more than one culture do not experience the same affinities with each of them (Devereux, 1967:204). When I collected reports from eye witnesses at the event where a legend got started, all eighteen reports (including my own) differed considerably, not only according to individual perception and background, but content and sequence of events had been experienced differently, too.

Part 1

Theoretical Considerations

Chapter 1
Who Is a Shaman?

1.1. Definition

Of all the terms used in this book, the word "medium"[1] is the most ambiguous. Who is a medium? Elliott, who studied Chinese spirit mediums in Singapore in the 1950s, said,

> The underlying assumption is that a spiritual being of vast and undefined powers possesses the body of a human medium and enables him to inflict injury upon himself without feeling pain, and to speak with divine wisdom, giving advice to worshippers and curing their illnesses (1955:15).

Is this definition still valid for mediums among our four ethnic groups?

Each year, during Thaipusam[2] and Timiti,[3] Tamil devotees fast and mortify their bodies (see Figs.1 and 3). They pierce their backs, cheeks and tongues with skewers. Before they walk on fire, they may even asked to be whipped but they are not mediums. They have vowed to perform an act of faith. They either thank or propitiate a god for help. May their mother be healed! May their brother pass his examination or be promoted! May their sister find a good husband. These are just a few reasons. (It is important to note that most of those who mortify themselves asked not a favor for themselves.)

Tamil mediums in Thailand, Malaysia, and Singapore may follow this tradition during festival time, however, mortification is no longer a required part of their work with clients. Similarly, most Chinese devotees do no longer expect the traditional tongue-cutting from their mediums. If necessary, red ink instead of blood may be used to write on charm paper. Mortification was, in the past, a dramatic phase of mediumistic performances. It proved that mediums were protected by their deity and it attested to the depth of their trance (see Fig.18). Mortification is practiced by Chinese and Tamil mediums today only occasionally. It was never practiced by Muslim or Buddhist mediums.

Mediums, though, may feel pain when their deity, e.g., Jesus Christ on the cross,[4] is suffering or when they are not prepared for the encounter with a spiritual entity. A deity may also punish a medium for disobeying instructions, e.g., by eating beef, having become polluted in other ways, or not wanting to serve the deity anymore.

In sum, in 1978–1979, mediums still invited deities into their body to fulfill the needs of their community.

For this book, we need a wider framework to reach a valid definition of Southeast Asian mediums because they act also as shamans and we need to know what distinguishes them from other practitioners.

Scientific studies of shamanism were first conducted in Northeast Asia where scholars developed a Siberian prototype. Later studies in other areas of the world provided us with the descriptions of different types of shamans and alerted us to a more critical approach. Bogoras (1907), Czaplicka (1914), Eliade (1946/1974), Lommel (1967), and Shirokogoroff (1935), for example, found that Tungus shamans were recruited from "excitable," "half crazy," and "deviant" individuals whose performances had ecstatic features. Ackerknecht (1949), who concluded that shamans were "cured" adolescent schizophrenics, based his findings on a rather simplistic cultural definition of normality. Summarizing current popular views, Howells (1956:129–144) saw shamans belonging to a "psychological type" which combines features of severe hysteria with that of schizophrenia (see also, Silverman 1967). Devereux (1956) was firmly convinced that shamans were psychologically disturbed. He posed the question whether a shamanic and/or ethnic psychosis (1) is the opening gambit of an idiosyncratic psychosis, (2) masks at a later stage an underlying idiosyncratic psychosis, or (3) represents the terminal restitutive manifestations of an idiosyncratic psychosis.

Kroeber found that not only shamans but the rest of the population of "primitive societies" were involved in psychopathology. He noted that "the psychopathologies which get rewarded among primitives are the mild or transient ones," particularly of the

> hysteric type, involving suggestibility of half-conscious volition . . . . The rewards seem to be reserved for individuals who can claim abnormal powers and controls, not for those *who are controlled* (1940:318)

Where shamans were sharing the psychopathology of their group, Kroeber admitted that they were better integrated and more effective than their contemporaries.

Who Is a Shaman?

This reminded me of Kris (1952) who said that artists use regression in the service of the ego. Levi-Strauss spoke of shamans who provided the sick members of their society with a language by which unexpressed and otherwise inexpressible psychic states can be immediately expressed (1963:167–185 and 186–205). Hardly any scholar attempted to explain why shamans, mediums, and healers function so well in their society while schizophrenics and hysterics do not.

Kakar finally recognized that non-Western systems may deviate from "Eurocentric positivistic norms" which, in psychological terms, are expressions of "poor reality testing" (1982:90–92). No attention, for example, was paid to the way individuals become shamans.

Eliade's four major criteria for a shaman are, a shaman

1. experiences dismemberment and rebirth during initiation;
2. goes on "magical flights" (ecstatic journeys) and may act as a psychopomp (see Glossary);
3. is the master of fire, and
4. has animal guardians or may assume animal form (e.g., based on totemistic views; 1946/1974).

Can these criteria be applied to mediums?

Let us look at the second criterium first. Eliade found later that shamans can also become "possessed" by spiritual entities and may act as mediums, while mediums claim that they can visit different realms like shamans. One medium I studied in Singapore, for example, told me that, while the deity is working through her body, her soul is taken to heaven where she visits other deities. During her "possession"[6] trance, the deity himself may have to return to one of the heavens to consult with higher spiritual entities. In this case, a mediumistic trance coincided with a shaman's flight. A medium's body was occupied by a spirit while the medium's soul was visiting different realms. This was not an exception, many practitioners, in my study, were not surprised about the coincidence of "possession" and "magical flight" and found this co-existence of a mind-expanding and a dissociate state quite natural. Possession, actually, ranked higher in the spiritual hierarchy because a deity was manifesting.

Mediums as well as shamans are expected to be "vehicles" of spiritual entities. This universal phenomenon is reflected, for example, in Thailand by calling a medium a *ma khi* ("mounted horse"). The Vietnamese expression *len dong* (Durand 1959:7) means literally "to mount a medium." In Haiti, a medium is a *cheval*

(French word for "horse"), and in West Africa, among the Hausa, a male medium is the "horse" and a female medium the "mare" of a spirit (Lewis 1971:58). In Thailand, Malaysia, and Singapore,

1. most mediums, like shamans, went through initiation at the end of their training period. The Chinese mediums could be initiated by a Taoist priest or by another experienced medium. Most mediums, however, said that they had been initiated not by a human master but by their spirit. Thai and Malay mediums could be initiated by an elder who represents a certain lineage of teachers. Only Tamil mediums were selected and "visited" by Hindu gods, without any previous initiation and training.
2. Most mediums can go on a "magical flight" and are intruded by spiritual entities simultaneously.
3. Tamil devotees who take a religious vow are able, for example, to walk on fire. Chinese mediums, e.g., during festivals for the Sky God or for the Nine Imperial Gods, may do so as well. Chinese mediums also put their arms into boiling oil (see De Groot 1910:1992 and Wolf 1976:142). No mastery of fire is expected from Thai or Malay mediums because they work in the framework of Buddhism or Islam.
4. Malay *bomohs*,[7] like shamans, can have animal guardians and can be possessed by animal spirits. It is, for example, believed that when a *bomoh* dies, he will be transformed into a tiger who teaches prospective candidates his art. Such spirit tiger may "enter" the body of a *bomoh* during trance (see Part 2, Case 14e). Spirit tigers are also known to Thai (Heinze 1977b). Chinese see the mountain god accompanied by a white tiger. De Groot (1910, VI:955) reported the Chinese belief that spirit tigers are great destroyers and expellers of ghosts, tear them apart and devour them. Such a white tiger is the symbol for one of the deified three sworn brothers of the Three Kingdoms. Five protective spirit tigers also appear on altars—the Yellow Tiger in the center, the White Tiger in the upper left, the Black Tiger in the upper right, the Red Tiger in the lower left, and the Green Tiger in the lower right (Durand 1959:179).

Tamil as well as Chinese can also be possessed by the Monkey God. For Tamil, it will be Hanuman who helped Rāma to rescue his wife Sita from the Demon King Ravana; for Chinese it will be Sun-heu-tze, the monkey who accompanied the monk Hsuan Tsang to India.

Who Is a Shaman?

Can we draw clear borderlines when we compare the functions of shamans and mediums with those of priests? Lessa calls a shaman

> a ceremonial practitioner whose powers come from direct contact with the supernatural by divine stroke, rather than from inheritance or memorized ritual; a "priest" is a ceremonial practitioner who often inherits his position and who learns a body of codified and standardized ritual knowledge from older priests and later transmits it to successors (1972:381).

My field data show that many shamans and mediums as well as priests inherit their "office." Most shamans and mediums are trained for their profession and have memorized long evocations (see Part 2, Case 14). Not recognized by "institutional" religion (Yang 1961), they, nevertheless, have institutionalized their performances. Chinese mediums may call a Taoist priest for certain functions (see Fig.19) but perform the functions of a priest at other times, e.g., when they convey the blessings of a deity.

To define who is a shaman and a medium, my explanations have to be wide enough to accommodate the different kinds of practitioners I encountered. We have to take into account also the alternate states of consciousness experienced and utilized. With these considerations in mind, I propose the definition that shamans and mediums are individuals who

1. respond to specific needs of their community that otherwise are not met;
2. mediate between different states of consciousness for those who seek immediate, personal experience of spiritual powers, i.e., they fulfill pragmatic, physiological as well as psychological, intellectual, social, and spiritual needs,

but most of all, they

3. provide access to "higher powers" and translate ineffable messages into a language which is understood by all.

These three definitions *do not include* individuals who occasionally enter different states of consciousness at certain festivals, e.g., walk on fire or carry a *kavadi*,[2] although deities may speak through them for the benefit of others. Fire walkers and *kavadi* carriers are usually not "called" by a deity. They voluntarily took a vow for a specific reason. They don't need an initiation and they undergo only a brief period of preparation, e.g., fasting, praying, chanting, drumming, asking to be whipped (to test and deepen their trance). They are supported by their family and friends and attended by *brahmins*. They use their alternate state of consciousness only for the benefit of their family at special occasions, i.e., they are not available to the public on a regular basis.

My definition *includes* all individuals who are able to enter a shamanic trance, i.e., they go on a magical flight or call spiritual entities into their body in a mediumistic trance, to serve their community on demand for altruistic reasons. This aspect will be discussed again in the Conclusions.

1.2. Historical Development of Shamanism

The practice of shamanism can be traced back to prehistoric times. Petroglyphs and cave paintings in southern France, Africa, Australia, and Asia show that the hunt of animals was ritualized. Broken skulls and grave offerings point to concerns about the soul of the dead. Shamans were, therefore, present already in hunting and gathering societies to assure success of the hunt and they propitiated not only the souls of the hunted animals but also the souls of dead members of their tribe. Shamans continued to work for the benefit of nomadic societies. In changed socio-economic settings, i.e., after tribes had settled down, in horticultural and agricultural societies, they evoked spirits to bring rain or stop a flood. Shamans were active during the formative period of each world religion and they continue to occur in the framework of the five religions we are concerned with: Buddhism, the popular forms of Taoism, Hinduism, Islam, and Christianity. Shamans were present in prehistoric forests and jungles, in rural areas and, today, they are active in urban areas as well.

How did it all start? We know that in prehistoric times man lived in small groups and had to come to terms with an apparently alien environment. The struggle for survival led to the development of means to manipulate natural and other unseen forces. When we want to understand the continued belief in "divine" intervention, we have to look for functional parallels.

When awe and fear arose in the face of natural powers, with them arose the need to supplicate the external powers. Awe and fear have been visualized as gnawing at the roots of a growing "tree." With its branches reaching out toward heaven and its roots deeply anchored in the earth, the "tree" continues to be the symbol for the ascent of shamans (Eliade, 1974).

Who Is a Shaman?

Shamans, mediums, and healers proved to be capable of materializing and internalizing power. They became the vehicles of spiritual power. They could tap this power and use it for divination, magic, and healing. Most of all they shifted attention of their clients from a seemingly hopeless situation to a level where change became possible and the unexpected could happen.

When, in Western thinking, spirits appear to be projections of fears and anxieties, it should not be forgotten that the belief and faith in spirits carries also its solution. Externalized fears and anxieties can be treated. It should, therefore, not surprise us when the fear of spirits is reinforced by the faith in spiritual intervention. Have we touched the life line of religions? Rituals to invoke, consult and manipulate spirits can well be "elementary forms of the religious life." It is important to keep these questions in mind, when we continue our investigation.

The highest goal became the stage where man has learned to manipulate himself. This is, indeed, the essence of *Theravāda* Buddhism. The last words of the Buddha were, "Be a lamp to yourselves . . . . work out your own salvation with diligence? (*Digha Nikaya, Mahaparinibbana Sutta*). These words were confirmed by Weber who said that "Discrepancies between normative expectations and actual experiences" will resolve as soon as man understands that salvation does not come through outside help but is cultivated by the individual himself (1965:L).

Religions are kept alive and carried by dynamic forces. We can no longer maintain that religious practices are static units. We should keep this in mind when we find names and forms of deities interchangeably used. We should look at their functions. Rituals to consult spirits occur exactly on the level where religions emerge from the formless stage.

What are the stages in between? Shamans, mediums, healers as well as priests have been tribal leaders. De Groot reported for *China*:

> Chinese sorcerers known as wu, were the real priests of China in the centuries immediately preceding our era . . . in them the spirits were believed to be incarnated so that they acted as intermediaries between men and the gods. They practiced magico-religious techniques, the arts of faith-healing, and claimed to be able to enter a state of trance in which they visited the transcendental world of the spirits and held communion with powerful gods, demons, fairies and deified cult heroes (Vol.2, 1919:1205).

Overmyer added, "*Wu* exorcised spirits of evil and illness, called down the spirits in sacrificial rituals, danced and chanted to ward off rain and disasters" (1976:164).

The descent of a *shen* (deity) marks the emergence of a *wu* (shaman). The shaman then proves his power of being able to call down deities and spirits, going on magical flights, interpreting dreams, conveying the wishes of spirits, and penetrating the future.

At the beginning of the Han Era (200 B.C.), the Chinese emperor decreed that *wu* from various parts of the country should assist with the sacrifices in the capital. But when, in the middle of the second century B.C., Confucianism became established as Chinese state religion, the *wu* were forced out of the Imperial Court and became practitioners of Chinese folk religion (Overmyer 1976:164).

Among other ethnic groups in Southeast Asia, e.g., Thai and Hindu, we know about shamanic practitioners of the upper classes, i.e., *brahmins* (priests) and *deva rajas* (god kings). Many *Malay-Muslim* sultans also acted as shamans. In the last century, for example, a sultan predicted the death of the British Commissioner who, indeed, died shortly after at sea (Winstedt 1961:11).

When division of labor led to specialization, shamans began to stay out of the political arena. Not participating in the formation of more complex forms of their society, they were less vulnerable. Their lack of direct involvement, however, was balanced by politicians seeking the advice of shamans. Newly evolving social systems did not develop institutions fast enough to answer all physiological, psychological, intellectual, social, and spiritual needs of their constituents, so the need for shamans continued.

Is the present interest in shamanic practices an "unheard cry for meaning?" Where the struggle for survival has subsided, the question "survival for what" continues. People have the "means to live," but "no meaning to live for (Frankl 1978:21). Victor E. Frankl spoke of the "existential vacuum," the loss of that "instinctual security which surrounds an animal." Instincts do no longer

> tell man what he has to do, nor do traditions direct him toward what he ought to do; soon he will not even know what he really wants to do and will be led by what other people want him to do, thus completely surrounding to conformism (Frankl 1961:20).

Problems have changed over time. Although we developed a wide range of coping mechanisms, the changes always stayed one step ahead of techniques to cope with them. Where alienation was experienced, many individuals found conformism to be their only protection, but others continued to ask shamans for assistance.

Who Is a Shaman?

Like never before, in our century, more changes occurred in every sector of life within a decade than in previous millennia. Changes are drastic and come fast, without allowing sufficient time to prepare the masses for shifts of attention. Who are the interpreters in transitional periods? Mass communication, especially Internet, is flooding us with overwhelming amounts of information. Do we have the means to check the reliability of each piece of information? These are not rhetorical questions, these are real issues.

Furthermore, solutions to existential problems may develop simultaneously in different countries. We should, therefore, not be misled by culturally conditioned variations, but look at what different ethnic coping mechanisms have in common.

1.3. Is Shamanism an Elementary Form of the Religious Life?

What do we know about elementary forms of the religious life? Geologists established theories about the evolution of the earth and biologists attempted to trace the development of life on earth. Many religions originated at a time when writing had not been invented and religious objects were perishable. The only religious records we have are early grave offerings, petroglyphs, and cave drawings.

"The notion that religion tunes human actions to an envisaged cosmic order and projects images of cosmic order onto the plane of human experience is hardly novel" (Geertz, 1966:4). However, not all religions have creation myths. The Buddha, for example, taught that questions about origin are unimportant for our present state of mind because we cannot change the past but we can cultivate our presence and our future.

So what is religion? Geertz proposed that religion be

(1) a system of symbols which acts to (2) establish powerful, pervasive, and long-lasting moods and motivations in men by (3) formulating conceptions of a general order or existence and (4) clothing these conceptions with such an aura of factuality that (5) the moods and motivations seem uniquely realistic (1966:4).

Melford E. Spiro defined religion as an "institution consisting of culturally patterned interaction with culturally postulated superhuman beings" (1966:94). He found that "the belief in superhuman beings and their power to assist or to harm man approaches universal distribution" (1966:92), calling "the corresponding functions of religion ... adjustive, adaptive, and integrative" (1966:109). The "main function of the higher religions . . . [is] to provide meaning for suffering (and some means to escape from or to transcend it)" (1966:110). According to Spiro, we can recognize the integrative function of religion when it allows

> the disguised expression of repressed motives, [and] serves a number of sociological functions. By providing a culturally approved means for the resolution of inner conflict (between personal desires and cultural norms), religion a. reduces the probability of psychotic distortion of desires, thereby providing a society of psychologically healthy members, b. protects society from the socially disruptive consequences of direct gratification of these forbidden desires, c. promotes social integration by providing a common goal (superhuman beings) and a common means (ritual) by which the desires may be gratified (1966:121).

These are powerful motivations. We can, however, only speculate about the nature of elementary religious forms, knowing they could not survive without change.

When people migrate, they take their old beliefs with them, but, in the process of adaptation to their new environment, invaders will incorporate beliefs upheld by the indigenous population, possibly to legitimize their conquest in the eyes of the conquered. This happened, for example, when Aryans invaded the Indian subcontinent, when Tibetan Buddhists incorporated the early Bon religion, and when Spaniards, for example, conquered South and Middle American territory. Elements of earlier religions were incorporated into the dominant religion.

Furthermore, constant regeneration kept belief systems alive.

> Concepts seem to move in a circular fashion—local beliefs are reinterpreted and codified by the elite and then, in a more elaborate form, superimposed on the original local beliefs. Thus, on the one hand, local beliefs gain legitimacy through acceptance by the elite, and, on the other hand, normative religions are kept alive by local practices (Heinze 1982:xi–xii).

Whenever I recognized "elementary forms of the religious life," they continued to have valid functions. Shamanic practices today may look differently, but they are, in their core, no relics of the past. We have to be aware of the changes caused by socio-economic developments and by shifts in the distribution of power.

Where religious forms survived thousands of years without much change, we may have found powerful *archetypes* (see, Glossary and, e.g., my essay on serpent mythology, 1995).

Who Is a Shaman?

New shamans appear when old value and belief systems break down. Whenever socio-economic and/or political changes force a society to move into unknown territory, needs arise and the demand for shamans is felt. Then, shamans emerge to recreate elementary forms of religion. We should, therefore, not be surprised when building blocks are taken from early oral as well as later codified religions. We can compare this process with using the best parts of a tested mechanism to build a more efficient tool. That means, the history of the parts can tell us something about parallel developments in different cultures and a functional analysis allows us to reconstruct "elementary forms."

What can we learn from a study of shamanic practices today? Kroeber said once

> Since we know nothing directly about the origin of totemism or other social phenomena but have information on these phenomena as they exist at present, our business is first to understand as thoroughly as possible the nature of these existing phenomena; in the hope that such understanding may gradually lead to a partial reconstruction of origins—without undue guessing (1920:48–55).

We have to determine the vital needs that are fulfilled by shamans, mediums, and healers. We have to define the role these practitioners play in their society. At the end, we may have learn something about the origin of religion.

I hope that theories and case studies presented in this book will contribute to our knowledge about re-emerging elementary forms of the religious life.

Chapter 2
The Social Setting

2.1. Thailand[1]

Thailand is located in Southeast Asia, between the 5th and the 21th degree of northern latitude and the 97th and 106th degree of eastern longitude. It covers 209,411 sq.m., an area about the size of France.

Thailand's central alluvial plain is traversed by the Menam River and its tributaries. The Salween River, flowing through the mountain forests in the west, is forming the border to Burma, while the Mekong River in the northeast and east separates Thailand's arid northeastern plateau from Laos and Cambodia. The western mountain ranges continue south into the Malaysian peninsula.

Seventy-five per cent of the Thai economy are based on agriculture (mainly wet rice, cassava and maize in central and northern Thailand), 9 per cent on industry and 7 per cent on commerce and services, the latter mainly around Thailand's two large cities: Bangkok, the capital with over 4 million inhabitants and Chiang Mai, the old capital of the north, with approximately 1 million inhabitants. The remaining 9 per cent include tin mining and rubber planting, mainly on the peninsula in the south.

Culturally, the Thai population is fairly homogenous. Eighty per cent of the 50 million Thai nationals are ethnic Thai, 15 per cent are Thai-Chinese, 4 per cent are Thai-Malay, and the remaining 1 per cent are either Indians (Tamil), hill tribes or belong to other ethnic groups.

At the end of the 13th century, after Thai had begun to move in larger groups from southern China into the present territory, a Thai kingdom consolidated around Sukkhothai in the north. Never having been colonized, Thailand remained an absolute kingdom until 1932. A coup d'etat led to a constitutional monarchy and, at present, the Thai government is headed by a prime minister, an appointed cabinet, and an elected house of representatives.

Constitutionally required to be a Buddhist (see Fig.44), the Thai king is also the protector of all other religions in Thailand. When 93.6 per cent of all Thai nationals claim to be Buddhists, ethnic Thai adhere to *Theravāda* and ethnic Thai-Chinese to *Mahāyāna* Buddhism. Religious affiliation seems to be connected with ethnicity. In mixed marriages, however, over time ethnically different partners may share social and cultural customs. Therefore, the clear distinction that ethnic Thai uphold *Theravāda* and ethnic Chinese *Mahāyāna* Buddhism can no longer be made in Thailand. Only a small number of Chinese consider themselves followers of *Mahāyāna* Buddhism today. The field data for this book confirmed that, with varying degrees of Chinese descent, all Thai follow more or less the *Theravāda* tradition, i.e., visit *Theravāda* monasteries and participate in *Theravāda* customs.

Hindu traders began to come in larger numbers to southern Thailand from the 2nd century A.D, on. They came by ship with the northeast monsoon and stayed at trading posts until they could return to India with the northwest monsoon. Half of the 20,000 Indians in Thailand today, live in the Bangkok area. They are Tamil from southern India. Vaisnavites are in the majority and Saivites in the minority. Some became Buddhist monks to follow the custom that young men, when reaching the age of 21, should ordain for one rainy season. The court *brahmin*, for example, had to become a Buddhist monk before he was permitted to act as advisor to the king and conduct royal ceremonies. He determines the auspicious time for events in the life of the royal family (coronations, weddings, etc.) as well as, for example, the correct time for signing a new constitution. The other 10,000 Indians in Thailand belong either to the Shri Guru Singh Sabha or the Namdhari Sangat sect.

In the 14th century, Islam entered the peninsula in the south (shared by Burma, Thailand, Malaysia, and Singapore) in the same way as Hinduism and Buddhism. It was introduced by traders from southern India and the Gulf of Bengal.

During the Ayudhya Period (1450–1767 A.D.) and even after the Thai capital had been moved to Bangkok in 1781, Muslims continued to come to Thailand from Malaysia in the south as well as from India in the west. The majority of Bangkok's Muslims, are, indeed, mainly descendants of Malay refugees (Scupin 1980).

In the middle of last century, other Muslim refugees from northeastern India (now Bangladesh) and from Yunnan (southern China)[2] entered northern Thailand on land routes and began to settle in Chiang Mai Valley.

Presently, 4 per cent of all Thai nationals are Thai-Malay who, with a few exceptions, are Muslims.[3] Four per cent seem to indicate a minority, but Muslims do not live evenly distributed in all provinces of Thailand. In the four southern provinces: Pattani, Narathivat, Yala, and Satun, approximately 80 per

The Social Setting

cent of the population are Thai-Malay, i.e., Muslims. In other words, of the approximately 400,000 inhabitants of Pattani, 320,000 are Thai-Malay, i.e., Muslims. They own rice paddies, fish, and actively participate in the commerce and trading of Pattani.

That we find a Thai-Malay majority in southern Thailand is not surprising because these southern states have been integrated into the Thai nation comparatively late. At the end of the 13th century, the great Sukkhothai monarch Ram Kamhaeng had already proclaimed that his realm extended far into the south, but the southern provinces stayed relatively untouched by decisions of Thai kings and were, at times, even ruled by Malay princes. At the beginning of the 20th century, Rama V changed the governmental structure. This affected also the position of Muslims in the south. They spoke little or no Thai and had no connections with the Thai ruling class. The new order put them educationally and economically into a weakened position. The proximity of the Muslim Federation of Malaysia and the strong affinities with the population on the other side of the Thai border led to separatist movements. Some Thai-Malay want either to join the Malaysian Federation or plan to form an independent state (Thomas 1982).

Since 1945, Muslim affairs in Thailand are administered by the National Council for Muslims in Bangkok. There are also Muslim councils and numerous other Muslim organizations in the south; e.g., each mosque has a *masjid* (mosque committee) of at least 7 up to 15 members who are presided by an *imam* (leader of a Muslim community). All Muslim organizations are ultimately under the jurisdiction of the Department of Religious Affairs in Bangkok which also supervises the administrative structures of Buddhist and Indian institutions. The 1980 report of this department mentions the presence of 347,494 Muslims and 431 mosques and prayer halls alone in the province of Pattani.

The approximately 250,000 hill tribesmen and -women: Karen, Meo, Yao, Lahu, Lisu, etc. live mainly in the north along the Burmese border and in the northeast along the border to Laos. They are predominantly animists. Some of them, e.g., the Karen, have begun to convert to Christianity and their conversion seems to ease their integration into the Thai nation.

2.2. Malaysia[4]

The Federation of Malaysia is located on the most southern peninsula of the Asian continent with the sheltered waters of the Straits of Malakka in the west and the east coast open to the northeast monsoon which blows from October to March.

Malaysia covers 127,315 sq.m. of which 75 per cent are dense jungle, including Sabah (18,460 sq.m.) and Sarawak (48,040 sq.m.), the latter two of the thirteen federal states are on North Kalimantan. The eleven states on the Malaysian peninsula are Johore, Kedah, Kelantan, Malakka, Negri Sembilan, Pahang, Penang, Perak, Perlin, Selangor, and Trengganu.

Close to the equator, the temperatures in Mainland Malaysia do not change much and it may rain anytime during the year.

For centuries, Malaysia has been ruled by local princes and sultans. During the Srivijaya Period (8th to 13th century), some of Malaysia's rulers were Indonesians. The Portuguese came to Malakka in 1511. In 1636, Malakka became Dutch, British in 1795 and Dutch again in 1801, British in 1807, Dutch for the third time in 1814 and, through the Treaty of London, it was ceded by the East India Company to the British Crown in 1824. The East India Company had already acquired the Island of Penang (Prince of Wales Island) when it separated from Kedah in 1786, By cession from the Sultan of Johore in 1824, the East India Company also obtained complete sovereignty over Singapore. The agreement of 1824 with Penang, Malakka, and Singapore was called the Straits Settlement. In 1858 the East India Company was replaced by the India Office but the Straits Settlement continued under a Governor General until 1867. At that time the India Office merged with the Colonial Office that, by 1914, ruled also Labuan (North Borneo), the Cocos Islands in the Indian Ocean and Christmas Island.

Labuan became a British colony in 1846 by cession from the Sultan of Brunei. Labuan joined the Straits Settlement in 1866. From 1890 to 1906, it was administered by the Governor of North Borneo. James Brooke obtained Sarawak in 1841 through cession from the Sultan of Brunei. By 1865, the British operated in North Borneo under various concessions that, in 1882, were transferred to the British North Borneo Company. Both Sarawak and North Borneo became protected states in 1888 and maintained this status until the Japanese invaded the area in 1941.

The first Malaysian Federation was formed in 1895 with the states Perak, Selangor, Pahang, and Negeri Sembilan. In 1909, a British adviser was appointed to Kedah, Lekantan, Perlis, and Trengganu. Johore agreed to accept a British adviser in 1914. The latter five states, however, remained outside the Federation until the end of World War II. The other Malaysian states never joined the Federation for fear of losing their power completely to the British.

On April 1, 1946, Malakka and Penang joined the other nine Malaysian states on the peninsula to form the Malayan Union. The Federation of Malaya Agreement of February 1, 1948, was a further step toward self-government. Malaysia's

The Social Setting

independence was declared on August 31, 1957, and Malaysia officially became a nation on September 16, 1963. The Federation of Malaysia included Singapore, North Borneo (renamed Sabah) and Sarawak. On August 9, 1965, Singapore separated to become an independent republic in the British Commonwealth.

Malaysia is a constitutional monarchy, headed by the Yang Dipertuan Agung who is elected for five years by the other sultans. He acts on government advice. The Federation has a bicameral parliament, i.e., a senate with 58 members each elected by the 13 state legislatures and 32 appointed by the Agung and the House of Representatives with 154 members elected for five years (114 from Mainland Malaysia, 24 from Sarawak and 16 from Sabah). The Cabinet is headed by the Prime Minister and consists of members of the legislature who are collectively responsible to the parliament.

Malaysia's sultans retained their pre-independence position except that they can no longer act contrary to the advice of the Executive Council (State Cabinet). Except Muslim courts and the native courts in Sabah and Sarawak, the judiciary is now federal. Judges are independent and may not be removed from office before the compulsory retirement age of 65, except on recommendation of a tribunal consisting of at least five judges and exjudges. The judiciary has the power to interpret the constitution and to declare laws invalid and executive acts unlawful.

The religion of the Federation of Malaysia is Islam. Each of the thirteen states is ruled by a sultan who is the head of the Islamic community in his territory. He is advised by a Religious Council. Islam has formally been declared state religion in Sabah in 1973, but Sarawak has not yet passed such a law. Freedom of other religious practices is constitutionally guaranteed.

Malaysia had, in 1975, a population of 12,250,000 of which 53.3 per cent were Malay (Muslim), 35.4 per cent Chinese (Taoist or Buddhist), 10.5 per cent Indian (Hindu or Sikh) and 0.8 per cent indigenous tribes (animist). Thirty-five per cent of all Malaysians live in towns with a population of over 5,000. In towns with 10,000 inhabitants or more the population increased during the last years by 52.6 per cent.

The distribution among the population of Sarawak (approximately 1.13 million) differs. Thirty-one per cent are Iban (Sea Dayak), 30 per cent Chinese, 19 per cent Malay, 8 per cent Bidayu (Land Dayak), 5 per cent Melanau, 5 per cent indigenous tribes and 2 per cent other races (Statistical Bulletin, 1972).

In Sabah, 31.9 per cent of the population (754,000) are Kadazan, 21.3 per cent Chinese, 18.2 per cent Malay, 11.7 per cent Bajau, 10.5 per cent other nationalities, 5.7 per cent Murut, and 0.7 per cent European (1960 Census).

The constitutional definition of a Malay is a person who professes the Muslim religion, habitually speaks Malay, conforms to Malay customs and (a) was born in the Federation or in Singapore before Merdeka (Independence Day) or was on Merdeka domiciled in the Federation or in Singapore or (b) is an issue of such a person.

Constitutionally, an ethnic Chinese is a Malay when he professes the Muslim religion, habitually speaks Malay and conforms to Malay customs. However, an ethnic Malay is not a Malay when he does not profess the Muslim religion. Also, an Indonesian who professes the Muslim religion, habitually speaks Malay and conforms to Malay customs cannot be considered to be a Malay when he was not born in the Federation or Singapore before *Merdeka*.

To be considered a native in Sarawak on Kalimantan, an individual has to be a citizen and belong to one of the following ethnic groups indigenous to Sarawak—Bukutan, Bisayah, Dusun, Sea Dayak, Land Dayak, Kadazan, Kalabit, Kayan, Kenyah (incl., Sabup and Sipend), Kajang (incl., Sekapan, Kejaman, Lahanan, Punan, Tanjong, and Kanowit), Lisum, Lugat, Malay, Melanok, Murut, Penan, Sian, Tabun, Tagale, and Ukit or, if of mixed blood, his/her parents must come exclusively from these ethnic groups.

In Sabah, a native is an individual who is a citizen and the issue of parents from ethnic groups indigenous to Sabah. Whether the individual was born before or after Malaysia Day does not matter, as long the father was domiciled in Sabah at the time of his or her birth.

The national language of the Federation of Malaysia is Bahasa Malaysia. Together with a script determined by federal law, it is used for all official purposes.

2.3. Singapore[5]

The Southeast Asia island of Singapore has a granite core with marshy lowlands full of tropical vegetation. It covers 230 sq.m., approximately the size of Chicago, and is situated just 85 miles north of the equator. Singapore is connected with the Malaysian Peninsula in the north by a causeway.

Singapore has an average rainfall of 90 inches per year but has no specific monsoon or rainy season. Mean maximum temperature is 87 degrees Fahrenheit and mean minimum 75 degrees Fahrenheit, with a high degree of humidity. The nights are usually cool with a light breeze.

Singapore was originally called Temasek ("Sea Town"). According to legend, Sang Nila Utama, a prince of Srivijaya, landed on the island that was occupied

The Social Setting

only by some fishing villages. When he spotted a strange beast, he mistook it for a lion and named the place *Singa Pura* ("Lion City").

Ruled by Malay sultans, Singapore was "rediscovered" by Sir Stamford Raffles at the beginning of last century and soon developed into a flourishing seaport.

When the Straits Settlement was dissolved in 1846, Singapore became crown colony. It was granted full self-government in 1959. On September 16, 1963, it joined the Federation of Malaya from which it withdrew on August 9, 1965, proclaiming itself a republic the next year. Singapore is now a city state in the British Commonwealth and a member of the United Nations.

It is governed by a president and a cabinet headed by a prime minister, the parliament of 69 members is elected by universal suffrage. In 1979, led by Prime Minister Lee Kuan Yew, the People's Action Party was the only political party represented in the parliament.

Although one of the smallest nations in the world, with a population of over 2.5 million in 1979, Singapore is a major trading and banking center. Located at major crossroads of Asia, it is the fourth biggest port in the world, the second biggest in Asia, and the largest in Southeast Asia. There are some two hundred shipping lines. Usually a ship arrives in or leaves Singapore every 15 minutes.

Singapore has a stable economy based on the Singapore dollar which is one of the strongest currencies in the world. Almost 23 per cent of government revenues are spent on education, 12 per cent on health services. Singapore's public housing project averages construction of one low-cost residential unit every 25 minutes. Approximately 50 per cent of the population live, at present, in HDB (Housing and Development Board) flats where the difference between income and rent is covered by the government.

Peter Chen wrote about Singapore that it "is a plural society with a heterogeneous population which is differentiated socio-culturally" (1978:1). According to the 1975 census, the three major ethnic groups are the Chinese (74 per cent), the Malay (14 per cent), and the Indian (11 per cent). Other minority groups constitute only 1 per cent of the population. The heterogeneity is further complicated by dialect groups. Among the Chinese, 42.2 are Hokkien, 22.4 per cent Teochew, 17 per cent Cantonese, 7 per cent Hainanese, and 7 per cent Hakka. Among the Malay, 85.8 per cent are Malay, 7.9 per cent Javanese, and 5.5 per cent Boyanese. Among the Indians, 66.3 per cent are Tamil, 12.0 per cent Malayali, and 8.4 per cent Punjabi.

Today, immigrants from Malaysia, Indonesia, China, India, and other countries are no longer in the majority. The following table shows the growing number of locally born Singaporeans;

Locally born Singaporeans
% of total population   year
          9   1821
        56   1947
        74   1970*

* That means, 77% of all Chinese, 75% of all Malay, and
56% of all Indians were born in Singapore.

Between 1931 and 1947, Singapore's population grew by 68 per cent. With the percentage of locally born Singaporeans rising constantly during the last fifty years, the age structure has also drastically changed. In 1979 over 50 per cent of all Singaporeans were under the age of twenty.

Before the mid 1950s, the ethnic groups represented in Singapore maintained their ethnic boundaries and sent their children to separate schools. By 1959, about half of the total enrollment was in English schools. English has become the first language with Chinese (Mandarin), Malay, and Tamil as the respective second languages. Making a foreign language, the *lingua franca* for the city-state indicates the general trend toward a Singaporean identity.

At least, five world religions are presently practiced in Singapore. Folk Taoism is permeating the belief system of Singaporean Chinese, though some of them converted either to Christianity, Islam, or follow Buddhist customs. Indians practice either Hinduism or Sikhism, while Malays are devout believers in Islam. Led by a Mufti, they have a Muslim Religious Council (MUIS) and a Shariah Court, e.g., for registering Muslim marriages. The rights of the Muslim World League (RABITTAH, based in Mecca) and other organizations are safeguarded by the Muslim Law Act of 1966.

2.4. The Complexity of Interlocking Social Systems

We have learned already that, in Southeast Asia, shamans, mediums, healers, their entourages and their clients live in the framework of multi-ethnic and multi-religious societies. This complicates our analysis and forces us to be more perceptive for differences as well as similarities.

Politically, a multi-ethnic country can be one nation. Sociologically, however, each nation is composed of complex systems of action in which, to different

The Social Setting

degrees, specific units of the population participate. Each of these complex systems of action is a social system by itself. It is

> an organized set of interdependent social persons, activities or forces. It is called a system because its organization includes mechanisms for maintaining an equilibrium or some other constancy in the relations between the units. From another perspective such mechanisms can be seen as boundary-maintaining mechanisms for systems can be isolated as separate entities only if they maintain some constancies in the face of environmental change, that is, if they maintain some boundaries vis-a-vis the environment. If every event within a system were a direct consequence of some event outside the system, it would be impossible to draw a boundary for the system, it would be, in effect, a mere unit in a large complex. The concept of a social system seems ideally suited for use in defining a society analytically, for it contains within it the crucial concepts of "unit" and "boundary" (Sills 1968:583).

In the following chapters, I will demonstrate how specific social systems and subsystems as units of action evolve around shamans, mediums, and healers. To understand the phenomenon, we have to look first at the elements of shamanism.

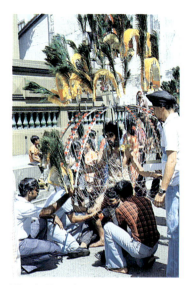

Fig. 1 *Kavadi carrier (Thaipusam), Singapore*

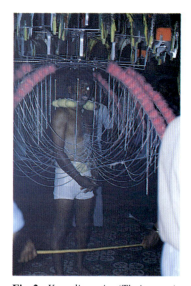

Fig. 2 *Kavadi carrier (Thaipusam), Singapore*

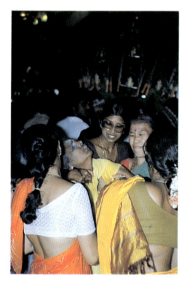

Fig. 3 *Overcome by ecstasy, Thandayuthapani Temple, Singapore*

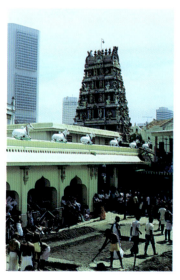

Fig. 4 *Preparations for fire walking (Timiti), Sri Mariamman Temple, Singapore*

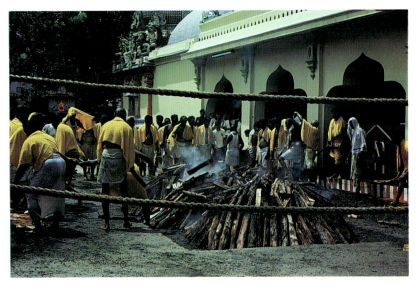

Fig. 5 *Preparations for fire walking (Timiti), Sri Mariamman Temple, Singapore*

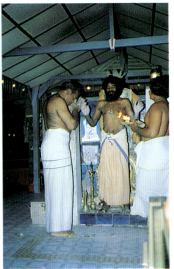

Fig. 6 *The God (Rāma) speaks, Snake Temple, Sembawang Shipyard, Singapore*

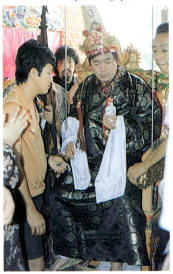

Fig.7 - Chinese medium in trance on a spike chair, after having consumed large portions of alcohol and opium, near Ord Bridge, Singapore

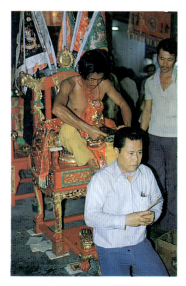

Fig. 8 *Chinese medium in trance on a spike chair, Ganges Road, Singapore*

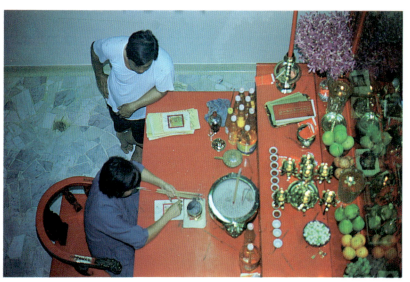

Fig. 9 *Chinese medium in trance, near Upper Thomson Road, Singapore*

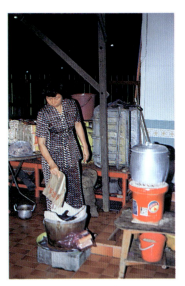

Fig. 10 *Chinese medium cooking food for a temple festival, near Upper Thomson Road, Singapore*

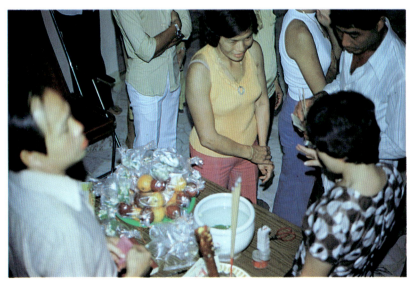

Fig. 11 *Entourage, assisting clients, near Upper Thomson Road, Singapore*

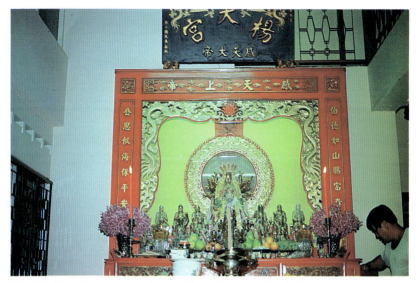

Fig. 12 *Altar of a house temple, near Upper Thomson Road, Singapore*

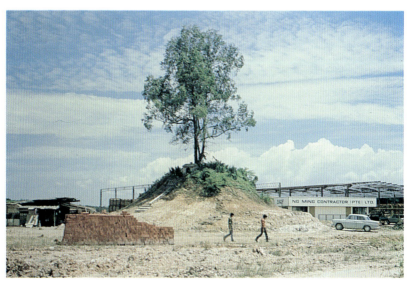

Fig. 13 *Small shrine under a tree, ball-bearing factory, Jurong, Singapore*

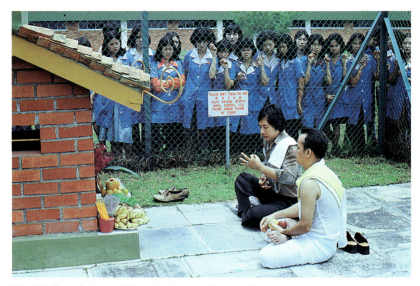

Fig. 14 *New shrine, ball-bearing factory, Jurong, Singapore*

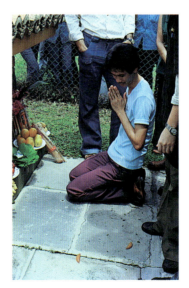

Fig. 15 *Using the* mu bei *in front of the factory shrine, Jurong, Singapore*

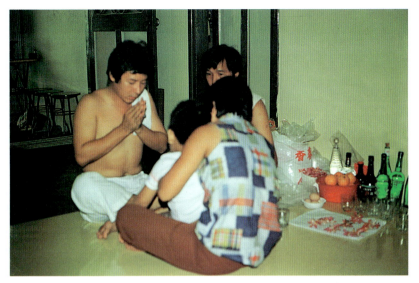

Fig. 16 *Chinese medium blessing clients, near Upper Serangoon Road, Singapore*

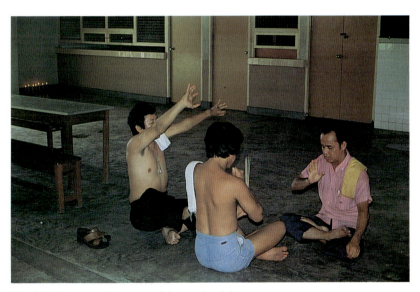

Fig. 17 *Chinese mediums exorcising a school, Singapore*

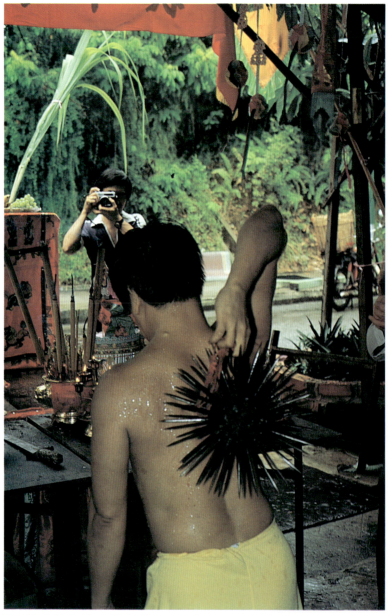

Fig. 18 *Spike ball used by a Chinese medium, Pegu Road, Singapore*

Chapter 3
Elements of Shamanism

3.1. The Shaman

3.1.1. Field data
Having conducted research on 122 shamans, mediums, and healers in Thailand, Malaysia, and Singapore for 36 years, the list below shows the distribution of practitioners I worked with, broken down by country, ethnicity and gender.

Thailand

Ethnic Thai		Malay		Hill tribe (Meo)			
M	F	M	F	M	F	M	F
14	17	6	1	-	1	20	19

Malaysia

Ethnic		Malay		Chinese			
2	-	9	1	-	-	11	1

Singapore

Ethnic Chinese		Ethnic Malay		Ethnic Indian			
52	15	1	1	2	-	55	16
						86	36

M = male F = female

3.1.2. Belief Systems
Of the 122 shamans, mediums, and healers, 43 were Buddhists, 65 believed in what has been called "religious Taoism," 10 were Muslims, 3 Tamils (Hindus), and one was a hill tribe animist. I did not collect more data on Muslim, Hindu or animistic shamans because, despite a few idiosyncratic differences, they still followed more closely the patterns of their tradition. Buddhists and Taoists appeared to be more inclined to adopt elements of other religions.

Let us now look at the belief systems of the different ethnic groups.

Chinese shamans, mediums, and healers followed mainly an oral tradition that, over time, had incorporated elements of other religions. They called themselves Taoists, (in a religious not a philosophical sense), but a large number of Chinese shamans in Singapore also claimed to be Buddhists or had been baptized. They went to Buddhist monasteries, Christian churches as well as Chinese temples. I observed, indeed, non-Christian rituals being performed in the Novena Church in Singapore. Although the rituals were conducted in silence, their nature was quite obvious. However, with the exception of glossolalia sessions at Our Lady of Lourdes in Singapore, trance performances of Christian shamans in Singapore were *not* conducted in churches but in individual homes or in Chinese (Folk Taoist) temples. The Mufti of Singapore also told me that quite a few Chinese converted to Islam, presumably to improve their business.

Thai shamans, mediums, and healers, with the exception of hill tribe animists, operated in the framework of Buddhism which tolerates *brahmin* (Hindu) and animist elements. Buddha's teachings are based on the Hindu concepts of *karma* and transmigration. (Hinduism, in fact, integrated Buddhism, approximately 600 years after the Buddha's death, by declaring Buddha to be the ninth reincarnation of Viṣṇu.)

Hindu shamans, mediums, and healers stayed within their own cultural world view.

Malay bomohs recited verses from the Koran, but their incantations included elements of nature religions, too. They all, however, emphasized that they were good Muslims. They prayed five times a day and went to the mosque on Friday.

3.1.3. Age

The age of the 122 shamans, mediums, and healers ranged from 16 to over 70 years of age. The majority were between 25 and 50 years old. They had become shamans either after puberty or in their mid-thirties when they were restructuring their life. My field data confirmed that, over 75 per cent of the shamans I studied in 1979, had accepted their vocation during the past seven years when they were over thirty years of age.

3.1.4. Gender

Of the 67 ethnic Chinese shamans, mediums, and healers, 61 were men and only 16 were women. Of the 31 ethnic Thai shamans, however, 17 were women (I will talk about Thai women taking care of clan spirits in Part 2, Case 20). The predominance of middle-aged male shamans became obvious when looking at the sample of the 10 Malay *bomohs*, only 2 of them were women. Among Hindus in Southeast Asia, shamanism is almost exclusively practiced by men, aside from women occasionally falling into trance during festivals (*Thaipusam* or *Timiti*, see Chapter 1, I, and Fig.3).

3.1.5. Occupation
Of the 122 shamans, mediums, and healers, 117 had day-time jobs. They were business men, clerks, contractors, car salesmen, truck drivers, farmers, fishermen, hawkers, housewives, etc. Among the five shamans without a regular daytime job, one was a retired business man and the other four had become full-time shamans, because the need for their services had increased.

3.1.6. Socio-economic Status
With three exceptions (high government officials in Bangkok, see Part 2, Case 18), the majority of shamans I studied, belonged either to the lower-middle or the working classes. Being a shaman, though, raised their status inside their own socio-economic network.

3.1.7. Character
The character profiles of the 122 practitioners differed considerably from outgoing worldly to religiously oriented and withdrawn. None of them showed pathological symptoms, i.e., was severely disturbed. I mention this because De Groot said that mediums, e.g.,

> must be a nervous, impressionable, hysterical kind of people, physically and mentally weak, and therefore easily stirred to ecstasy. The strain on their nerves cannot be borne for many years, and hence they all die young (1910, VI:1296).

I know only of one case where somebody died because he had *refused* to become a shaman. Less than 10 per cent of all shamans I interviewed, whether Chinese, Thai, Malay or Indian, were suffering of poor health before they accepted the "call." All said that their health had been significantly improved, since they were serving their deities and 90 per cent felt they had been "selected" for their good behavior in previous lives. They maintained that it had taken several life times to prepare themselves for becoming a vehicle of the Divine.

All shamans I studied were able to go smoothly into and out of trance. They used their alternate states of consciousness[1] to fulfill the needs of their clients. It became apparent that it takes a healthy, almost robust mind to enter trance "voluntarily under controlled circumstances" (Lewis 1971:56). Even after long sessions, practitioners seemed to emerge refreshed. Case 16 (Part 2) reports on a medium who regularly healed and advised three days and three nights without getting up from her seat. She observed the phases of the moon which conform with *wan phra* (like our Sunday, the day for Buddhists practices). She healed, therefore, on the days between *wan phras*.

There were, however, practitioners who depleted their own energy, because they had not been fully trained or because they had "not been called" and were "forcing the issue." So lack of training and lack of calling may, indeed, lead to an untimely death.

Durand, who studied shamans in Vietnam, reported that none of them had a nervous condition, however, among the predominantly female Vietnamese shamans there were some deceived lovers, divorcees, widows, and women without children. Most women seemed to have experienced some emotional trouble (1959:15). This could not be verified for the 36 female shamans I studied in Southeast Asia. With one exception (Phrom Mali, see Part 2, Case 16), they were married, had children, and led a satisfactory home life.

Chinese mediums in Singapore are called *tang-ki* (Hokkien, "divining youth") or *ki-tong* (Teochew, reversing the syllables), or *kong t'ung* (Cantonese, "youth into whom a spirit descends"). Straitsborn Chinese may call a medium *loh-tang*. Elliott found in the Singapore of the fifties that men under twenty

> are the most suitable candidates — particularly those whose horoscopes . . . do not include a proper weighting of the more stable elements. Such people are expected to lead blameless but unhappy lives, and to die young (1955:46–57).

Chinese mediums in Singapore, however, were much older and of both sexes. In 1979, approximately 82 per cent were men and 18 per cent were women.

Chinese and Thai traditions maintain that individuals may accept the "call" to prolong their lives. They believe the time spent in trance is added to their life span. Also, in "serving" the spiritual world, they feel protected.

Most shamans, mediums, and healers were unassuming. Nothing, outside their work, indicated their connection to the spirit world. Most of them, however, had natural charisma.

Elements of Shamanism

To remove another stereotype, I want to stress that none of my male shamans was effeminate. Furthermore, when it is said that shamans will be "possessed" by and even marry spirits of the opposite sex, this is not always the case in Thailand, Malaysia, and Singapore. Only a few men were "visited" by female deities (e.g., a sea or an earth goddess), the majority of women, however, was "visited" by male deities. Male-oriented societies seem to have difficulties in tolerating the manifestations of powerful female spirits. The Indian goddess Kālī is the exception. When I contemplated on a painting which depicted Kālī dancing on the corpse of her consort Śiva, I suddenly understood that her fierceness is important. She is supposed to fight the most powerful demons. For Hindus, therefore, the Great Mother Kālī is the last resort in calamities.

Delaney, who conducted research on spirit mediums in northern Thailand, confirmed that it is necessary for spirits to be male and of noble lineage.

Otherwise upper class women would be forced to admit they are seeking counsel and advice from lower class female practitioners. The ideology of mediumship keeps the status differences between client and practitioner from becoming a problem. Upper class women are simply being helped by high level male spirits who happen to possess lower class mediums (1977:15).

3.1.8. Differences Between Thailand, Malaysia, and Singapore:

3.1.8.1. Thailand

I found three kinds of practitioners who were consulted in crisis situations. Such mediators to the spirit world were selected according to individual needs. The three groups distinguished themselves by the source on which they based their authority.

1. *Buddhist monks* are supposed to keep the *dhamma* (Pāli, "Buddha's teachings") alive. They become *ong* ("sacred") at the time of their ordination. Monks need not claim any authority or divine revelation other than the spiritual insights they have gained during their years of cultivation. They are the teachers of the *Sangha*, the Buddhist community. Ahjan Man, an *arahant* ("enlightened one") of the 20th century (1871–1949), spoke to his disciples as well as deities and nature spirits who came to listen to his sermons (Heinze 1977b). A prominent abbot in Bangkok (presently the Sangharaja, highest authority in Thai Buddhist affairs) told me that monks

should not refuse to "cater to the needs of the people." In the canonical literature, Buddha sanctioned "useful means" (*upaya*), when insights gained during cultivation have not yet set an individual free. Therefore, when asked to do so, monks will dispense *nam mon* (blessed water) and provide charms (*khryang raeng*, see also Tambiah, 1968, 1970, 1973, 1984). Monks exorcise individuals (see Part 2, Case 17 and Fig.43) as well as Buddha statues and houses possessed by unwanted spirits. My personal observations in Bangkok (1972 and 1979) were confirmed by a report in the *San Francisco Examiner*:

> A Streetside Exorcism To Appease The Spirits
> Bangkok, (Thailand (UPI) - Buddhist monks and Chinese dragon dancers were called in to exorcise restless spirits at a busy Bangkok intersection where several people died recently in traffic accidents.
> Nine saffron-robed monks chanted and sprinkled holy water on the pavement Tuesday following complaints the spirits of dead accident victims caused nightmares for people living near the dangerous intersection . . . .
> The religious rite, a Chinese dragon dance and the burning of symbolic gold and silver colored paper stopped traffic at the busy junction of Rama IV and Saphan Lueng Roads.
> But instead of honking horns or complaining about the stalled traffic, motorists bowed reverently and prayed for the mercy of the traffic spirits (November 9, 1983).

2. *Brahmins*[2] draw their authority from being the legitimate mediators to gods of the Hindu pantheon (mainly Viṣṇu, Śiva, and Śiva's son, Murgam). In 1979, they were invited to cast horoscopes, e.g., they determined the auspicious time for important events in the life of individuals (e.g., weddings) as well as for affairs of state (e.g., opening of public buildings). Because their services were more expensive, they were consulted mainly by the elite, but they were ready to advise, bless or exorcise anybody who was willing to pay their fees. They also assisted the faithful who fell into trance during festival time (see Fig.3).

3. *Monks* are not supposed to become "possessed" and brahmins rarely are, but there are *laymen and -women who learn how to monitor their trances*. These practitioners are closer to the people because they live among them.

They are believed to have a "hot" line to the spiritual world. So they draw authority from the spiritual forces who speak and act through them. In 1979, some shamans also guided the souls of the dying into the other world, others recalled the wandering spirits of the living. Thai shamans mastered these feats to varying degrees and some specialized on certain services. Distinguishable by the degree of control they had over their spiritual contacts, I found the following three sub-groups in Thailand:

a. The *ma khi* ("horses of the spirit") become *fully possessed* and do not remember what transpires during possession. It is believed that a spirit takes over the body of a shaman whose soul may be visiting the heavens in the meantime (see Part 2, Case 1). Spirits may also be in need of a body through which they can help others to improve their own *kamma*, i.e., the quality of their next rebirth (see also Zuehlsdorf 1972).

Hinderling found in Thailand that not only

did the intruding spirit take care of the affairs of the medium concerned but also the fact that having been "chosen" by the spirits together with the attention that this person receives from the surroundings could have a therapeutic effect (1973:22).

To be intruded by spirits of a higher level, i.e., deities, sages and highly evolved monks, even former kings of Thailand (see Part 2, Case 16), certainly raises the status of a medium.

Most practitioners in my sample did, however, not suffer from an initial illness and did not fit Hinderling's findings that, in the case of *khon song*, (mediums), mental crises are regulated by religious patterns. With one exception (see Part 2, Case 16), my practitioners also contradicted Lewis' observations that vocation is "announced by an initially uncontrolled state of possession: a traumatic experience associated with hysteroid ecstatic behavior" which leads "to a state where possession can be controlled and can be turned on and off at will" (1971:55).

We should not forget that shamans and mediums do not really "possess" their spirits, they are possessed by them.

b. Over the years, most practitioners in my sample *developed, to a certain degree, control* over their possession, but they continued to rely on the help of assistants in cases when an unwanted spirit may take over.

c. Other individuals *decide to become shamans* and *do not use a possession state*. They seek training from respected elders (see Part 2, Case 18) and may be telepathically advised by spirits.

In sum, the majority of shamans, mediums, and healers I studied had not suffered from an illness from which they were cured the moment they accepted the "call." All claimed, however, that they enjoyed good health and good fortune after they had begun to serve spiritual entities and had become "instrumental" in "salvation work."

3.1.8.2. Malaysia

Applying the above statements to *Malaysia*, i.e., Malay-Muslims, a *bomoh* is a medicine man who uses the knowledge of traditional medicine. He may also foretell the future and raise spirits by reciting verses from the Koran, e.g., *berkat, el fatehya, terang hati, sembahyang haja* (see Danaraj 1964; Gimlette 1974:18–19; Hartog 1973:352–372; Mustapha 1977; and others). A *bomoh belian* is a spirit-raising exorcist, and a *bomoh gebien* a spirit medium. A *bomoh mok peh* cures the sick. He also finds lost and stolen objects, and divines, with a bundle of small canes. He can tell whether a witchcraft charm has been hidden under the house. A *bomoh patah* is a doctor who treats fractures, a *bomoh pesaka* is a hereditary medicine man, and a *bomoh puteri* raises *puteri* ("princesses," higher spirits) for curing purposes.

3.1.8.3. Singapore

In Singapore I found among the shamans, mediums, and healers Buddhist monks, *bomohs*, and *brahmins* as well. To them I had to add

3.1.8.3.1. Taoist priests

Taoist priests who were consulted by Chinese for specific purposes. Taoist priests based their authority on lineages where teachers select and authorize only one successor from a large group of disciples. The secret scriptures, the ritual texts for making charms and the instructions for exorcism are all lineage-specific. Like Buddhist monks and *brahmins*, Taoist priests are advised by spirits. They read petitions or dance the pattern of the Big Dipper (see Fig.26) to contact spirits but, in 1979, they rarely went into trance.

3.1.8.3.2. Shamans, mediums, and healers

Shamans, mediums, and *healers* in all three countries differed due to their personal faculties and techniques developed either through trial and error or through divine inspiration.

Some shamans spent time talking with clients; others spent more time with performing elaborate rituals and reciting formalized evocations and prayers. Some employed magic (including sleight of hand) or performed other inexplicable feats. Some shamans stressed the moral aspects of "divine" advice. Some became experts in exorcism. Some were famous for "removing bad luck" (Chinese, *kuay oon*). Most of them divined and provided spiritual protection in form of blessings, amulets, charm papers, lustral water, etc. Some shamans cultivated their faculties of curing and used their herbal knowledge, massaged and suggested a bath with blessed water. Some did all of the above.

Some shamans had many clients and received considerable donations; others remained poor although they had a large number of clients. Donations were often minimal. Some practitioners developed cults, others were unimpressive, but worked successfully on subtle levels. "But almost all the ones I observed shared one particular clinical characteristic; they were skilled at responding quickly to exigent intra- and inter-personal *crises*" (Kleinman 1980:233).

In brief, ethnic differences determined the predominance of certain religious elements. Where, however, shamans added elements from other religions to their rituals, these elements seemed to blend in quite well and appeared to be supplementary and supportive. Idiosyncracies were a combination of the shaman's own character, the characteristics of the "possessing" deities, and the expectations of the devotees.

Most shamans developed a followership on their own and generally tried to avoid a competitive stance toward other shamans. Where not sufficient physicians were available, shamans became the most respected members of their community (see Hartog 1972:355 for *bomohs* in rural Malaysia). Some shamans ran regular weekly clinics in their home where patients could come without appointment. Some even made house calls.

It is important to keep in mind that I found a wide range of shamans, mediums, and healers in Thailand, Malaysia, and Singapore. The needs and functions they fulfilled will be documented in Part 2.

Trance and Healing in Southeast Asia Today

3.1.9. How Does One Become a Shaman?

3.1.9.1. Hereditary

All ten Malay *bomohs* and two of the 67 Chinese shamans in my study inherited their faculties, the two Chinese shamans and the two Malay *bomohs* in Singapore from their grandmother or an uncle from their mother's side, the eight Malay *bomohs* in Malaysia and Thailand from one of their grandfathers. Of the remaining 110 shamans, no previous case of a practicing shaman was known in their families. When the care of clan spirits is inherited matrilineally in northern Thailand (Heinze 1982a), this does not imply that the women in charge are shamans. They may occasionally fall into trance, but they do not work with clients outside their family on a regular basis.

3.1.9.2. Revelations or visions

Most shamans and mediums in my sample experienced visions at the beginning of their career. In the case of Malay-Muslim *bomohs* (see Part 2, Cases 11–14), the grandmother on their mother's side or the grandfather on their father's side appeared in dreams and informed them of their mission.

In several Chinese cases, individuals became "possessed" during festivals while witnessing other shamanic performances and hearing the chanting and beating of drums (see IV:3–4 of this chapter). Encouraged by experienced shamans, they then apprenticed themselves to a master.

Reports of how Chinese become shamans and mediums are presented in Part 2, Case 1, 3, and 4. Case 2 reports on revelations which led to the mediumship of a Tamil dock worker. Cases 15, 16, and 20 illustrate developments in Thailand.

3.1.9.3. Decision

Mainly in Thailand, I came across cases where individuals decided to become shamans (Part 2, Case 18). They meditated and were taught evocations to access alternate states of consciousness. Their spirits — Phra Narai, deified heroes or famous monks — did not enter the body of shamans. They stayed behind them and advised what to say and what to do. (Incidentally, the Bangkok group I conducted research on was training only male shamans.)

In sum, in the first two categories, shamanic practices were preceded by visions. An "intrusion" indicated that a spiritual entity had selected an individual for altruistic reasons. In all three categories, the attainment of shamanic faculties was confirmed by other shamans. After needs had been fulfilled and positive results had been observed, public recognition was instantaneous. The process followed the rules of natural selection. Effective shamans were sought, ineffective shamans faded away fast.

3.1.10. Preparation

3.1.10.1. Solely advised by spiritual entities

In the majority of cases, be they Chinese, Thai, Malay, or Indian, shamans and mediums were *solely advised* by *spiritual entities*. Their clients expected to come into the presence of spiritual forces who speak to them, cure and answer questions. This belief naturally supported the work of the practitioners they consulted. People need more than just medicine. People want moral advice and the blessings of a higher authority. This view was shared by the hundreds of clients I interviewed.

Most shamans and mediums maintained they had no recall of what transpired during trance. Most of them said that the spirits taught them how to change their life style and how to make decisions outside of trance. Some received instructions during meditation, telepathically.

3.1.10.2. Formal training

Only a few Chinese and Thai but none of the Malay and Indian shamans and mediums interviewed went through any *formal training*. In Singapore, there were at least four traditional Chinese schools for *tang-ki* and a group of approximately fifteen young men who work up to and perfect their mediumship mainly through meditation under the guidance of a charismatic leader.

In 1979, four men were also trained at the Red Swastika Society to develop their skills for holding a T-shaped stick during sandbox writing (see Part 2, Case 8 and Figs.28 and 29).

When selected, new shamans remember other shamans' performances. They had been brought to mediums by their parents and, later on, had consulted mediums on their own. Nobody had difficulty in emulating the culture-specific models, though most of them later developed a style of their own.

3.1.11. Initiation and Change of Life Style

Dore (First Part, Vol.I:150) mentioned De Groot's report on initiations in the China of the past. Mediums would keep funerary urns that each contained the soul of a deceased person. An applicant would approach one of the urns. When it was unsealed, it was believed that the imprisoned soul would escape into the body of the novice and stay with him or her from there on.

In the case of Singapore Chinese, a Taoist priest might conduct a series of initiations. In Thailand, the leader of a spirit medium lineage has to introduce each novice officially to the lineage. (During the spirit dances, held in June each year in Northern Thailand, only members recognized by their lineage were allowed to participate, others had to be officially invited; see Part 2, Case 19).

Malay *bomohs* and Indian *swamis* did not require any initiation other than being selected by an ancestral spirit, the spirit of a dead shaman, or a deity.

Because nobody talked about initiations to outsiders, it could not be verified whether candidates in Southeast Asia go through dismemberment and rebirth experiences, but all reported that their lives changed considerably since they began to practice. Some chose a life of celibacy, although their spouse still stayed in their house or apartment. Most of the shamans and mediums became vegetarians, this meant they did not eat beef, at least, not on the days they practiced. They also began to meditate regularly.

When outsiders wonder why some shamans or mediums drink or smoke during sessions although they never would do so in daily life, it is said that they want to put the "possessing" spirit, e.g., a deified general, "into a good mood" (see Fig.7).

Jordan told us that he observed on Taiwan an appearance of the Living Buddha which was

> vigorous to the point of rambunctious. In song and story the Living Buddha of Salvation is an idiosyncratic bonze whose orthodox behavior shocks his fellow priests but contributes to the salvation of souls. This alarming unpredictability is represented in Gau's performance by constant smoking of cigarettes (sometimes several simultaneously) while in trance and the consumption of an entire bottle of rice wine at the onset of trance (1977:10).

In January 1979, I observed an almost identical performance on the Malay island of Penang (see Fig. 20). "Possessed" by the Living Buddha, the Chinese medium drank and smoked to the delight of his clients. In Singapore, I saw another Chinese medium in trance consume large amounts of rice wine, whiskey and opium within a comparatively short time. Without any visible signs of intoxification, the medium continued to advise, divine, and cure for hours (see Fig.7). In another case, a middle-age housewife, "possessed" by a deified general from the Three Kingdoms, drank liquor when in trance, although she was a diabetic and had a

Elements of Shamanism

strong dislike of any form of alcohol (see Part 2, Case 1). Delaney (1977:11) confirmed for northern Thailand that Thai shamans smoke, drink, and dance to show the traits of their spirits. The display of human weaknesses seemed to increase the popularity of the spirits.

3.1.12. Reasons to Continue

3.1.12.1. Altruistic

The majority of shamans, mediums and healers had day-time occupations. They practiced in their spare time, e.g., the 1st and 15th day of the lunar month or once a week on Saturdays, or twice a week on Tuesdays and Fridays, or three times a week on Mondays, Wednesdays, Fridays, or all evenings with two sessions held on Saturdays and Sundays (see, Case 1, Part 2). Their reasons to continue are truly *altruistic*.

There would be donation boxes or small red envelopes (called *ang pow* in *Chinese*), left voluntarily by clients on the altar. These envelopes contained, in 1979, from 10 cent up to 2 dollars, seldom more. The money was collected either by the temple keeper but mostly by the temple committee who, advised by deities, as they said, would spend the donations for

1. the upkeep of the temple: incense, candles, oil for the altar lamps, charm papers (when clients had not bought these supplies already in a special shop or from the temple keeper),
2. the temple keeper (when he was living in or close to the temple),
3. paraphernalia (see 4.2., this Chapter),

When large sums had been accumulated,

4. dinners were organized for devotees on festival days and, in the Chinese case, lion dances and operas would be performed opposite the main altar to entertain the deities, or
5. donations were made to welfare organizations (e.g., orphanages and old-age homes).

3.1.12.2. Gain in status

Shamans in Southeast Asia enjoyed a *gain in status*, not so much in the greater society but inside their own social system, e.g. among their family (who usually was large), entourage (attendants and regular devotees), and clients. The reputation that certain shamans' services were effective brought about not only a rise in social status but ranked the shamans also higher in the spiritual hierarchy. In the case of Chinese female shamans, a husband would kneel in front of his wife when deities manifested in her body, while outside the sessions the same husband did not hesitate to exert his rights as head of household (see Part 2, Case 1).

3.1.12.3. Other reasons

There were *other reasons* to continue. For example, some shamans, mediums, and healers had fixed rates. One Singapore Chinese medium expected, in 1979, a donation of Singapore $36 (approximately US$18) together with a bottle of oil, joss paper, and fruit for "changing luck" (*kuay oon*). Or the age of clients was converted into dollars when they wanted the deity to produce precious stones. These gems appeared miraculously when the medium bit into a piece of fruit the client had brought. The gems, mainly jade, were then set by a jeweller and worn as amulets on a gold chain.

Stories were told how shamans, mediums, and healers lost their power when they became too greedy. Where, however, *prosperity* of shamans and their families became visible, it was said that it proved not only the gratitude of clients but the gratitude of the "possessing" deity who rewards faithful servants. It is certainly difficult to refuse donations of enthusiastic clients who, for example, insist on landscaping the garden of a house temple or who want to redecorate the house of the shaman to increase their own merit. In 1979, individuals did continue to show their gratitude to deities and included those who possessed "special healing powers" because they had the "ability to communicate with the spirit world" (Frank 1961:58).

3.1.12.4. Exploited by others

Even when shamans stayed altruistic, they may be *exploited by others*. I came across several cases where temple committees set the fees and took personal advantage of the shaman, for example, by "borrowing" money from the donation box (see Part 2, Case 2).

3.2. Entourage (see also, introduction, note 7)

3.2.1. Characteristics

At the beginning of a shaman's or medium's career, the entourage consisted of relatives, friends, and colleagues who agreed among themselves when they would serve during the sessions. Later, assistants were recruited from the group of regular devotees. After their involvement had been "approved" by the deity, they continued to serve on a voluntary basis. Even where official temple committees had been formed, their members stayed loosely organized. (The situation differed considerably, however, when a clan organization or, e.g., in Singapore, a former secret society, was sponsoring temple and mediums.)

Temple committees met regularly on the eve of festivals to

1. set up different altars outside the temple,
2. put up gates to pass or bridges to cross. Such crossings symbolize walking away from bad luck and entering a new and brighter future (see van Gennep's "rites of passage" 1909/1960 and Blacker 1975:19–33).

Differences in age and socio-economic status played no role when assistants carried out their sacred tasks. A lawyer or a physician might serve a deity on equal terms with a dock worker. The time they had been serving a deity determined their rank in the hierarchy developing around a shaman. All enjoyed a rise in status, because they were more intimately related to deities and they always claimed they had been appointed by the deities to do "salvation work."

It should be noted here that, in the cases I observed in Singapore, most attendants and temple committee members were male, even when the shaman was female. The male temple committee members also cleaned the temple after the sessions. Women were supposed to prepare the meal after the session (see Fig.10).

Fluctuations in size and enthusiasm of the entourage were indicators whether a cult was born, growing, flourishing, dying and moribund or reviving (Elliott 1955:126–133). The status of entourage and clients depended on the shaman's, i.e., the spirit's, effectiveness. Most practitioners I worked with in 1979, however, did not encourage the development of a cult, they stayed humble and did not seem to seek glorification.

Yang reported on developments in China where "someone from time to time among a large number of worshippers had prayers fulfilled," this maintained the prestige of the god and the temple continued to exist (1961:353). His statement is valid for most of the shamans, mediums, and healers mentioned in this study. Where local governments did not appear to be in favor of growing religious groups, most shamans, mediums, and healers kept a low profile and relied on loosely structured communities. They were flexible and concerned about diffusing suspicion.

3.2.2. Functions

Shamans and mediums, when in trance, sometimes spoke another dialect, e.g., medieval Hokkien, or even a different language (Mandarin, Indonesian, Tamil). These dialects or languages were not always intelligible to each client and required the presence of a translator. Most clients were too awed to understand the words of a deity anyway. They were glad when a translator offered interpretations. When, during my fieldwork, an answer appeared to be inappropriate, the assistant readily admitted he had made a mistake in his translation. Translators even answered before a deity had spoken. Clients did not object because the presence of a deity lent sufficient justification. It was unthinkable that a translator would take liberties, overstep his responsibility and deviate from the "divine word," without being severely reprimanded by the deity.

The number of attendants grew with the reputation of a shaman. A translator might continue to wipe the altar clean during a session. He might also give ritual objects to the shaman, but other helpers are needed to

1. distribute numbers among clients to establish the waiting order,
2. keep records, especially when herbal medicine is dispensed,
3. explain how charm papers have to be used by burning them and mixing the ashes with water for drinking and/or bathing or folding them to be worn as amulets, or affixing them to the front wall of one's house or apartment,
4. instruct
   a. how the deity has to be evoked, and
   b. how many joss sticks, for example, have to be lit and put into different urns, in what sequence, when entering and leaving a temple (see Fig.11).

It is essential to perform a ritual correctly. Rituals are, therefore, institutionalized after the first successful performance. I had the opportunity to observe the process of ritualization at a Chinese house temple in Singapore. Deities had given the instructions how they wanted to be addressed and how they expected to be treated, but the members of the entourage seemed to have been given differing instructions. Not to contradict each other and to meet the clients' expectations, they had to get together and coordinate their answers. Even when mistakes were made inadvertently or out of ignorance, it was believed that the efficacy of the ritual had been jeopardized.

So when a ritual failed to yield the expected results, it was often blamed on mistakes made by the ritualist. Other reasons for failure were impurity (e.g., women entering the temple during their monthly illness or the shaman having eaten beef). Opinions differed. A Chinese medium told me that she continues to perform during her monthly illness, but a female client, entering the temple during her monthly "illness," would pollute the "sacred space" (see Part 2, Case 1).

When the services of a shaman proved to be effective, the number of clients kept growing, so did the amount of donations. In the Chinese case, a temple committee may offer the management of a temple to the highest bidder. Assisted by some volunteers, he would care for the temple, e.g., take all incoming money to pay monks and Taoist priests for certain functions, finance festivals, and cover all other expenses connected with the temple's maintenance. Other temples were run as free enterprise by shamans and their families or by a temple community (Nyce 1973:94 and Elliott 1955:41).

In general, even when a shaman had hundreds of clients, the donations were modest and barely covered expenses. Only four of the 122 shamans I studied displayed some wealth.

3.3. Clients

3.3.1. Characteristics

All men and women who consulted shamans, mediums, and healers were, in 1978/1979, adults. They belonged to a wide range of age groups. Having accompanied their parents when they were children, they were brought by younger relatives when they could not come on their own anymore. I observed, though, that the majority of clients were between 18 and 45 years of age, with women being slightly in the majority.

Each society is composed of a wide range of socio-economic groups, the lower-middle and the working classes being the largest in number, with professionals usually in the minority. The clients of the practitioners I studied, showed the same distribution. They belonged predominantly to the lower-middle and working classes, but a few professionals came to consult the deities too. To whatever socio-economic group they belonged, all clients sought protection and help of spiritual powers, manifesting in the shaman or medium of their choice.

3.3.2. How Do Clients Meet Shamans, Mediums, and Healers?

When shamans began to practice, their first clients would be relatives, friends and colleagues. The word spread fast when protection and advice given by the deities turned out to be effective. Wherever and whomever I asked about practitioners, no matter which ethnic group in Singapore, Malaysia or Thailand, everybody knew at least somebody who had contact with shamans, mediums and healers, if s/he had not already visited a practitioner in a personal crisis him- or herself.

In general, shamans did not advertise. There was no need for it. They preferred to work within their individual networks and respected the networks of others. Working strictly by word of mouth, the danger that false claims were made was reduced. Incidentally, practitioners never claimed their help would be successful. They considered it preposterous to outguess the decisions of spiritual powers. Practitioners suggested solutions to the clients' problems and everybody prayed for a positive outcome of the ritual.

3.3.3. When Are Shamans, Mediums, and Healers Consulted?

The main reasons were very pragmatic. Shamans, mediums, and healers were consulted in matters of

1. health, including exorcism and the blessing of medicine prescribed by "modern" physicians, or
2. family problems, e.g., between spouses, parents, children, in-laws, or problems with colleagues or supervisors,
3. concern about professional careers, job changes or not knowing whether to start a new business or whether to buy or sell a house.

Clients may also be concerned about

4. fertility, longevity, and wealth, e.g., asking for a lottery number.

Practitioners may, furthermore, be asked

5. to determine the right location, e.g., for a house and an altar, and
6. to provide divine blessings for various reasons.

The therapeutic effects of a shaman's intervention are demonstrated by the following two examples:

In Singapore, I met a physician who monitored the life-saving equipment at a large hospital. He went regularly to a Chinese medium to secure the protection of a deity for his work. He told me that a surgeon may blunder during an operation, but a failure of the life-saving equipment would be fatal for the patient. He strongly believed that, with the protection of a deity, he does perform his professional duties with a better peace of mind.

In another case, a physician informed a worker that his brain tumor required operation. Mortally afraid of such drastic measure, the worker consulted a Chinese medium. The deity, through the medium, told him that the tumor was too advanced to be removed spiritually. The worker had to undergo surgery within two weeks to stay alive. When still not ready for the tumor operation, the deity announced he would go with the worker into the operation room and guide the surgeon's hands. If the worker should be "pure," he even would be able to see the deity. The hospital staff was surprised by the sudden calmness of the patient. The operation turned out to be comparatively easy and the worker recuperated within an unusually short time.

These two cases prove how the belief in spiritual protection and help activated the self-healing powers and the confidence of two clients.

Do shamans, mediums, and healer refuse cases? I agree with Frank who found that they "are usually adept at distinguishing illnesses they can treat successfully from those that are beyond their powers and they manage to reject patients with whom they are likely to fail" (1961:56). I was present, at several occasions, when practitioners declared it was not the right time for treatment. They all recommended frequently to see a Western-trained physician.

Where public health facilities are available, shamans in Southeast Asia send their clients to see a physician first. To give an example of the caution taken by shamans, I remember an incident when a dying man was brought to a medium on Ganges Road. The practitioner took one look at the old man and announced that he would go up to heaven to plead for him. If, however, his time should be up that is all he could do. The dying man and his family were satisfied that somebody was pleading the case and the shaman had gracefully avoided the situation of pretending to cure a dying man. He gave the assurance that a natural process was going on. The dying man felt protected and, accompanied by the love of all concerned, he "knew" he could continue to "go to the light" (see the *Tibetan Book of the Dead,* Evans-Wentz 1960).

It was usually the client who decided to supplement modern medicine with "traditional" treatments. Another dimension was added to "complete" the healing process. I will discuss this point more extensively in Chapter 4.

3.4. Shamanic Performances

3.4.1. Operational Base
Chinese shamans usually practiced in temples. Comber estimated that, in the fifties, there were about 500 Chinese public places of worship in Singapore. He said,

> They are known by a variety of names, depending less upon the nature of the buildings than upon the imagination of their founders. The following names are found in use in Singapore: Kung, Tz'u, T'ing, Miao, Tien, T'ang,[3] and Szu. There is no significant difference for our purposes between these exotic sounding names. They may all be translated "temple," "shrine" or "monastery".... They range in size from tiny roadside shrines and attap huts to imposing carved wood and stonework buildings (1958:1).

The number of Chinese places of worship in Singapore was much larger in 1978/79. To count Chinese temples in Singapore was impossible because many shamans practiced in front of a house altar in their own home. When their reputation had grown, their apartment in a high-rise building or their rented or owned house was progressively converted into a temple where worshippers could come anytime to pray. Shamans may move into a larger house where the lower floor was used for temple purposes. When temple committees began to collect money and private donations came in large amounts, sufficient to build a new temple,[4] only then the license required for temple operation was secured and this place of worship became countable in the registrar's office.

While, at certain times, in some temples up to three shamans may be working, many Chinese temples in Singapore had no medium anymore. The reasons given in 1979 were that mediums lost their power, moved away or died. Freelance mediums or mediums from other temples may be invited on festival days. During the rest of the year, these temples stayed open for worshippers. Those who wanted answers from their deities used divining blocks (*mu bei*, see Fig.15).

Furthermore, when city planners ordered the demolition of old Chinese temples, mediums returned to practicing in their homes which may be Housing

Development Board (HDB) flats in high rise buildings.[5] Or donations by high city officials allowed the building of a new temple at a different location.[4]

Hindu, *Malay*, and *Thai* mediums practiced usually in their own home.

3.4.2. Paraphernalia

In 1979, Malay-Muslim *bomohs* practiced in their daily clothes and used a minimum in equipment, i.e.,

1. water and flowers, blessed while chanting verses from the Koran[6] and to be offered while evoking familiar spirits;
2. limes (*limau nipis*), cut into four pieces for divination. When more than two pieces fell cut side up (*buka*), the question had been answered positively. When more than two pieces fell cut side down (*tutup*), the answer was "no";
3. a wooden knife, put between the toes of clients to diagnose the nature of their ailment and to find out whether an evil spirit caused the illness; and
4. herbal medicine.

Indian male shamans wore a white *dhoti* (loin cloth), leaving the upper part of their body bare. They also used limes to exorcise and *nim* (margosa, pomegranate) leaves to sprinkle blessed water. And they distributed *vibhuti* (cow dung ashes) to mark the clients' forehead or to be applied externally or internally for healing purposes.

One of my *Thai* male shamans followed the Indian tradition and wore a white *dhoti*, draping a shawl like the sacred cord of *brahmins* across his upper body. The other Thai shamans wore either street clothes or Burmese attire (see Part 2, Cases 19 and 20, and Figs.45 and 46). The Thai hill tribe shaman had her eyes covered with a black cloth. When she was riding through the spirit world, she sat on a bench, like a horse, and shook metal objects in a rhythmic fashion.

Most *Chinese* shamans required more elaborate equipment (see Elliott 1955:57–58). Attendants wore sometimes white clothes during festivals to distinguish themselves from the devotees or to indicate that they were keeping special vows of purity. Male Chinese mediums usually wore yellow pants and put on ceremonial robes when the deity "entered" their body (see Fig.8). Important was

> a kind of apron (Hokkien, *siu to*), called a "stomacher" by de Groot, which fastens across the front of the body. This is made of coloured, embroidered silk, and proclaims

the identity of the *shen* (deity), the name of the temple, and probably the name of the donor as well. A temple must possess stomachers suitable for each one of the *shen* that is likely to make an appearance (Elliott 1955:51).

In Singapore, I met only one male Chinese medium who practiced in his street clothes. Female Chinese mediums will either wear suits of subdued color (see Fig.9) or long white dresses and crowns when visited by Kuan Yin (see Fig.21).

A black flag with the Eight Trigrams printed or embroidered in yellow or gold was placed in a huge incense urn in front of a Chinese temple when a medium was working inside (see Fig.23). The *Pa Kua* (Eight Trigrams) were supposed to ward off evil. Legends say the trigrams has been "invented" by the mythical ruler Fu Hsi to warn ghosts (Elliott 1955:51). Inside a temple, black flags were used for blessing adults and yellow flags for blessing children.

A *lung wei* (dragon throne) had to be ready for the shaman to sit in front of the altar when in trance. The dragon throne was a heavily built, portable, wooden chair with dragon heads carved at the end of each arm rest and each end of the back rest (see Fig.8). The chairs were usually painted red though blue and green chairs were also kept in reserve for other deities. On the Malay Island of Penang, I found that Chinese shamans sometimes simply used a "Lotus Chair" (usually a simple stool).

On the main altar and the different side altars, there were urns into which lighted incense sticks were placed at the beginning of each session by assistants or the shaman. Devotees added their own incense sticks when they entered the temple. During the session, benzoin was burned, e.g., to support the trance of the medium. Red ink and brushes to write on charm paper (*fu*) had to be ready, together with at least one dragon whip which would be used during exorcism. There were two kinds of exorcising whips. One consisted of a tuft from a horse's tail, fastened to a wooden handle about 18 inches long. The other, known as a "method cord," was a long plaited rope, attached to a shorter wooden handle in the shape of a dragon's head (Elliott 1955:52, see also Fig.24). To ward off evil spirits, blessed water with pomegranate leaves and crushed rock salt mixed with uncooked rice were kept at hand.

Indispensable were the *mu bei*, made out of kidney-shaped pieces of bamboo root (divining blocks, see Fig.15). Between 6 to 8 inches in length, they had been split lengthwise into two halves, each with one flat and one convex side. The

> bamboo should be taken from a plant where the living root was able to throw several stems, showing intense vital and productive power ... strongly animated by a shen.

also by constantly lying on an altar, the blocks are thought of being imbued with the spirit of the god who is worshipped there. Spirituality may be increased by passing them through the smoke of incense sticks which the questioner piously places in the urn in front of the statue of the god. When a question is asked, the blocks are piously lifted flat faces upward towards the idol and then dropped on the ground. If they lie there with the two convex sides uppermost, the answer is called "double yin," or "full yin"; if both flat faces are uppermost, it is "double yang" or "full yang," and in both cases it is negative, but one flat and one convex side is an affirmative answer, called "perfect" (De Groot 1910:1285).

De Groot (1910:1288) told us that such blocks were used as early as the 11th century B.C.[7] The literary name for these blocks, *kiao*, did not occur in Chinese classics. Some scholars think that originally pieces of jade may have been used.

Where shamans and mediums were not available, sortilege (divination with bamboo sticks) might be practiced in Chinese Taoist or Thai Buddhist temples.

Most temples have among their furnishings bamboo tubes holding a set of sticks, varying from 20 to 103 sticks in a set. Each stick is marked with a number, and each number is identified with a slip of printed verses in a file of slips. The person requesting divine guidance kneels in front of the image of the god; he shakes the bamboo tube holding the lot sticks until one stick drops out. He gives the stick to the temple priests, who pulls a slip out of the file according to the number, and reads and explains the verse (Yang 1961:262).

Based on Confucian or Buddhist thought, the verses were supposed to provide words of guidance.

Because *chanting* and *music* were frequently used to induce trance and to evoke the deities, drums and gongs had to be at hand. They would be played by members of the temple committee or regular devotees who took over when necessary. And there would be a *muh-yu* (wooden fish, a skull-shaped block) beaten during chanting. Even small children may join in the chanting or play an instrument.

In some Indian temples or wherever *Indian* shamans and mediums performed, the devotees would sing *bhajans* (devotional songs) at the beginning of the session.

Thai khon song or *Malay bomohs*, when entering a trance, did not require any music other than perhaps a chanted evocation. Only in northern Thailand, I observed a Meo shaman chanting and shaking metal objects in each hand while "riding through the spirit world" (see Part 2, Case 21) or a Thai orchestra was accompanying the spirit dances in Chiang Mai (see Part 2, Case 19).

Swords may be used by *Chinese* mediums to cut their tongue and draw blood to write on charm paper. They would slash their backs with large swords to demonstrate that a deity was protecting them from injury. Or they used the swords in a dance to exorcise evil forces and to fight with invisible intruders. Chinese mediums would also use a prick ball (*teng k'au*) on their back and later sit on it during trance. A prick ball has 108 metal spikes, radiating from a central core, varying in diameter from 6 to 18 inches. Sometimes there was a network of colored yarn between the spikes or the ball was packed with yellow paper so that only the sharp ends protruded. The ball was held on a short chain or cord, swung over the head and then rolled across the shaman's back (see Fig.18). Blood would drop from superficial wounds, but after the blood had been wiped away, the scratches healed soon and left only minor scars if any (Elliott 1955:53).

Chinese temples had portable altars for festivals and processions. There were also portable wooden bridges (*p'ing an ch'iao*) over which believers walk into a better future (for symbolism about bridges between different worlds, see especially Blacker 1975:19–33). And there were sedan chairs for carrying the images of deities during processions. Other chairs are equipped with iron spikes (*teng-kio*) or knives (*to-kio*, see also Elliott 1955:54). The spikes were on the seat, the back, the arm and the foot rests (see Figs.7 and 8). Mediums may also use skewers, each with the head of one of the Five Generals, the protectors of the five directions (see Fig.24). They pierced their cheeks, tongues and upper arms at special occasions.

Indian devotees did the same to fulfill a vow. Indians also fastened lemons with hooks to their body and carried *kavadis* attached to their body with 108 hooks (footnote 2, Part 1, Chapter 1, and Figs.1 and 2). *Kavadi* carriers were, however, laymen and *not* shamans.

In 1979, most shamans and mediums just used water and flowers for blessing and did not mortify themselves at all. *Thai-Buddhist* and *Malay-Muslim* shamans never mortified themselves, because their religion did not expect self-immolation.

Important still were the charm papers in *Chinese* temples. They were either brought by clients or sold inside the temple by the temple keeper. It is believed that the deity, through the medium, writes magical characters on the paper with a writing brush, dipped into red ink to which blood has been added, drawn by the medium cutting his tongue. We are reminded of the belief in the magical quality of blood which survived also in the Christian Church where wine symbolizes Christ's blood during Holy Communion.

Dore told us that the

> earliest word employed by the Chinese for denoting a charm or spell is *Chuh*, which means to implore, invoke spirits, supplicate the gods for blessing, hence prayer combined with some exorcising formula summoning the gods to come to the assistance of man (1914–1929).

Dore reported that, in the works of Mencius (B.C.372–289), the character *fu* (bamboo slips made to tally with a corresponding part) occurred and was used for charms "of any form on wood, metal, linen or paper, written or engraved."

Frequently, written charms were called *luh*. Later writers combined these two words to *fu-luh*, "meaning all kinds of magic script for expelling demons, curing diseases and conferring happiness."

Dore considered a charm to be "an official document, a mandate, an injunction, coming from a god and setting to work superhuman powers who carry out the orders of the divinity." Because the Chinese world of spirits was modelled after the administrative system of the country with its higher and lower officials, higher gods would issue commands and lower gods would carry them out.

There always was an ample supply of charm papers in a Chinese temple, waiting to be activated by the medium in writing magical signs on it with red ink or dabbing it with an incense stick to heighten the potency of the charm. Bad luck can be removed by brushing a client from head to toe in front and in the back with a bundle of charm papers. Charm papers were also taken home to be affixed to the front wall of one's house, shop, apartment or they were folded and worn as talismans. Charm papers were, furthermore, burned, the ashes mixed with water and drunk for internal protection or used for bathing.[8]

All four ethnic groups used, in 1979, still blessed water for healing and protection.

Thai shamans provided many kinds of magic to influence and protect people. Their talismans (*khryang raeng*) may be Buddha images. Often several small terra-cotta depictions of Buddhist scenes or portraits of high ranking monks, individually gold-framed were lined up on a gold chain. Men usually wore necklaces under their shirt, so that the amulets could not be seen by others. Verses from the Buddhist Canon were also written on small pieces of paper, rolled up in small cylinders, and worn on these necklaces, not to speak of the many charms made out of wood and other substances (see, e.g., Tambiah 1984). Furthermore, in Southeast Asia, police men and soldiers may ask for magical tattoos, because they believe these tattoos would protect them against knives and bullets.

Malay may wear small metal pendants containing words of the Koran. They called these talismans *azimat* or *jimat*. *Tangkal* are other kinds of Malay talismans. Malay charms, in general, were called *pengaruh* or *pangaroh* and *pelian*.

Indians used the Sanskrit word *kavaca* for amulets which were made of bark or birch leaves and inscribed with mystical words.

It would go far beyond the scope of this book to discuss the making and use of charms and talismans in more detail. Let us, therefore, turn to the kind of trances experienced by shamans, medium, and healers.

3.4.3. Varieties of Trances

We all experience alternate states of consciousness, e.g., when we are dreaming or during the hypnagogic state preceding sleep or the hypnopompic state dispelling sleep. Of all the scholars who have attempted to establish a typology of alternate states of consciousness, I will mention only three, Fischer (1971), Krippner (1972), and Cohen (in Pelletier and Garfield 1976:87).

Fischer (1971) developed a diagram where states of (1) increasing arousal lead to hyperarousal and dysfunctional states while (2) increasing tranquility leads to hypoarousal, functional states, and complete stillness.

Krippner (1972) spoke of twenty semiautonomous states of consciousness: (1) dreaming, (2) sleeping, (3) hypnagogic state, (4) hypnopompic state, (5) hyperalertness, (6) lethargy, (7) state of rapture, (8) hysteria, (9) fragmentation, (10) regressiveness (inappropriate for the individual's age), (11) meditation, (12) trance, (13) reverie, (14) day-dreaming, (15) internal scanning, (16) stupor, (17) coma, (18) stored memory, (19) expanded conscious state, and (20) normal waking consciousness.

Cohen offered three main categories: (1) psychotic, (2) drug-induced, and (3) meditative or mystical states. He saw psychosis as a "pressured withdrawal from external reality with an incomplete return." Drug-induced states were for Cohen "more voluntary and elected with potentially less permanent disability," and mystical states were "consciously chosen, experienced, and then usually followed by a higher order of cognitive integration and sense of well-being" (1967; quoted in Pelletier and Garfield 1976;87).

These attempts of mapping states of consciousness alert us to the wide range of alternate states. I became aware that terminologies, used by experts (e.g., psychologists and psychiatrists), need refinement.

Furthermore, the effects of alternate states of consciousness on our autonomic nervous system have not yet been sufficiently studied. Only fairly recently it was recognized that a wide range of physical changes may be triggered during trance. Wallace and Benson (1972 in Zinberg 1977:137), for example, found that in wakeful relaxed states reductions in oxygen consumption occur together with changes in carbon dioxide elimination. The rate and volume of reduced respiration causes a slight increase in the acidity of arterial blood, marked by a decrease in the blood lactate level. The heart beat slows down and there will be a considerable increase in skin resistance and in alpha brain-wave patterns with occasional theta waves. These findings were confirmed by a physician at General Hospital, Singapore, who is prescribing meditation for high blood pressure cases. He used the polygraph to measure the change in skin resistance, i.e., the physical effects of meditation, practiced by his clients.

Jilek (1982:339–340) talked about the "endogenous opiod agents enkephalin and beta-endorphin and possibly other neuroendocrine peptides, such as neurotensin and bradykinin" which may "play an important role in the integration of pain information." Jilek mentioned Kline who described antidysphoric, antidepressant, anxiolytic, analgesic, and disinhibiting effects of beta-endorphin occurring within 5 to 10 minutes after injection and lasting from 1 to 6 hours. Kline (in Jilek) speculated that "beta-endorphin, produced by the anterior pituitary, may be the body's own way of producing and controlling affective states." More research on these processes is needed to assist us in teaching individuals how to monitor and to produce, for example, beta-endorphins, so that they can enhance their self-healing powers.

Shamans, mediums, and healers know how to access different states of consciousness. They use these states to fulfill the needs of their clients. The capacity to trance has them singled out for this task. Although, in curious ways, trances may manifest in individuals whom we least suspect to be susceptible, there must be a reason why some individuals can access trances more easily than others. One possible explanation may be that they are more sensitive (fine-tuned) and have a permeable ego axis. In other words, the strength of shamans manifests on a level where there is no ego.

Among the techniques to induce trance, I recognized the role of rhythmic sensory stimulation which had been studied already in the thirties by Adrian and Matthews and, in the forties, by Walters and Walters who came to the conclusion that rhythmic stimulation of the organ of hearing as a whole can be accomplished only by using a sound stimulus containing components of supraliminal intensity over the whole gamut of audible frequencies — in effect a steep-fronted sound such as produced by untuned percussion instruments (cited in Jilek 1982:327).

The Walters found

Stimulation of other receptors gives even more convincing results, particularly when very large group of sensory units can be excited simultaneously and rhythmically, for then the central electrical response is correspondingly larger and the subjective reports more assured (1949:37–58, 82, cited in Neher 1961:152).

The effect of drumming on the central nervous system has been known for over 20,000 years (e.g., petroglyphs document the use of drums in rituals). Prince (1968) considered the possibility of auditory driving a commonly used portal of entry into dissociative states. Neher (1961) exposed clinically and electroencephalographically normal individuals to low-frequency high-amplitude acoustic stimulations, produced by instruments similar to the deerskin drums used by North American Indians. He observed that different sound frequencies were transmitted along different nerve pathways in the brain (1961:152–153). (He did, however, not control for the flashing lights he had used to reinforce the low-frequency drumming.) Jilek reported that

auditory driving responses were elicited at the fundamental of each stimulus frequency (3, 4, 6, and 8 beats per second), and also at second harmonics and second subharmonics of some stimulus frequencies. Subjective responses similar to those obtained with photic driving were obtained in Neher's (1961) experiments, including visual and auditory imagery. According to Neher (1962), responses are heightened by accompanying rhythms reinforcing the main rhythms and by concomitant rhythmic stimulation in tactual and kinesthetic sensory modes. Susceptibility to rhythmic sensory stimulation is increased by stress and exertion, with resulting adrenalin secretion, also by hyperventilation and hypoglycemia (1982:327–328).

Jilek listed several techniques for the production of altered states of consciousness: focussed suggestive attention, pain stimulation, hypoglycemia, dehydration, forced hypermotility, hot or cold temperature stimulation, acoustic stimulation, seclusion

Elements of Shamanism

and restricted mobility, visual-sensory and sleep deprivation, kinetic stimulation, and hyperventilation (1982:335–339, see also, Heinze 1993:200–209).

Dissociative techniques are obviously not only used by shamans, mediums, and healers, spiritual exercises trigger similar physiological and psychological experiences. Kakar spoke of two

> that depend largely upon producing dissociation in the seeker-disciple: "rebirthing," generated with the help of quick deep breathing; and the "energy darshan" in the ritual initiation into the cult, where dance, rhythmic music and variation in lighting masterfully combine dissociation techniques from different shamanic traditions (1982:106).

Alternate states of consciousness experienced by shamans, mediums, and healers in 1979 differed not only in depth but varied also according to the characteristics of the "possessing" spirit, the faculties of the individual practitioner, and the purpose of the trance. Other differences arose from the situational and sociocultural context (Jilek 1982:326). Table 1, below,

1. lists the characteristics of alternate states of consciousness relevant to this book;
2. indicates whether these states are used for the benefit of others or are part of the process of self-cultivation;
3. distinguishes between "full possession," during which the "spirit is the actor," and "out of body experience" (OBE, also called "magical flight"), during which the "shaman is the actor";
4. observes increasing gain or increasing loss of control where the practitioner requires assistance.

In *Table 2*, the cross in the middle of the working model indicates everyday consensus reality. Increasing mind expansion is plotted on the upward vertical line, increasing dissociation on the downward vertical line. On the horizontal axis, increased gain of control moves toward the right and increased loss of control moves toward the left. The development of an individual will be plotted on the diagonal, from left bottom to right top.

During the research for this book, it became apparent that *possession* states were preferred by Southeast Asian practitioners. It is, therefore, necessary to say more about the wide range of possession states that have been scientifically studied so far.

Possession has been defined by Rouget

Table 1

Alternate States of Consciousness (ASC) Characteristics and Uses

1. *Possession* (based on the belief in spirit intrusion) - spirit is actor (D)
   a. professionally produced and used by shamans and mediums or
   b. uncontrolled, requiring exorcism and other treatment.
   Full possession where even shamans and mediums need assistance differs considerably from possession of lesser depth, different quality, and shorter duration.
   Individuals may be possessed by
      1) minor deities (seldom a high god) of an institutionalized religion,
      2) deified heroes, ancestor spirits, and restless spirits of the dead,
      3) nature spirits, and
      4) animal spirits, e.g., tiger spirits (souls of dead Malay shamans), horse spirits (e.g., Kuda Kepang, requiring initiation and some degree of professionalism; now mainly performed for entertainment at Muslim weddings and circumcisions, etc.).
      5) Non-professionals are usually possessed by low-ranking spirits who want to draw attention to their plight.

2. *Magical Flight* (out of body experience, OBE) - shaman is actor (M)
   a. spontaneously experienced or when close to death (NDE) or
   b. professionally produced to retrieve information.

3. *Other Dissociative (D) or Mind-Expanding (M) States*
   a. startle syndrome (mass hysteria (D) - not controlled, requires treatment;
   b. hallucinations (D/M) - if uncontrolled, requires treatment;
   c. effect of hallucinatory drugs (D/M) - used for mind-expanding or recreational purposes, not fully controlled;
   d. orgiastic trance (D) - produced by stimulants: drugs, alcohol, singing, drumming, dancing in a community setting, has cathartic effect; if uncontrolled, requires assistance;
   e. fire walking trance (D) - practiced by individuals as test of their faith or in fulfillment of a vow, in a community setting; not used professionally; requires assistance;

f. kavadi-carrying trance (D) - see III:5; requires assistance;
g. glossolalia (D) - practiced by individuals, mainly in community settings;
h. automatic writing (D/M) - used for private divination;
i. sandbox writing (D/M)* - used for professional divination;
j. extrasensory perception, ESP (M) - used privately and professionally;
k. hypnosis (D/M) - used privately and professionally.

4. *Aftereffects of ASC*
   a. shamans repeat and interpret for others what spirits have said (M);
   b. shamans have been taught by spirits how to help others. The presence of a spirit is no longer required (M).

5. *ASC Used for Self-Development*
   a. hypnagogic, hypnopompic, and dream states (D/M);
   b. active imagination (M);
   c. autosuggestion (M);
   d. different kinds and degrees of meditation (M);
   e. ecstasy, experienced either alone as the result of intense meditation or in community settings, e.g., when entering a sacred enclosure (D/M);
   f. visions (M);
   g. intuitive knowledge, full access to information from all levels of consciousness (M).

* It is believed that the writing implements become "possessed."

Table 2

Alternate States of Consciousness (ASC)
Working Model

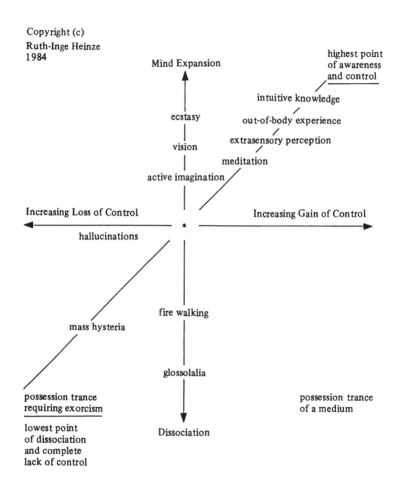

* state of being fully awake

as a state of consciousness composed of two components, one psychophysiological the other cultural. The universality of trance indicates that it corresponds to a psychophysiological disposition innate in human nature, although, of course, developed to varying degrees in different individuals. The variability of its manifestations is the result of the variety of cultures by which it is conditioned (1985:3).

Rouget also made another interesting distinction, in equating

1. *ecstasy* with magical flight, immobility, silence, solitude, no crisis, sensory deprivation, recollection, hallucinations.

He saw

2. *possession* [as] movement, noise, in company, crisis, sensory overstimulation, amnesia, no hallucinations (1985:11).

When individuals in Southeast Asia become "possessed," it is believed that an intrusion has occurred. It is, then, determined whether the possession is desirable or undesirable. The latter requires exorcism by an experienced medium because the possessed are not able of handling the intrusion themselves. Mediums never said they were "possessed," they claimed they were "directed" by higher spiritual beings who, in the Chinese case, were called *shen*. The lower spirits (in the Chinese case, *kuei*) possess for mischievous reasons and to draw attention to their plight. For example, they may not have living relatives who bring offerings and perform the prescribed rituals. They can be appeased by the possessed individual in performing the required offerings and rituals.

To contrast possession in Southeast Asia with occurrences in other parts of the world, I decided to quote from Jones' research (in Hitchcock 1976:1–5). He mentioned four types of spirit possession known in the Nepalese Himalayas. He used the distinction of time and space. Borrowing the term from Lewis (1971), he called

1. *peripheral possessions* all those forms which are not necessarily defined in terms of a particular time or particular space. That implies the uncontrollability of *peripheral possession* which may happen only once in a lifetime and cannot be predicted.
2. *Reincarnate possessions* are for life and are experienced by full-time religious practitioners who are connected with a religious institution or a

designated sacred space. Being the focus of power, reincarnates are involved in rituals, curing, healing, divination, predicting and preventing misfortune.
3. *Tutelary possessions* are just the opposite. Time is designated but space is not. "An individual calls upon a tutelary spirit during a session or ritual to possess him or take over his body for the duration of the ritual or ceremony. The individual ... is never relegated to an institution such as a church, temple, or monastery. His possession is periodic and specific, but the place in which he conducts his activities as a result of possession is sporadic and unspecified and is determined solely by individual choice and situational demand."
4. *Oracular possessions* by a spirit, god or goddess occur at a designated time and space (e.g., the Dalai Lama's Oracle, Jones in Hitchcock 1976:4)).

I call Jones' *peripheral possessions* "undesirable" or "uncontrollable" because individuals experiencing them are not prepared for the event, require assistance, and may not be encouraged to be trained to become a medium. *Reincarnate possessions* rarely occur in Southeast Asia, at least not in the sense Jones is using the term. This leaves us with *tutelary* and *oracular possessions* which also are rarely found in Southeast Asia. Even my terms "desirable" and "controllable" versus "undesirable" and "uncontrollable" possessions do not include all phenomena I encountered during my fieldwork. What is important here is that Southeast Asians distinguish quite well between pathological phenomena and those which can be developed to access different states of consciousness with the goal to fulfill needs of the community.

Frigerio, conducting research among the Umbandistas in Argentina, recognized three levels of possession: *irradiacion, encostamiento* and *incorporacion* (borrowing these terms from the Portuguese).

> Irradiacion (irradiation) means that some of the entity's energy is reaching the medium, but does not have full control over his body; the medium may experience strange sensations in certain body parts, or may have intuitions about certain problems, but is still basically himself.
>
> Encostamiento (to be beside) means that the spirit is leaning against the medium ... touching him and in this way controlling his body. It may also cause the medium to forget some of what he is witnessing. In daily usage, these two terms, irradiacion and encostamiento, are frequently used interchangeably, to denote a state of half-way possession.

Elements of Shamanism

> Incorporacion (incorporation) . . . means that the entity has fully entered the body of the medium and he is therefore completely possessed (1989:2).
>
> I found that clients expected to talk to the god and not the medium. Mediums, therefore, claimed to be "fully possessed not to disappoint their clients" (Heinze 1991:161–162).

In a paper on "Variety of Possession Experiences," Etzel Cardena described three states:

> 1. transitional: dizziness/light headednes, precarious equilibrium, somatic alterations, cognitive disorganization (common to state transitions: sleep, anesthesia, hypnosis; pre-reorganization);
> 2. with discrete identity: change of one identity to another, co-identities, unusual behavior and experience (multiplicity of being, dissociation, expression of forces/entities);
> 3. transcendent: total involvement, consciousness expansion, energy, organismic (breakdown of self/body; alternate modality of experiencing; 1989:120–135).

Cardena's "transitional" state corresponds to Frigerio's *irradiacion* and *encostamiento* states. Cardena's second state has been described by others as "full possession" and Cardena's "transcendent" state can be compared with "magical flight" and other "mind expanding" experiences (Heinze 1991:163).

Furthermore, trances in Singapore, Malaysia, and Thailand, differed considerably from the trances of Siberian shamans. Using the Siberian model as the prototype for comparing shamanic performance, has put researchers off the track because it leaves out the wide range of other shamanic trances.

What trances are used by folk practitioners in *Singapore, Malaysia* and *Thailand*?

> The masters of alternate states of consciousness in Malaysia seldom go into full possession trance, except during horse or tiger possession . . . . The trances of Thai shamans are often so light that physical changes are not visible . . . . Clients of Singapore Chinese mediums, however, expect to come into the presence of the deities . . . . They want to "see" the deities, talk to them or be talked to directly (Heinze 1991:163).

For a description of alternate states of consciousness mentioned in this book, the reader is referred to the Glossary. Examples of alternate states of consciousness are also given in Part 2. For possession, see Cases 1 to 7, 11, 12, 15, 16, 18 to 20; for tiger possession, Case 14; for horse possession, Case 10; for magical flight, Cases 13 and 21; for automatic writing, Case 8; for glossolalia, Case 9; and for aftereffects of alternate states of consciousness, see Case 17.

Thai and *Malay* shamans entered trances after a brief period of meditation or some chanted evocations, moving seemingly effortless into a different state of consciousness. *Indian* shamans were carried into trance mainly by *bhajans* (devotional songs), chanted by their followers to evoke Hindu deities. Most of the *Chinese* mediums I observed developed elaborate techniques of "working" themselves into trance. These techniques were quite similar to those Carmen Blacker described for Japanese shamans (1975:276–277). Japanese induced trances by loud rhythmical sounds, produced by drums, conch shell trumpets, bells, iron-ringed croziers, chanting of words of power, dancing, and inhaling of incense. The smoke of incense was also seen as carrying messages to heaven. Some of the Japanese trances have orgiastic features.

In Singapore, members of a Chinese medium's entourage purified the air around the altar and the dragon throne with incense before each session. Dragon whips (see Fig.24) were wielded inside and outside to prevent evil spirits from entering the temple and the medium. While devotees beat drums and gongs to accompany the chanting, the medium stood in front of the altar, yawning and making retching sounds which traditionally indicated onsetting trance. It was obviously activating a reversal of the breathing pattern. In ever faster movements, a medium rolled his head up to a climax where his body stiffened. This pattern seemed to have remained unchanged. My observations in Southeast Asia 1978–1979 confirmed de Groot's description of the "descent of a spirit into a medium" in early China.

> Drowsily staring, he shivers and yawns resting his arms on the table and his head on is arms, as if falling asleep. As the incantation proceeds with increasing velocity and loudness with the accompaniment of gongs and drums, "eye opening" papers are being burned. The medium suddenly jumps up to frisk and skip about (1910:1274).

When a shaman or medium had fully entered a trance state, he paid first respect to the "arriving" deity. While he stood, sometimes shaking, in front of the main altar, his assistants clothed him with the stomacher (see Section IV:2 of this chapter). The stomacher carried the name of the "possessing" deity and perhaps the name of the temple and its donor(s). The dragon throne was pulled up and the medium sat down, ready for consultation.

Chinese on the Malay Island of Penang called the inviting of spirits *chianh sin*. The medium's assistant started the session with knocking three times with the handle of the authority whip from left to right on the front edge of the altar. Then the medium worked up a frenzy, whirling his head around until

> he strikes a significant pose on the chair, resembling the pose of the deity. This is the signal for the assistant to put on the medium the robe of the deity. The convulsive movements will continue for a short while until the medium utters a shout and jumps up to face the statue of the deity. He asks for his authority flag, whip and lighted joss sticks and pays homage to the gods before he turns and allows himself to be addressed by the assistants or the clients. During the trance, the medium will continue to shake . . . (Wan Hooi Poh 1979:34–38).

Wan Hooi Poh's description confirmed my observations of "possession trances" among Chinese in Singapore.

However, one of my Chinese female mediums in Singapore entered her trance by silently praying in front of the main altar (see Part 2, Case 1). Her toes locked the moment she was entering trance. The degree to which her toes were locked, became, indeed, the indicator for the intensity of her possession. Once in a while, she would slightly relax her toes and then tightened the lock again. (It is difficult to maintain a deep trance for a long period of time.) Her clients looked the "god" into his face and saw no difference in her performance.

Why do trances differ in depth? Temple committee members said that a deity does not fully enter the body of a medium. Such energy would be too much to bear for a human body. Deities, therefore, take only command of four out of seven vital points of mediums and of one third of their soul. It also has to be taken into account that other mediums may have invited the deity at the same time. The phenomenon of multiple appearances of deities never has been fully explained to me. Mediums said that no deity stays long in a human body, i.e., not for an entire session when there are many clients. Deities come and go. Should one deity leave in the middle of a session, an assistant deity will take over. Deities have supposedly numerous deputies for this purpose. However, the assistant deity may be less powerful and may not be able to protect the medium against mischievous spirits. The medium's assistants then have the duty to immediately recognize the change. They chant, burn charm papers, and throw uncooked rice mixed with salt into the air to prevent further pollution (see also Wan Hooi Poh 1979:28).

I observed that mediums in "possession" trance are insensitive to pain and seem to hear no other sounds than the questions directed to the "possessing" deity. When I asked mediums whether I could take a photo of their trance session, they told me to wait until their trance had deepened. They confirmed later on that they had, indeed, not been aware of the flash of my camera right in front of their face.

Trance answers may be incoherent,

> but the interpreter translates the divine language with the greatest fluency into the intelligible human while another brother writes these revelations down on paper. But the moment comes for the spirit to announce in the same way its intention to depart. An assistant spurts a draught of water in which the ashes of "eye-opening papers" were dropped into the face of the medium and a third burns some charm paper money for the spirit in order to reward it for its revelations and to buy its forgiveness should it have been involuntarily displeased or impolitely treated (De Groot 1910:1274).

I watched mediums sink into the arms of their helpers. The assistants closed the medium's "third eye" by pressing their thumb on a point right between the medium's eye brows. The medium relaxed, opened his eyes and smiled. He had returned to his body.

At the end of each session in 1979, an *Indian* shaman in Singapore asked his assistants to put burning benzoin on his tongue and the flames filled his mouth. Not being hurt, proved to the clients that the departing deity was protecting him. The burning benzoin also protected the deity against pollution during departure.

Coming out of an alternate states of consciousness was less dramatic for other shamans. *Thai* and *Malay* shamans woke up like from a good sleep. Delaney (1977:10) saw Thai shamans becoming drowsy, putting their head for a few minutes on a pillow and then waking up to ask what had happened.

To fake shamanism and mediumship is easy. The culturally expected patterns are known to everybody. The partitioners are professionals who always "deliver" an "effective" performance. Success validates the authenticity of each shaman. Only a deity could have known the answer. Only a deity could have brought about the turn for the better. Only a deity can set a troubled mind at ease. What shamans and mediums believe is not so important as long as they are able to instil faith in others.

Sometimes, shamans and mediums may also be forced to "act" during their trance performance, e.g., when their "possession" begins to weaken. Prolonged deep trances are rare. It is not expected that deities are present all the time. When they return to their abode, they may either send another spirit to replace them or leave some of their energies with the shaman.

It would go beyond the scope of this book to describe the different phases and the various trances in more detail. Additional information can be found in Part 2, Shamanic Practices: A Case History Approach, and the Glossary.

3.4.4. When Trances Are Used

Among the four ethnic groups and the five world religions I studied, trances are important because they facilitate the manifestation of spirits. The presence of spiritual entities is necessary to retrieve information and to cure.

I agree with Olson (1982) who studied the possession of a Chinese-Mexican shaman. Possession trances occur in front of audiences and "benefit from the opportunity of conducting the possession drama." On the other hand, audiences need the experience of possession to "assure themselves of their assumptions . . . about the supernatural." Audiences "gain help for themselves through spiritual channels, perhaps hear their own grievances articulated through the mouthpiece of the spirits" (1982:26). Deities, speaking through the medium, assess problems and reduce them to socially and ethnically acceptable units. Olson found that the belief in spirits is a culturally-provided compensatory device which represents initial resolution of intrapsychic stresses in using the symbolism of opposing emotional forces. In other words, individual conflict is expressed in a language and a symbolism clients as well as the entire community can readily understand (Olson 1982:2). The nature of spirits and deities reflects the kind of complexes repressed by the clients and the "divine" messages "contain clues toward understanding disturbances" (Olson 1982:20). It is the "healed healer" (Halifax 1982) who initiates therapeutic recovery by symbolizing conflicts and distancing emotions.

Are spirits, as Jung suggested, "unconscious autonomous complexes which appear as projections because they are not associated with the ego" (1960:95, 99). No outsider, only the individual, experiencing the presence of spirits, can determine what they are. This dilemma reminds us of a Buddhist legend where the Buddha suggested to pay attention to what is needed in the moment, any investigation, for example, from where "an arrow came," "what material the arrow was made of" or "who shot it," would be completely irrelevant. Whatever spirits are, we can learn from the techniques of shamans and mediums who access unknown areas of our mind.

Practitioners may add their own moral advice in saying they can help only individuals who are honest about themselves and their situation and who have no intention to harm others. In Asia, shamanism, mediumship, and healing are traditionally anchored in the clients' religious ethic (see also, Delaney 1977:15–16). When a deity already knows individual problems, it is interpreted to be the proof of Divine omniscience. Clients are led to search their conscience and suggestions are made about how their attitudes toward others can be mended. Among the penalties imposed may be retribution and prayers. In Catholicism, an individual confesses and God, through the priest, determines the punishment. In Southeast Asia, deities tell individuals where they have failed. This includes a wide range of cases where individuals may not yet be aware of or have not yet confessed their trespasses. They are then taught a lesson in self-criticism.

In cases of physical illness, practitioners in 1979 diagnosed whether the ailment was physical, psychosomatic, spirit-inflicted or the result of magic. *Malay bomohs* put a knife between the toes of a patient to find the cause of illness (see Part 2, Case 12). Most of the practitioners of the four ethnic groups prescribed herbal remedies, used massage and suggested bathing with blessed water.

Bad luck was removed by waving charm papers around a client and cracking the dragon whip to chase mischievous spirits away. Sometimes it was suggested that clients, preferably in early childhood, should have been adopted because their real parents were astrologically not good for them. Dore (First Part, Vol.I, 1914:23) mentioned this *han-tsin* (nominal adoption) which is not a contract and does not establish the right to inherit but deflects the influence of unfortunate constellations. I myself was repeatedly asked "how many parents I have." I understood the question only when somebody explained to me the underlying rational.

Aside from divine messages, received by mediums, the main function of a trance is to channel power, energize clients, and convey protection and blessings. Protection is, then, taken home in the form of blessed water, flowers, charm papers, amulets and, in the Indian case, *prasad*, left-overs from the food offered to the gods.

3.5. Nature of Spiritual Beings

In the following, we will look at the spiritual entities who seek communication with man and with whom man has been in contact since time immemorial.

None of the practitioners I interviewed claimed to be an expert on spiritual beings. They said that deities and spirits live in realms of which human beings have only limited knowledge. Spiritual beings are neither good nor evil. Spiritually advanced practitioners stressed that it was ignorance which led to the creation of dichotomies. Southeast Asian practitioners, in general, do not talk about evil forces who tempt the faithful and fight the good. Buddhists, for example, said that, during our spiritual development, ignorance decreases at the same rate as knowledge increases, depending on the degree of responsibility an individual is willing to take. People believe that a "good" spirit may become enraged and will punish individuals for trespassing and a so-called "evil" spirit may grant benefits so there is no need for exorcism. All depends on the kind of knowledge a practitioner has developed. In general, it is believed that spirits from higher heavens are less inclined to harm without cause while spirits from lower levels are more mischievous "by nature," because "they have not seen the light," i.e., lack spiritual development.

Malay-Muslim bomohs were the most hesitant to disclose the identity of spirits with whom they work. Muslim are supposed to believe only in one god. They pray to Allah five times each day and go to the mosque on Friday. Allah, however, is a distant god who last spoke to Moses. When Allah conveyed the Koran to Muhammad, the Archangel Gabriel was his messenger. To whom can a pious Muslim turn in a crisis situation? The Mufti of Singapore told me in 1979 that Muslims should increase their prayers or go to an *imam* (leader of a Muslim community) who will help them pray. However, when an acute problem remains unsolved, "useful means" can be resorted to as long as they are employed in the name of Allah. This sounds very much like the *upaya* ("useful means" in Buddhism).[9] Muslim will use verses from the Koran, either to pray or to activate the magic power of the divinely inspired word (Tambiah 1968). With the belief in supernatural powers, the belief in pre-Islam spirits[10] persisted. Even the orthodox Sunni affirm the existence of spiritual entities and believe that devotees can communicate with them.

A *bomoh* in Singapore, who as a young man came from Java, told me he is "directed" by the Earth Goddess. Other *bomohs* in Malaysia and Thailand claimed they had tiger, horse, and nature spirits and were "visited" also by Javanese ancestors and familiars they created themselves (e.g., by using substances from the brain of a corpse). A shaman in Pattani suggested that he would "make" such a familiar for me and was surprised that I declined his offer.

Basically, Malay know of two kind of spirits — bounded and unbounded ones.[10] One of the unbounded spirits is the *jinn*, a genie or elemental made from fire.[11] The white *jinn*, for example, lives in the sun and guards the gates of the sky.

He has a brother with seven heads, called Maharajah Dewa (Śiva). *Hantu raya* live in the three major realms of earth, water, and jungle, and *hantu pemburu*, as well as *hantu rimba*, in the roughly bounded realms of mines and fishing grounds. The *hantu tinggi* and *hantu berok* live in trees and animals. Bounded spirits are the *dato* (tutelary spirits, e.g., souls of Muslim saints), the *belian* (weretiger), *pelesit* (familiar spirit, soul of somebody, who suffered a violent death) and other spirits who can be generated at the will of man.

The situation is different with *Hindu* and *Buddhist* practitioners who believe that

1. spirits may "select" human beings because they are unable to reincarnate themselves. They need a human body through which they can perform good deeds and improve their own *karma*.

Aside from this class of spirits, there are

2. higher spiritual entities who do not reincarnate any more. They want to "possess" human beings for altruistic reasons.

It is believed that

3. minor deities may manifest also as messengers of higher gods.
4. "Undesired possession," on the other hand, may be interpreted as punishment by deities who are dissatisfied with the conduct of their followers

or, it is said, that

5. mischievous lower spirits want to draw attention to their plight. They may have become restless because they have suffered a sudden and/or violent death or they have not received the offerings due to them. Without any living descendants to "send them off," they hover around the place they have died. Confused and in desperation, they may attach themselves to passers-by. After a shaman or medium has diagnosed the case and suggested the necessary rituals, they can easily be appeased.

In *India,* approximately three thousand years ago, the *muni* (sages) of the Vedas rode on the chariot of the winds (Rg Veda X:136), gathering information from different realms of existence. Some thousand years later, Patanjali collected and codified the knowledge of ancient *yogis* (ascetics) in 196 *sūtras* that explain how we can cultivate ourselves to come to "know God (Prabhavananda 1953).

Tamil (Hindu) today distinguish between *bhuta* (nature spirits and demons), *pitr* (ancestor spirits), *devata* (deities), and *Brahmā* (the Supreme Consciousness). Tamil can communicate with these spiritual entities with the help of *brahmins* (individuals who inherit their priesthood) or they consult shamans and mediums (lay practitioners belonging to different castes or even being casteless).[12]

Looking at the facial expressions, the movements, and the objects a shaman uses during "possession," everybody can recognize whether Hanuman (the virile monkey general of Rāma), Rāma (the seventh incarnation of Viṣṇu, see Fig.6), Murgam (Śiva's son) with his three-pronged *vel* (spear) or Mahākālī (the fierce aspect of Śiva's consort) have manifested. Some spirits may also pay surprise visits, so the assistants have to announce each time which deity has arrived (this is valid also for the other three groups of this study).

In sum, Indians become "possessed" by deities from the Hindu pantheon, ancestor and nature spirits to fulfill individual or group need. We have, however, to exclude the occasional "possession" of young girls or frustrated women who have problems with lovers or in-laws, have been abandoned by their husbands or have become widows. Allowing themselves to be possessed by nature spirits or deified heroes gives them an opportunity to act out their frustration in a seemingly hopeless situation. The community will rally to their support and they become temporarily the focus of attention. The exorcism then facilitates their reintegration (see, Claus 1975).

Thailand is a Buddhist country where, by constitution, the king has to be a Buddhist and Buddhism has been the state religion for over seven hundred years. Raised in the Hindu tradition, Buddha taught the Four Noble Truths, the fourth being the Way to Eliminate Suffering. Early Buddhists, i.e., the *Theravadin*,[13] spoke already about the hierarchies of the Three Worlds.[14] Hindu deities became the guardians of the *dhamma* (teachings of the historical Buddha, the Universal Law) and may seek to improve their *kamma* (footnote 1 of Introduction) by protecting and helping other sentient beings, but they have to be reborn as a human being to work toward *mokṣa* (final release from worldly existence). In Buddhism, this state is called *nibbana* ("blowing out," enlightenment).

Followers of later forms of Buddhism, e.g., *Mahāyāna* (see Glossary), focussed on the metaphysical aspects of the Buddha's teaching and began to worship *bodhisattvas* (Buddhas-to-be) who forego their entry into *nibbana* to save all sentient beings. A *bodhisattva* can be evoked for help. Those who call the name of Amitābha Buddha at the time of their death, for example, will be reborn in the "Western Paradise" where they have a second chance to cultivate themselves.

Thai Buddhists today recognize basically three kinds of spirits,

1. spirits of the dead (souls of spiritually advanced individuals who have been reborn in one of the many heavens: prominent monks, powerful individuals, deified heroes and kings) and astral bodies of the living;
2. nature spirits, e.g., *krut* (Garuda, mystical bird, vehicle of Viṣṇu, enemy of snakes), *nāgas* (mystical serpents, guardians of the Buddha and his esoteric teachings); as well as tree and mountain spirits;
3. spirits who exists on their own. Although they are never seen nor heard, it is believed that they can influence the fate of humans, e.g., Yama (King of Death and ruler over the various hells, in Hinduism, Buddhism, and Taoism). (See also Irwin 1907, and Heinze 1982:119–222).

Bangkok mediums called in 1979, for example, the spirit of Phra Narai (Part 2, Case 18 and Fig.44) or the spirit of a monk who had lived in the last century and become famous for converting salt water into water fit for drinking (see Part 2, Case 15). The spirit of a follower of Moggallana, one of the Buddha's closest disciples, helped a monk shaman to exorcise vengeful ghosts (Part 2, Case 17) and the spirit of King Chulalongkorn who died in 1910, empowered another medium to heal three days and three nights in a row without getting up, i.e., as long as there were clients in the hall (Part 2, Case 16).

In 1979, *Chinese* practitioners in Singapore manifested the largest number of spirits (from nature spirits to local deities, the Kitchen God and the God of the Walls and Moats, Star Lords, and Gods who decide the fate of humans, etc.). They included also deities from different belief systems (e.g., Christian saints and Buddhist bodhisattvas).

Wolf explained the logic of the Chinese pantheon in his essay on "Gods, Ghosts, and Ancestors" (1974) and Johnson (1985) examined

> the evolution of a new class of deities, the City God (Ch'eng-huang shen). He connects the spread of City God temples during the late T'ang and early Sung dynasties to two factors: the values of a newly emerging class of urban merchants, and

a change in the attitude of the government toward the cults of the populace (quoted in Teiser, 1995:384).

The cult of the city gods was first known in the Yangtze area. During the reign of the Tang dynasty (618–906 A.D.), city gods were still rather uncommon, but, during the Sung dynasty (960–1179 A.D.), more worthy men of the past were deified for their virtuous deeds and city judges were, after their death, appointed to preside over courts in hell (Eberhard, 1968:191–192). The Chinese belief system became more and more syncretic[15] and more and more gods populated the heavens. I refer to Hansen (1990) who discussed the relationship between the pantheon and the commercial revolution of the twelfth and thirteenth centuries. Chard (1990), for example, examined the history of the God of the Stove (Tsao-chuen) and Kleeman (1988) traced Wen-ch'ang's career from a local hero to a stellar deity who also became the Emperor of Literature (Wen-ti) in the state-sanctioned pantheon. (See, also T'ien-hou, Queen of Heaven, discussed below, and Teiser's more detailed review, 1995).

The most popular deity among Singapore Chinese is *Kuan Teh*, *Kuang Kong* or *Kwan-yu*. A full account of this legendary general's exploits is told in *The Romantic Story of the Three Kingdoms* (San Kuo-Chih Yen-i), composed by Lo Kwan-chung at the time of the Yuen (Mongol) Dynasty (1270–1368 A.D.). The story is told in four volumes with 120 chapters. An English translation in two volumes by C.H. Brewitt-Taylor appeared in 1925 (republished by Tuttle 1990). It is based on actual events during the troubled period of the Three Kingdoms (220–280 A.D.: Shu 221–264; Wei 220–265, and Wu 220–280), following the fall of the Late Han Dynasty in the 3rd century A.D. Kuan Teh and his blood brothers, Liu-pei and Chang-fei, took the famous oath in the peach garden and joined expeditionary forces to combat insurgents who, belonging to a secret militant sect, the Yellow Turbans, threatened the Dragon Emperor. After having performed many heroic feats, Kuan Teh was captured by Sun Ch'uan and put to death in 219 A.D. Nine hundred years later his merits were officially recognized. He was canonized during the Sung Dynasty in 1120 A.D. and became *Chung Hai Kong* ("Faithful and Loyal Lord"). Eight years later he was elevated to the rank of *Chuang Mu Wu An Wang* ("Martial Emperor and Pacifier") and, in 1594, during the Ming Dynasty, he became the God of War (*Kuan Kong* or *Kuan-ti*). (Different names and honorific titles may be used in Singapore for his two sworn brothers, Liu-pei and Chang-fei.)[16] Kuan Kong, the red-faced and black-bearded Chinese God of War is not so much worshiped for his martial success but his readiness to defend the weak and helpless. He is also the patron saint of non-warlike trades, e.g., the literati, and he is the patron of secret societies (Comber 1958:16).

Toa Peh Kong is the red-cheeked Grand Old Man with a white beard, gold ingots in one hand and, in the other a walking stick. He is the tutelary deity of Straits Chinese, that means, he is not known in China. He can be evoked by a shortened version of his name, *Peh kong* or a longer version, *Toh Peh Kong Tolong*. Some say he is identical with the local deity *Fu Tak Cheng Shan*. *Topekong*, in the Standard Malay-English Dictionary, means a Chinese household deity. *To* is probably an abbreviation for *dato* (a honorific title). The Malay word *tokong* (Chinese temple) may also be connected with his name. His devotees do not eat a local fish, *ikan talang* (Malay; chroninemus sp.) which has five black marks on his body, allegedly the imprints of *Toa Peh Kong*'s fingers. In Chinese, the fish is called *Toa Pe Kong Yu*. Some devotees also do not eat durian which is considered to be *Toa Peh Kong*'s fruit.

Legends, told in Penang, report that an old Hokkien scholar named Chang Li who had connections with secret societies, was forced to flee to Malaysia during the reign of Emperor Ch'ien Lung (1736–1796). He settled in Penang and became a school teacher. Other stories maintain that Chang Li and his two sworn brothers, Chao-Chin and Fu-Ch'un, were Hakka pioneers who, coming from China, landed at Tanjong Tokong in 1786. They were later buried at the same place and local residents prayed at their tomb for protection against epidemics. All three pioneers were later deified and the name *Toa Peh Kong* became a generic term for pioneering heroes.

Some scholars suggest that Chang Li was not a proper name but a rank held in the Triad or Heaven and Earth Society. The rank was similar to that of Elder Brother, Tiger General or White Fan in secret society hierarchy. A powerful Chinese secret society was, indeed, established under the name of Toa Peh Kong Society at Jelutong, Penang, at the end of 1844 and played a leading Part 1n the Penang Riots of 1867.

Other scholars saw the Grand Old Man as "simply a deity worshipped by seafaring people . . . second only to the Queen of Heaven" (Comber 1958:32–35; also Eberhard 1952).

Toa Peh Kong is evoked to bring prosperity, to cure diseases, and to avert danger, e.g., to calm the ocean. His first shrine was built in Tanjong Tokong in 1792 by Hakka and Hokkien. Every year in October, Singaporeans go on a pilgrimage to another of his shrines on Kusu Island.

Elements of Shamanism

Nor Cha Sam T'ai Tze, the Third Prince, is represented in Chinese temples in Singapore as well as in Malaysia (including Sabah and Sarawak). General Lee Ching, his father, was deified as the God who Supports the Pagoda in His Hand. *Nor Cha Sam T'ai Tze* himself was general and commander of the Ch'en Tang Pass under the ruler Chou whose crimes caused the downfall of the Shang Dynasty in 1122 B.C. The Third Prince is one of the most frequently mentioned heroes in Chinese legends. Chapters 12 to 14 of the Chinese novel, *Metamorphoses of the Gods* (Feng-shen yen-i), written during the Ming Dynasty in the 16th century by an unknown author,[17] contain the prince's life story. In iconography, the Third Prince is a minor, child-like, but nevertheless important deity. He usually holds a magic bracelet in one hand and a magic sword in the other while he has "wind-and fire" wheels under his feet (see also Dore, Second Part, IX, 1931:11–122).

Equally popular is *Sun-heu-tze* (Ts'oi T'in Tai Seng Yeh), the Great Sage of all the Heavens, irreverently in English called the Monkey God. He is the mythical monkey who accompanied the Buddhist monk Hsuan-tsang to India in 629 A.D. After 17 years, Hsuan-tsang returned to China, bringing with him 657 Buddhist scriptures. His story can be found in *A Record of Travels in the West* (Si-yiu-ki), written by Wu Ch'eng En (1500–1582 A.D.). For details about the Monkey God's mythical origin, how he stole the peaches of immortality and how he was subdued by the Buddha, see, among others, also Dore (Second Part, VII, 1926:553–562). In a temple on Bukut Timah Road in Singapore, some of his devotees healed, in 1979, in front of his altar.

The Nine Imperial Gods, *Kau Wong Yeh*, are worshipped especially during the first nine days of the ninth lunar month. *Kau Wong Yeh* is their Cantonese name, Hokkiens will call them *Kau Ong Yah* or *Kew Ong Yeah*, the latter form is also used in Ampang (Malaysia) and in Amoy (China). The Nine Imperial Gods are further called *Chiu Huang Yen* or *Chiu Wang Yeh*, depending on which dialect group supports the temple. The nine gods are the sons of *Tou Mu* (Goddess of the North Star). Their names are *T'ien Ying, T'ien Jen, T'ien Chu, T'ien Hsi, T'ien Ch'in, T'ien Fu, T'ien Ch'ung, T'ien Jui*, and *T'ien P'eng*. It is believed that each of the nine resides on one of the seven stars of the Big Dipper and on two invisible stars nearby. One of their temples stands on Upper Serangoon Road in Singapore, but other communities in Singapore and Malaysia (e.g., Ampang) celebrate the birthday of the gods with equal pomp (see Part 2, Case 7). During the festival, organized in 1978 by the Geylang Community on a huge space allocated by the authorities of the city of Singapore at Mountbatton Road, a medium, clad as Kuan Yin, led a crowd of over ten thousands for nine days through the different stages of the ritual (see Fig.21).

Kuan Yin is among Chinese the Goddess of Mercy. She is the female form of Avalokitesvara, the *bodhisattva* of Amitābha Buddha who can manifest in 84 different forms. Singapore and Penang Chinese maintain she was a princess in the closing years of the Chou Dynasty (approximately in the 3rd century B.C.). Her father ruled over the Western Kingdom, Hsing Lin (presumably India). The Chinese writer Chung Shan K'e told us in his book, *The Birth of Kung Yin*, that her mother Pao Te, during her forty years of marriage to King Miao Chuang, produced only two daughters. Her third child, *Miao-shen*, again was a daughter who did not marry like her sisters but excelled in modesty. When she entered a nunnery against the wishes of her father, he ordered the nunnery to be destroyed and his daughter executed. Miao-shen was, however, rescued and carried off by a tiger. Later she healed her father from a fatal illness by cutting off both of her arms. - The desire of *Miao-shen's* mother for vegetarian dishes during pregnancy is reflected in the custom of Kuan Yin's devotees keeping a vegetarian diet on the three days during the year which are devoted to her worship (see Comber 1958:21–26 and Wong 1967).

Miao-shen was deified by the Jade Emperor and became *Kuan Yin*. Some say she is identical with the Ceylonese god Dumana, but there is no evidence for this assumption. Others think she is the son of Amitābha Buddha. The *Miao-shen* legend was written down by the monk P'u-ming in 1102. Dore (Second Part, VI, 1920:134–233) did not think Miao-shen became *Kuan Yin*.

Kuan Yin is considered to be an emanation of the *bodhisattva* Avalokitesvara who appeared first in the Christian era. (In the 6th century A.D., he was depicted in Tantric Buddhism together with Manjusri and Vajrapani.) Little is written about *Kuan Yin* in earlier times. She is mentioned in the Lotus Sūtra which was translated into Chinese in 417 A.D. *Kuan Yin* is also sometimes confused with Hariti who in Northern India is the giver of children (Dore, Second Part, VI, 1919:203) or with the Queen of Heaven, *T'ien Hou*, who allegedly was the sixth daughter of a subdistrict magistrate in Foochow. Born in 979 A.D., *T'ien Hou* became later a sea goddess who was mainly worshiped by southern sailors. (One of her principal images can be found on P'u-to Island.) The worship of a deified subdistrict magistrate's daughter may have merged with the worship of an earlier sea goddess to later become a stellar deity (see Part 2, Case 7).

Kuan Yin's full title is *Nan Wu Ta Tz'u Ta Pei Chiu K'u Chiu Nan Kuang La Ling Kan Kuan Shih Yin P'u Sat* (The Most Merciful and Compassionate Bodhisattva, Protector of the Afflicted, Exalted Spirit who Hears the Cries of Mortals). Singapore Chinese will use this title as an evocation. They also call *Kuan Yin* affectionately "Third Aunt" (Comber 1958:21).

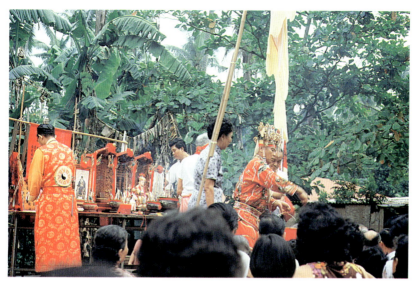

Fig. 19 *A Sea Goddess speaks through a Chinese medium while a Taoist priest recites from the Taoist Canon, Changi, Singapore*

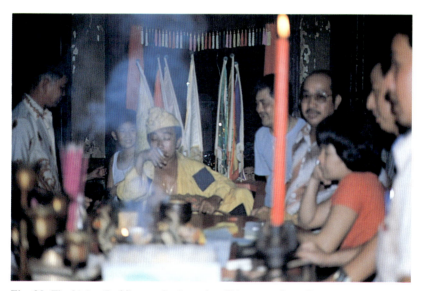

Fig. 20 *The Living Buddha speaks through a Chinese medium, Penang*

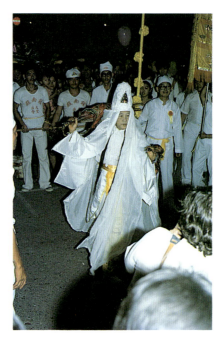

Fig. 21 *Chinese medium, clad as Kuan Yin, at the Festival of the Nine Imperial Gods, Singapore*

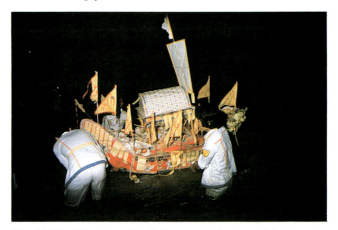

Fig. 22 *The Nine Imperial Gods are sent back to their heavenly abodes at the end of their festival, Singapore*

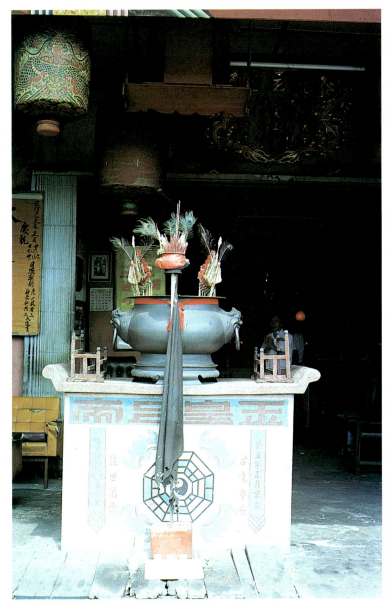

Fig. 23 *Altar with the eight trigrams. The black flag indicates the presence of a medium, Chinese temple near Ord Bridge, Singapore*

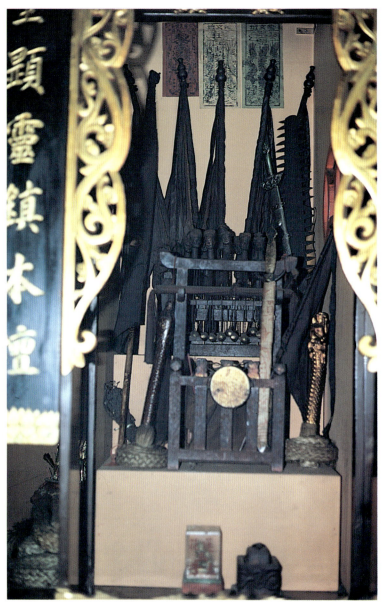

Fig. 24 Dragon whips and Four General skewers, Chinese temple near Ord Bridge, Singapore

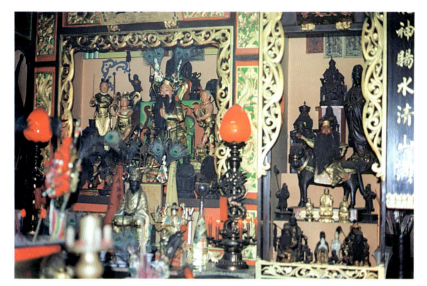

Fig. 25 *Typical Chinese altar, Singapore*

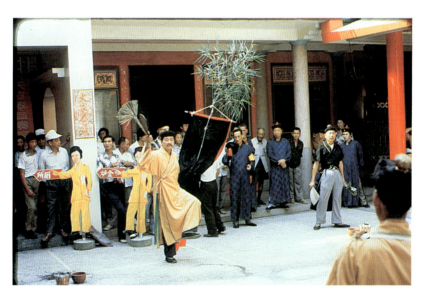

Fig. 26 *Taoist priest dancing the pattern of the Big Dipper, Taiwan*

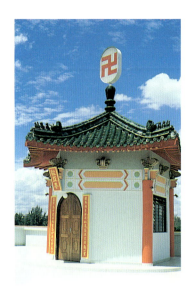

Fig. 27 *Temple dedicated to receiving messages from the Highest God, Red Swastika Society, Singapore*

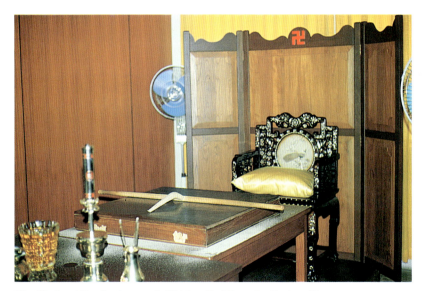

Fig. 28 *Sand Box for Automatic Writing, Red Swastika Society, Singapore*

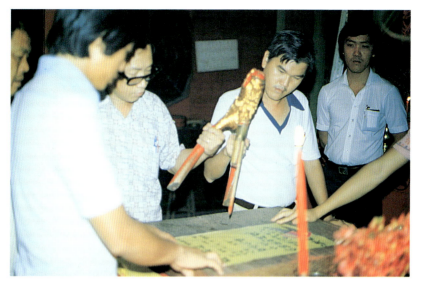

Fig. 29 *Automatic Writing, Keng Yeo Taoist Association, Jurong, Singapore*

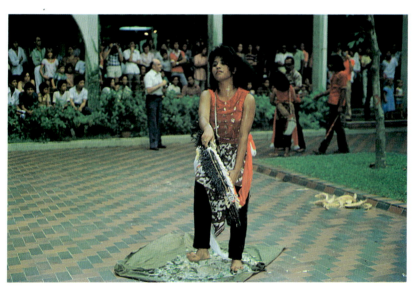

Fig. 30 *Kuda Kepang, Rasa Singapura, Singapore*

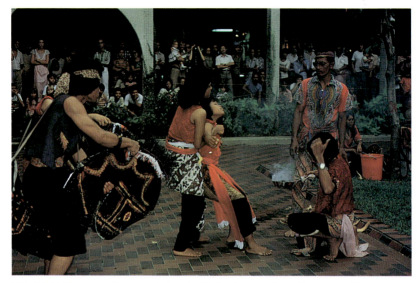

Fig. 31 *Falling out of trance during the Kuda Kepang, Rasa Singapura, Singapore*

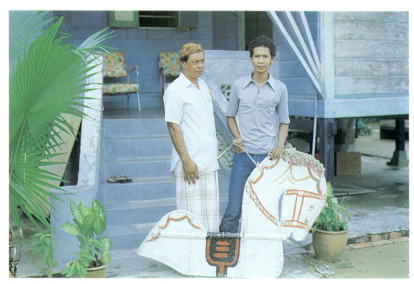

Fig. 32 *Kuda Kepang trainers, Changi, Singapore*

The Kuan Yin temple at Waterloo Street in Singapore had, in 1979, no resident mediums. *Kuan Yin* herself manifested in Singapore mediums only for blessings on special occasions. It was said that she sends, for example, one of her assistants who may be the deified general *Kam T'ien Siong Teh* (see Part 2, Case 1) to do "salvation work."

Amitābha Buddha and Kuan Yin may occasionally "come down" (see Chapter 1.1. and Part 2, Case 4), but Chinese mediums in Singapore are not visited by spiritual entities as high as the Jade Emperor, Lord of Heaven, or Sakyamuni, the historical Buddha of the sixth century B.C.

We know so much about Chinese belief systems and customs because the Chinese kept written records for more than two thousand years in contrast to other ethnic groups who transmitted their traditions orally and were motivated to establish written records only fairly recently. Oral traditions have the advantage that they were transmitted selectively while written records "froze," i.e., did not change with time, became public domain and can be misrepresented by outsiders.

Some of the *Chinese* practitioners I worked with, were baptized. In Christianity, God spoke to Adam and Moses and, later, saints acted as intermediaries between man and the Creator. But there were also some Christians who came "to know God" (Prabhavananda 1953) while praying, in meditation or ecstasy or when speaking in tongues (see Part 2, Case 9). In 1979, Chinese Christians continued to follow Chinese customs and silently performed shamanic rituals in the Novena Church in Singapore, for example. Or they experienced Christ on the Cross during their shamanic trance (Part 2, Case 5). Therefore, a crucifix and the Holy Mary may appear side by side with Hindu, Buddhist, Taoist, and local deities on Chinese house and temple altars (see Fig.25). All deities serve similar complementary functions.

3.6. Interethnic Overlap

In Singapore, Malaysia, and Thailand, members of the four major ethnic groups — Chinese, Malay, Thai, and Tamil (Indian) — may go to shamans, mediums, and healers of other ethnic groups. When individuals sought help and protection from spiritual beings, they followed the recommendations of relatives, friends and colleagues and selected practitioners who were considered to be the most efficacious in solving their specific problems.

The process of interethnic and interdenominational overlap in multi-ethnic and multi-religious societies keeps elementary concepts alive, so basic concepts are active in different contexts. A researcher should not get overly concerned when legends told about deities differ from temple to temple. They may even differ among members of the entourage of one temple. Where we have written versions, we will find parts left out in the oral versions, not so much out of ignorance, but because certain features lost relevance. Knowledge about deities from other groups led to adding desirable "new" features to one's own belief system. The new features were superimposed on a seemingly different system with surprising ease. Yang observed already in China, that

> cults of local heroes which succeeded in surviving for generations appear to have developed in a cyclical pattern of three successive states. First, the founding of the cult was characterized by a crisis and the dominance of such values as patriotism, courage, and extreme self-sacrifice required to meet the critical situation. Secondly, in its subsequent existence through a long period of normal times, the cult was sustained by common magic and mythological lore. In the third stage, a new crisis would again bring out the ethico-political values which by now were deeply interwoven with the magical and mythological aspect of the cult, and the cycle would be repeated (1961:172).

I witnessed at several occasions the birth of legends. Already during the session, different stories were told by the witnesses of the miracle and the "deity's words" were individually reinterpreted. Over time, the stories were embellished and became more elaborate, as they reflected the expectations fulfilled by the presence of a deity. Elements from world religions were woven into the fabric of the story to legitimize the legend and to strengthen the growing belief.

Westerners, facing the growing number of variations, should not expect to ever discover the "original" story. Chinese people do not share this scholarly concern. Yang found in China of the past already a "chaotic mass of functional gods" (1961:20) and Weber offered an explanation for this phenomenon in his *Religion of China*.

> The great spirits of nature were increasingly depersonalized. Their cult was reduced to official ritual, the ritual was gradually emptied of all emotional elements and finally became equated with mere social convention. This was the work of the cultured stratum of intellectuals who left entirely aside the typical religious needs of the masses (1951:178).

Chinese in Southeast Asia are not taught any "Chinese religion," neither at home nor at school. Only a few Chinese may apprentice themselves to a Taoist priest. Chinese children accompany their parents or grandparents to temples and remember, at times of crisis, how deities can be approached through shamans, mediums, and healers.

For pragmatic *Chinese*, the power of a deity has to be constantly reconfirmed and confirmation comes through manifestation. People want to experience the presence of a deity. They believe divine power can be accessed through mediums who, with their paraphernalia, are judged by effectiveness and not their provenance. There will, therefore, be a wide range of deities on Chinese altars, whether at home or in a temple (see Fig.25) and deities from other belief systems will be among them.

Indian practitioners have not yet broken out of the classic brahmanical mold. Their mediums, though of lowly birth, usually emulate brahmanical rites. They all firmly believe in manifestations of Hindu deities.

Thai operate in the framework of *Theravāda* Buddhism. When asked about "useful means," they will quote passages from the Buddhist Canon, believing that the inherent power of verses from the scriptures will protect them and cure the sick. Thai practitioners often work in front of house altars on which Buddha statues stand next to those of Hindu deities. Although Hindu deities in Buddhism are in need of "salvation" themselves, they live on levels which are spiritually higher than the level we live on and they are imbued with sufficient spiritual power to guard the *dhamma* and to help us whenever and wherever they are evoked.

Malay bomohs use verses from the Koran and have memorized traditional evocations. Because Islam does not allow any representation in anthropomorphic form, *bomohs,* who all claim to be good Muslims, display only verses from the Koran in their house and no altars or statues will be seen neither in mosques nor in prayer halls nor in the houses of pious Muslims.

The overlap of belief systems in 1978/79 was, therefore, most obvious with Chinese. However, all four ethnic groups — Chinese, Thai, Malay, and Indian — consulted shamans, mediums, and healers also from other ethnic groups because the degree of effectiveness was most important to them.

Chapter 4
Socio-Psychological Considerations

4.1. Introduction

In April 11, 1975, at a Symposium on Neurological Sciences in Kuala Lumpur, Professor Taib Osman confirmed that there would not be any shamans, mediums, and healers, "if there were no need for their services."[1]

In 1979, I found that clients were deeply moved when they witnessed the trances of folk practitioners. "They experience a process of transformation, a catharsis, a purification and ordering of the psyche, an increase in self-confidence and security" (Lommel 1967:101; also Demetrio 1977). Shamans, mediums, and healers transmit their own experiences during trance. They facilitate the conditions under which hidden fears can safely be brought to consciousness. I observed, for example, the surfacing of several "possessions" in the safe presence of an expert (see Part 2, Case 17, also Fig.41). Externalized fears were treated and clients could release their suppressed or repressed problems. They felt understood.

Trust was established and practitioners could activate the self-healing powers of their clients. Clients felt protected. They were taught how to endure the strains of every-day life. This alerted me to paying attention to other dimensions of the healing process. James, for example, gave three alternative explanations for the success of "mind curers":

1. *Theistic* explanations speak of "divine grace" which creates a new nature so that the old nature is disbanded.
2. *Pantheistic* explanations describe the "narrower private self" merging with the "wider or greater self."

James equated our own subconscious self with the spirit of the universe. "The moment the isolating barriers of mistrust and anxiety are removed," the union is completed. James found that

3. *medico-materialistic* explanations are simpler, cerebral processes ... act more freely when they are left to act automatically.

Seeking to regulate the "experience," physiological processes "only succeed in inhibiting results." James doubted whether his "third explanation might, in a psycho-physical account of the universe, be combined with either of the others" (1941:11–12). In 1979, the needs of individuals who consulted shamans, mediums, and healers appeared to be predominantly pragmatic but closer inspection confirmed that the needs had more than one dimension.

Shamans, mediums, and healers have operated in changing societies for thousands of years (see Chapter 1.2., and Heinze 1991:131–137). They solve problems which go beyond the knowledge of Western physicians and the limiting dogma of world religions. Physiological, psychological, mental, social, and spiritual imbalances are all seen as the result of inappropriate acts and unethical behavior. Therefore, folk practitioners are more than curers. They cut through the complexity of problems, touch the core, and point to causes beyond the physical realm.

Man has lost the acuity of his senses which early man, in his struggle for survival, developed in an alien jungle. In prehistoric times, everybody had to be his or her own shaman.

Over time, certain members of a tribe proved to be more successful than others and so shamans carved out their role inside their tribe. Do the needs they fulfilled in nomadic, hunting and gathering societies differ from ours? When the survival of a group depended on the outcome of a hunt, the souls of hunted animals had to be propitiated. Basic fears also led to the placating of nature and ancestor spirits.

When nomadic tribes settled down, the developing horticultural and agricultural societies, however, needed shamans to produce or to stop rain and avoid floods.

With larger groups of people, living together in ever growing villages and cities, the environment became increasingly complex and division of labor had to be institutionalized. Shamans were no longer leaders of their tribe, politicians took over. To govern the growing population effectively, they had to create administrative institutions.

When we continue to trace shamanic beliefs, we find that shamanic activities continued under the umbrella of developing world religions. *Buddhism* evolved from *Hindu* beliefs and both systems are based on the concept of *karma* and transmigration — the belief that individuals may have neglected or cultivated their faculties in previous lives. Without a dogma, shamanism was so all-encompassing

Socio-Psychological Considerations

that folk practitioners had no difficulties to work comfortably inside the framework of world religions. Shamans told me, for example, that they remembered having been ascetics or monks in previous lives. They considered themselves fortunate of having had the opportunity of several life times to develop a greater sensitivity for other dimensions, so they could become eligible for "divine grace," that means, they believe they have been selected by spiritual beings to do "salvation work."

After Buddhism had been introduced to China and, after the collapse of the Han Dynasty in the second century A.D., indigenous *Chinese* religions (including Taoism) adopted the concept of *karma*, too, and Chinese began to focus on deities who could be approached for help. Revelations (which continue into our century) supported these beliefs. We find, therefore, many messianic cults in China.

Man had become alienated from his natural environment and began to look for the forgotten purpose of human existence. According to Weber, man has always attempted to surround himself with a meaningful cosmos. Confusion arose when man suddenly felt overwhelmed by fears about his and his family's health, about losing his means of income, about feeling misunderstood, not appreciated, and having lost his sense of purpose. Why have we forgotten how to tap our own resources? Why did we make ourselves dependent on help?

Malay-Muslim bomohs, for example, kept intimate relationships with the invisible world since time immemorial. Most of them still inherit their faculties from their ancestors (see Part 2, Cases 11–14). When they converted to Islam, it became important to them, not to offend any of the strict rules for Muslims.

Bomohs in Malaysia, though, are still called to prevent rain from falling. Such occasions may be royal weddings or football matches. They say that no *bomoh*

> can really "stop the rain," against the law of nature, but they can prevent it from falling at a particular site by means of powerful incantations. One of the experts in this field is 61-year old Bomoh Lebai Abdullah bin Omar who baffled thousands of spectators at a cricket match. It was the beginning of the rainy season in Malaya. The Commonwealth Cricket Team jointly led by Mr. Willie Watson and Mr. Colin Ingleby Mackenzie of England was to play Selangor and All Malaya for three days from October 6th, 1962. The organizing committee of the Malayan Cricket Association engaged Bomoh Lebai from Kuala Lipis, Pahang, as this Bomoh had previously gained the reputation for having kept the rains away for the Merdeka Football Tournament and Celebrations. Before the start of the match, on the last day, Bomoh Lebai came out of concealment in the Selangor Club where he had been in constant

meditation for three days when he had kept the rain away from the padang . . . . Amidst thunderous applause by thousands of spectators, he walked steadily holding a bat horizontally . . . to the wickets . . . . Rain clouds darkened the skies around 3:30 p.m.

All that Bomoh Lebai did was to pull a handkerchief out of his pocket and loosen a large knot on it and utter incantations quietly. The knot, according to the Bomoh was to signify that the rain had been "tied up." True enough, no rain fell on the padang although there was rain in several surrounding areas. . . . Members of the Team rushed up to the Bomoh and offered congratulations and asked for his autograph. One of them even asked the Bomoh to accompany him to England (Danaraj 1964:20–21).

The increasing demand for *bomohs* in transitional times is further documented by so-called cases of "mass hysteria" which continue to occur among Malay children and women in schools and factories in Malaysia and Singapore.[2] In 1970, the newspapers mentioned at least fifty cases. One shoe factory in Malakka experienced forty cases in two years. The *Wall Street Journal*, Friday, March 7, 1980, reported recent cases in companies such as Texas Instruments, RCA, Harris Semiconductor, and Motorola. Each of these companies employed up to 6,000 young women. "Mass hysteria" among them certainly "doesn't increase productivity." Quoting from the above-mentioned issue of the *Wall Street Journal:*

> mass hysteria has struck other countries . . . . Europe witnessed the mewing nuns of Loudun and the barking girls of Oxford. Housewives in Matoon, Ill., complained in the 1940s of a nighttime prowler who sprayed them with anesthetic gas. In the later 1960s, a textile mill in the American South had to close when its women workers said they were being bitten by June bugs . . . .
>
> But Malaysia's events are more dramatic, perhaps for good reason. Freud said hysteria was a symptom of thwarted sexuality, and Malay culture, formal and subdued, doesn't permit women much outlet. In the new factories, they face Western values and are often drawn into production-floor conflicts. Their frustrations can only be channelled toward the supernatural and, in Malaysia, spirit possession is socially acceptable; confrontation is not.
>
> "Hysteria is an expression of hostility without physical violence," Dr. Teoh Jin Inn says. "It is the *hantu* that does it, not the victim."
>
> Dr. Teoh . . . has made a study of hysteria and has been called in as an emergency consultant to several stricken factories. He sees the malady as a sign of deeper turmoil there.

"We're moving from tradition into modernization," he says. "The Malay are pushed from 16th Century *kampongs* into the computer age without a chance to make adjustments. They dare not introspect. Education, industrialization, the rapid pace have created a transient personality. It isn't weak-mindedness. they are put into an intolerable situation."

At the shoe factory in Malacca that blew up 40 times, two down-to-earth researchers found that mass hysteria may also have something to do with industrial peace. Pay was $1.50 a day. The place was mismanaged. It had no medical benefits, no grievance procedures and, of course, no unions . . . the women explained of an atmosphere of intimidation. Outbreaks of hysteria followed rumors of layoffs, including some rumor that men would replace the women to put a lid on hysteria.

. . . Westerners have tried Valium and smelling salts to quell an eruption but Dr. Teoh, the psychiatrist, offers this advice: "Close the factory down. Call a *bomoh*. Sacrifice a goat."

Kalifah Nordin Junid, licensed healer, agrees. The bomoh . . . has handled many factory jobs. "Once upon a time there was jungle," he says, "and all of a sudden they start cutting with no ceremony to take the spirit. Then they build new factories. The area suffers. It is a common thing."

(For occurrences of mass hysteria at the time I was conducting my fieldwork in 1978/1979, see Part 2, Case 3 and Fig.17.)

In multi-ethnic and multi-religious societies like Malaysia and Singapore and, to a lesser degree, Thailand, traditional social systems are breaking up. Extended families do no longer live together. After they have moved into high-rise buildings, people do no longer interact with neighbors. They can no longer rely on the support of their old socio-cultural systems and begin to search for points of reference and systems with which they can identify and connect. When newly evolving social systems do not yet cover all functions traditional social systems would fulfil, individuals will look for alternative solutions to their problems.

For example, in Malaysia, where in the seventies not enough Western trained physicians were available in rural areas, *bomohs* were invited to treat ailments which did not require modern techniques. In Singapore, today, self-improvement courses are very popular and have high attendance rates. People want to learn how they can cope with their own problems. In cases of emergency, however, individuals continue to look for outside help and go to shamans, mediums, and healers when

1. they feel a need for love, attention, empathy, and assurance;
2. their healing forces have to be activated and when
3. spiritual protection and reinforcement beyond the physical realm have become vitally important.

This answers the question about the role of shamans, mediums, and healers in three modern Southeast Asian countries today. Practitioners fulfill urgent needs and are available "where two worlds meet" (Miller 1979:184–185).

The practitioners we are talking about are not so much "concerned with maintenance or restoration of social order when it is endangered or breaks down." They leave these tasks to government officials. Priests of world religions attend to the institutionalized worship of gods, preside over rites of passages at the time of birth, marriage and death (van Gennep 1960) and, sometimes, even legitimize state power. Physicians administer "modern medicine" and, similar to government officials and priests, operate "safely on this side of the boundary between the visible and invisible world" (Miller 1979:185). Shamans, mediums, and healers are the link between both worlds.

Some basic information about the access and use of spiritual power has already been offered in Chapter 3.4.3 and 4. In Section I:2, I talked about how individuals become shamans, mediums, and/or healers and why some individuals are "called" and others not.

Researchers have to admit that they stand on the other side of the fence. They look for the visible and measurable and leave out the vast complex of the invisible and immeasurable. We have to move beyond the many existing stereotypes to understand the nature of shamanism and traditional healing.

When I introduced colleagues to shamans, mediums, and healers with whom I had established close relationships, they were surprised about the practitioners' simplicity and earthliness or, in other cases, their degree of sophistication and high level of spiritual accomplishment. Shamans, mediums, and healers have a wider range of personality characteristics than previous researchers have led us to believe.

Except Malay-Muslim *bomohs* who inherit their faculties, all of the shamans, mediums, and healers I observed during my fieldwork had been in a personal crisis situation, either accumulative latent or acute, when access to "spiritual" forces opened up. Harmony was restored, between themselves and their environment and they decided to share this newly gained harmony with others so that everybody could lead a more effective life. They devoted their lives to fulfilling the needs of

Socio-Psychological Considerations

others, even when it entailed personal sacrifices. They needed, for example, daytime jobs to support themselves and their families.

At this point, I have to say something about the importance of rituals. Shamans, mediums, and healers cultivate rituals so that their clients can overcome fears and receive divine nourishment. The discrepancies between the clients' own design and reality are resolved during the *communitas* experience at a sacred space and time.

Each ritual requires, therefore, the creation of a sacred space and sacred time so that the unexpected can happen. Participants have to purify themselves and then enter the sacred space ceremoniously. The Divine is invited and becomes manifest and participants mutually reinforce the experience of the sacred union. Imbalances are balanced and the interconnection is celebrated. After gratitude has been expressed for the spiritual presence, the ritualist has to send off the Divine. This is necessary because a prolonged stay would overwhelm the untrained participants. The Divine also has to be protected from becoming polluted by staying too long in a secular environment. After the ritual closure and after all have left the sacred space, the ritual then has to be processed to confirm the experience (Heinze 1990, and, among others, Turner 1966).

The functions of folk practitioners require, therefore, a high degree of professionalism. The stereotype of a hysteric or schizophrenic becoming a "healed healer" cannot be applied to the wide range of practitioners of the 20th century I met in 1979 in three Southeast Asian countries. People knew the difference between mentally disturbed and mentally developed individuals. The results spoke for themselves. Shamans, mediums, and healers fulfilled more than ever before not only physical but also psychological, mental, social and spiritual needs. People stopped going to those who were less gifted because they were not effective.

In sum, the field data I collected, during 1978–1979, in Thailand, Malaysia, and Singapore, on 122 shamans, medium, and healers, their entourage (between 8 to 20 members) and, sometimes, several hundreds of clients, showed that the needs ranged from very pragmatic concerns about health, problems inside the family and "on the job," longevity, fertility, to the search for meaning. Important was the accessibility and local availability of "spiritual power" (see also Chapter 3.3.3.).

I would like to cite Weber who wrote about the impediments to the development of monotheism. There was always

> the religious need of the laity for an accessible and tangible familiar religious object which could be brought into relationship with concrete life situations or with definite

groups of people to the exclusion of outsiders, an object which would above all be accessible to magical influences. The security provided by a tested magical manipulation is far more reassuring than the experience of worshipping a god who — precisely because he is omnipotent — is not subject to magical influence (1965:25).

My data strongly confirmed the need "for an accessible and tangible familiar religious object."

James mentioned, at the beginning of the 20th century already, that different types of religions respond to different types of needs. Somebody who lives more habitually on one side of the pain-, fear-, and misery-threshold might need a different sort of religion than one who habitually lives on the other (1941:135).

> How irrelevant remote seem all our usual refined optimism and intellectual and moral consolations in presence of a need for help like this! Here is the real core of the religious problem . . . . .No prophet can claim to bring a final message unless he says things that will have a sound of reality in the ears of victims such as these (James 1941:162).

I agree with James who said,

> We cannot divide man sharply into an animal and a rational part. We cannot distinguish natural from supernatural effects; nor among the latter know which are favors of God, and which are counterfeit operations of the demon. We have merely to collect things together without any special *a priori* theological system, and out of an aggregate of piecemeal judgments as to the value of this and that experience — judgments in which our general philosophic prejudices, our instincts and our common sense are our only guides — decide that *on the whole* one type of religion is approved by its fruits, and another type condemned. "One the whole," — I fear we shall never escape complicity with that qualification, so dear to your practical man, so repugnant to your systematizer! (1941:327).

Let me repeat: Shamanism, mediumship and healing in Singapore, Malaysia, and Thailand are presently practiced in multi-ethnic settings. Clients in Southeast Asia may consult shamans, mediums, and healers not only from their own but other ethnic and religious groups as well. Even entourages of one shaman may belong to different ethnic groups (see Chapter 3.4.6.). Furthermore, all three countries are in the process of modernization and urbanization, that means, they experience rapid social change. Present social systems differ from those in which shamanism, mediumship, and healing originated, but the different forms of shamanism, mediumship, and healing should not deceive us, they still fulfill basic human needs.

Shamanism, mediumship, and healing today are more than ever based on faith. Their belief systems operate on a level where religion is in a preconscious, uncodified, and non-institutionalized stage. That means, "elementary forms of the religious life" emerge from this dynamic stage and are constantly regenerated to fit individual needs arising in changing environments.

We have to pay more attention to the multi-dimensional aspects of daily life in the 20th century. Most practitioners of modern medicine still uphold the Cartesian world view and perceive mental and physical phenomena as distinct entities (see, among others, Frankl 1961:131).

Tillich, for example, spoke about the multidimensional unity of life which calls for a multidimensional concept of health (1967:3–12). He suggested the exploration of the following dimensions,

1. *Mechanical* and *physical* dimensions require knowledge of the adequate functioning of what constitutes man. Dis-ease is non-functioning.
2. The *chemical* dimension is concerned with the balance of chemical substances and processes in a living organism.
3. Balance in the *biological* dimension is achieved by self-alteration and self-preservation, while
4. the process of *psychological* growth demands not only self-alteration but also cultivation of self-awareness and understanding.
5. The *spiritual* dimension, finally, does comprise meanings and values inherent in morality, culture and religion. The self-actualization of man occurs in this dimension and prepares him/her for the encounter with others (1967:3–12).

Tillich asked not to subject ourselves to a law allegedly coming from God or man, but to actualize what we potentially are. A distorted self-identity can lead to a "lawless explosion of all possibilities," where psycho-therapeutic problems can become moral problems.

> [H]ealing is the power of overcoming both distortions. But the healing of the spirit is not possible by good will, because the good will is just that which needs healing. In

order to be healed, the spirit must be grasped by something which transcends it, which is not strange to it, but within which is the fulfillment of its potentialities . . . . Spirit is the presence of what concerns us ultimately, the ground of our being and meaning. This is the intention of religion but it is not identical with religion (1967:9–10).

Tillich knew of the magic influence of healers on patients and of patients upon themselves. Magic is actually the impact of one unconscious power upon another. Reliance on a certain religion (accepting authority, going through a conversion experience) may work in some cases, it is of limited use in others.

The different stages in the life of individuals and the different situations they are exposed to are intimately connected with each of the above-mentioned five levels of human existence. The well-being of individuals depends on unobstructed communication with all dimensions. That means "complete healing" is multi-dimensional.

To come to a better understanding of the factors involved in shamanism, mediumship, and traditional healing, we have to look at the differences between belief and knowledge. A belief appears to be a reality for the believer, but escapes scientific verification. The value of a belief can, therefore, only be judged by its results. Knowledge, on the other hand, requires verification, not only intuitively but also by scientific means (see INTRODUCTION).

On what kind of knowledge do those who are concerned with healing base their actions?

Keeping the multi-dimensional concepts of health and of healing practices in mind, we will investigate three categories which are concerned with belief and knowledge. They are belief in and knowledge of modern medicine, belief in and knowledge of traditional medicine, and belief in and knowledge of the Divine Source.

4.2. Belief in and Knowledge of Modern Medicine

Who are the people who *believe in modern medicine*? They are the untrained patients who seek medical and psychological help. Those who *know modern medicine* are the physicians and psychiatrists who seldom admit the limitations of their trade. A well-known physician once told his graduating class that he had a confession to make: Half of what he had taught them was wrong and he could not even tell them which half (personal communication, December 1978).

Socio-Psychological Considerations

In cases of physical illness, all clients interviewed during the fieldwork for this study had first seen representatives of modern, i.e, Western, medicine, but had difficulties in communication. They found modern doctors to be too impersonal and businesslike, giving patients very little information about the actual situation, charging high fees, and prescribing expensive medicines.[3] Patients were especially apprehensive about modern miracle drugs where unpleasant side-effects were discovered after treatment. (In Southeast Asia, patients usually go to a shaman and have the prescribed drugs blessed to avoid negative influences.)

In sum, it was felt that modern doctors seemed to know only of two alternatives: drugs or operation and were not interested in traditional healing methods. Clients found that modern doctors treat the illness not the patient. They treat the symptoms not the cause of illness. Similar complaints were voiced about psychiatrists who may send patients to mental hospitals because they neither had sufficient time to listen nor had their patients sufficient means to pay for expensive psychotherapy. Medical staff and social workers were, indeed, facing an overload of cases.[4]

On the other hand, clients received immediate personal attention and empathy from shamans, mediums, and healers. Charges, if any, were low, this applied to the diagnosis as well as the treatment (e.g., herbs, massages, steam baths). Patients were not isolated in hospitals and separated from relatives and friends who could cooperate in the healing process (Miller, 1979:179, note 20). Expectancy prepared the ground for "divine intervention" and deities responded to the clients' needs. When doors to self-healing powers were opened, clients were ready to be healed (see also Torrey (1986).

Having shown the differences between modern and traditional medicine in Southeast Asia. I will now discuss the second group.

4.3. Belief in and Knowledge of Traditional Medicine

Those who *believe in* and *rely on traditional medicine* base their trust on the fact that traditional medical *knowledge* went through the process of trial and error for a considerably longer period (i.e., a couple of thousand years), while practitioners of modern medicine still discover undesirable side effects of new drugs they prescribe.

With respect to traditional medical systems

1. *Indian* practitioners referred to *ayurvedic* knowledge. The Atharva Veda as well as the Susruta and the Caraka Samhita were both codified in the first

century A.D., but had been the basis for medical practices already for more than two thousand years.
2. *Thai* practitioners cited Indian sources. Books in Buddhist monasteries, for example, claimed Jivaka, Buddha's physician (6th century B.C.), as the author. Over the centuries, knowledge from local herbalists and other sources has been added, but Thai healers maintained that the ancient Indian knowledge is the most effective. Legends reported that Jivaka's teacher sent him into the jungle to explore the properties of herbs. After years of solitude, Jivaka returned and announced that, if used wisely, all herbs could successfully been used in healing.
3. *Chinese* practitioners based their knowledge on the *Pen T'sao* ("Book on Herbs") by the mythical Shen Nung. The *Pen T'sao*, used today, was composed during the Ming Period (1368–1644 A.D.). The *Nei Ching* ("Inner Book," i.e., Book on Internal Diseases), ascribed to the mythical Yellow Emperor (Huang-ti) was codified in the first century A.D. Practitioners frequently display portraits of Shen Nung or Huang-ti next to the altar where they go into trance. In Spring 1979, I saw a painting of Shen Nun hanging left of the altar of a Sino-Kadazan medium in Sabah on Borneo (see Fig. 48). She told me that she painted it after Shen Nung had appeared to her in a dream.
4. *Malay bomohs* may use fragments of the books of Luman al-Hakim, a historical figure who also appears in Arabian fables.

All ethnic groups discussed in this book were performing healing rituals.

Healing rituals move through three separate stages. The sickness is labeled with an appropriate and sanctioned cultural category. The label is ritually manipulated (culturally transformed). Finally a new label (cured, well) is applied and sanctioned as a meaningful symbolic form that may be independent of behavioral or social change (Kleinman 1980:372).

Furthermore, "healing ceremonies are highly charged emotionally" (Frank 1961:66). Environmental or bodily stress and feelings of estrangement and isolation fade away. Healing is not an intellectual process. Clients enter what Turner (1969:97) called "*communitas*," a stage where ordinary time and space are suspended. This temporary suspension of daily worries allows participants to distance themselves from the cause of pain. If detached properly, they can emerge refreshed.

Although certain elements of the social systems around shamans, mediums, and healers may locally differ, the understanding and reassurance offered is common to all. Faith is generated. The belief that, when approached correctly, forces greater than man will intervene is an important factor.

In *Singapore* of 1979, clients as well as practitioners did not confuse modern medical treatment with those of traditional medicine. They did not believe that one could substitute for the other. Deities "supervised" modern treatments. Blessed water, flowers, and charm papers carried divine blessings and protection. Deities also were able to plead for clients even when they could not change an individual's fate. This answer was given to an old man when he was brought in a comatose state to a traditional Chinese medium working at a temple on Ganges Avenue. The deity announced, through the medium, that the man was possessed by a "coffin spirit" and performed a dramatic exorcism. The relatives were then advised to return with the patient in three days. In the meantime, the deity would go to heaven and plead for him. If, however, it should turn out that this man's time was up, the deity could not change his fate (personal observation, January 8, 1979). Relatives and the dying man himself were satisfied because somebody was pleading the cause.

Traditional forms of treatment have only recently been tested and used by modern physicians. Acupuncture, for example, was, in 1979, performed at General Hospital in Singapore and patients with high blood pressure were taught meditation to reduce, e.g., the blood lactate level, and establish a calmer disposition toward their illness. The government of Singapore also recognized and was supervising the services of traditional physicians. There were in Singapore, for example, three major organization of Chinese physicians, i.e., the Chinese Physicians Association (CPA), the Thong Chai Medical Institution (TCMI), and the Chinese Acupuncture and Cauterisation Centre (CACC). Each had its own school of Chinese medicine and its own outpatient clinics. In 1976, the CPA alone had 387 members, 120 of whom were on duty at the three branches of the CPA-managed Chung Hwa Free Clinic. About 75 per cent of the qualified Chinese physicians in Singapore were represented by the CPA (Quah 1977a and 1977b). Acupuncture was also practiced at a Free Clinic in the Geylang District, funded by money coming from Arab states. I was allowed to practice acupuncture at this clinic under the supervision of my Chinese teacher. This gave me the opportunity to observe practitioner-client relationships first hand.

In spring 1979, 400 *bomohs*, *sinsehs* (Chinese healers) and *ayurvedic* practitioners, including delegates from Indonesia and Brunei, met in the Malaysian capital, Kuala Lumpur. The convention on traditional medicine had been called by the

United Malays National Organization. The traditional healers claimed they can cure venereal diseases, high blood pressure, piles, diabetes, paralysis, hysteria, backache, kidney and heart diseases, and ailments of the urinary tract. They demanded official recognition. Raden Supathan reported on the success of Indonesian *bomohs* who already marketed their traditional medicine called *jamu*. After the two-day convention, the Malaysian government set up a medical institute for *bomohs* with a modern laboratory to test roots and herbs and the manufacture of traditional medicine. Minister of Culture Datuk Samad Idris, a staunch supporter of folk medicine, told the *bomohs* that more research and training were needed before official recognition can be accorded. He suggested that *bomohs* combine their practice, handed down for generations, with those of Western trained doctors.

Bomohs had been credited already with successful rehabilitation of 800 drug addicts under a program sponsored by the United Malay Organization. This program was not included into the institute because the treatment for drug addiction varied among individual *bomohs* and could not be standardized. This decision supported my point about the merits of individualized treatment.

In *Thailand*, a rehabilitation program for drug addicts was, for example, conducted at Wat Tham Krabod near Saraburi. The abbot (see Fig.39) was, in 1978, 52 years old. He had left his wife and two children in Lopburi at the age of 26 to become a Buddhist monk. Since 1959, he was curing drug addicts with herbal potions and steam baths. The monastery records showed that his treatment cured over 10,000 addicts in three years (between 1959 and 1962). At public rehabilitation centers in Thailand, more than 95 percent of the addicts, released as cured, return. According to one of the supervising monks, less than 20 per cent of the addicts who came to Wat Tham Krabod have fallen back into their old habit. The abbot added that when the environment to which cured addicts return is supportive, the relapse rate will even be less than 10 per cent.

Before starting the ten-day treatment, addicts had to take a religious vow. The next three days they were given an emetic to clean their system. Fellow patients cheered when they took the potion and supported the individual lovingly through the painful days of purging. Steam baths and herbal concoctions after the ordeal restored the patients' strength.

The roster for December 30, 1978, reported 20 cures for that day, 57 were newly admitted, and 33 patients decided to stay longer. The cured addicts worked on agricultural projects and new buildings for this Buddhist rehabilitation center. The following statistics speak for themselves.

1963	7,219 cures	1968	1,472 cures	1973	2,435 cures
1964	5,016 cures	1969	1,451 cures	1974	3.125 cures
1965	3,221 cures	1970	1,290 cures	1975	5,281 cures
1966	1,402 cures	1971	1,153 cures	1976	5,623 cures
1967	1,700 cures	1972	1,171 cures	1977	3,025 cures

The number of addicts the monastery can admit depends on the amount of private donations. In 1979, patients did not pay more than 20 baht (US$1) per day. So far, the abbot refused government support because he does not want to violate the trust of his patients (the government may ask him to open his files for inspection). He also did not disclose the composition of his herbal potion an aunt of his has taught him.

It is not the purpose of this book to discuss the traditional systems of healing in more detail. All practitioners recommended natural cures, i.e., herbs, massage, and bathing. Divine blessings and protection were added to restore the inner balance of a client's mind, body, and soul. They were truly holistic. Such *natural means are less limited and intrusive than modern drugs and operations.*

4.3. Belief in and Knowledge of the Divine Source

The *belief in* and the *knowledge of the Divine Source* are *unlimited*. Knowledge of the Divine Source goes beyond the capacity of human understanding, but the Infinite Source can be tapped by experts. Divine powers are trusted more readily, because they are based on universal laws.

Indians call these laws, *dharma*. Everybody has to live according to his or her *dharma*, i.e., the duties s/he is born with, the duties of his/her station in life (I use the term "station in life" for "caste," because the caste system has been abolished in India, after independence, in 1948).

Hindus, as well as *Chinese* and *Thai Buddhists*, and *Chinese Taoists*, furthermore, believe in the law of *karma* where the quality of each thought, word, and action determines the quality of present and future existences. *Malay-Muslims* speak of the law of *taqdir*, i.e., the will of Allah. This adds the factor of providence. It is believed that universal laws and decisions of God are binding. Where infractions occur, amendments have to be made. On the other hand, rewards can be expected for right behavior.

To quote Weber,

> Our everybody experience proves that there exists just such a psychological need for reassurance as to the legitimacy or deservedness of one's happiness, whether this involves political success, superior economic status, bodily health, success in the game of love, or anything else (1965:107).

Ironically, the more we know the more we become aware of the limitations of our knowledge. Indeed, less than ten per cent of the information reaching our organs of perception rises to consciousness. Our autonomic nervous system blocks off a wide range of inputs "to avoid systems' overload," but, more importantly, during the process of socialization, at home, at school, being trained for an occupation and specializing in a field, more and more doors are closed under the pretext that certain information is irrelevant. As a result, only a small part of the information actually perceived is processed. However, there are individuals who have kept channels open. They have learned to use this unlimited and seemingly chaotic information productively. We call these individuals shamans, mediums, and healers.

Studies to explore the communication processes are still in progress. At the moment, photons are considered to be the carriers of information. They are tuned in vibrational patterns. Alterted to this process, we can observe how we are tuned and we can become aware of the process by which we tune others, e.g. with the sound of our voice.

We have to continue our work and check our results carefully. At this point, however, we must admit that shamans, mediums, and healers are opening doors we unfortunately have closed in the past.

James reminded us that ordinary people who follow the conventional observances of their culture, whether they are Hindus, Buddhists, Taoists, Christians, or Muslims, believe in religions which were made for them by others. Communicated by tradition, forms were fixed, imitated and habitually transmitted.

It is of little use to study second-hand religions. When people want original experiences, they have to look for "the pattern setters to all this mass of suggested feelings and imitated conduct. These experiences we can only find in individuals for whom religion exists not as a dull habit" (James 1941:6).

Shamans, mediums and healers provide their clients with personal, religious experiences. They operate on different levels of consciousness. Whether spiritual entities are present or not, experiences are provided which support faith and faith facilitates beneficial effects.

Socio-Psychological Considerations

Social systems evolving around practitioners are relevant as long as they remain meaningful and produce unique experiences. External components may differ, however, having looked closely, we see that practitioners from different ethnic groups show a striking similarity in pattern.

4.5. Are Shamans, Mediums, and Healers Beyond Criticism?

The answer is "no." Practitioners depend on their entourage. Practitioners as well as entourage cannot continue to operate without clients. That means, inefficient or fraudulent practitioners are weeded out by the process of natural selection. When they do not produce satisfactory results, clients and entourages lose faith and leave.

In some cases, entourages may become selfish. For practitioners it is not easy to avoid the pressure of their assistants. Entourages set the pace, codify the rituals, and handle promotion. It is believed that disagreements between shamans, mediums, healers, and their entourages will be solved by the deity. Sometimes, however, conflicts linger on and test the tolerance and determination of all involved.

Institutionalization can become destructive and routinization of mystical experiences carries its dangers. Jordan (1977), writing about successful Chinese mediums on Taiwan, reported that some could not resist the temptation of collecting large sums of money. The accumulation of wealth led to self-destruction. Mediums built temples and headed large organization, but most of them lost their faculty of manifestation and delegated many functions, i.e., they did not act as mediators to other realms anymore.

Modern physicians and psychiatrists, in questioning the qualifications of traditional practitioners, may criticize their lack of formal education. Shamans rely mostly on oral knowledge which has been transmitted for several thousands of years. If to-day's culture does not provide this knowledge anymore, their intuition can excavate the forgotten wisdom from their DNA. In any case, the possibility of spiritual intervention cannot be excluded!

Modern physicians and psychiatrists should compare the success rates of folk practitioners with their own. A cooperation between modern and traditional practitioners could be mutually stimulating but, feeling responsible for the health services in their country, governments hesitate to recognize alternative services and have not yet created avenues necessary for cooperation.

On the other hand, sufficient health facilities may not always be available and they may also be insufficiently equipped to fulfill the pragmatic physical, psychological, mental, social, and spiritual needs of the people. In most cases, public services are also too expensive for clients from the working classes. When, at this point, traditional practitioners emerge and have results, the question can be asked:

> What right have we to believe Nature under any obligation to do her work by means of complete minds only! She may find an incomplete mind a more suitable instrument for a particular purpose. It is the work that is done, and the quality in the worker by which it was done, that is alone of moment (Dr. Maudsley, quoted in James 1941:19).

I mentioned above that most of the clients I interviewed for this study had seen a physician before they decided to consult a medium, shaman, or healer.

Clients maintained they needed physiological, psychological, mental, social, and spiritual help which modern medicine did not afford them. Traditional practitioners, on the other hand, did not underestimate the merits of modern medicine and sent clients to modern physicians when necessary. They never took cases they could not solve.

I observed practitioners successfully working with emotional problems (Part 2, Case 3). I watched the cathartic effect of exorcism on frustrated minds (Part 2, Case 17). All twenty-one case studies in Part 2 attest that practitioners gave clients the reassurance necessary to face their daily tasks.

The work of shamans, mediums, and traditional healers has been called a coping mechanism. It is more than that. The greatest service traditional healers can render is the restructuring of their clients' psyche. They suggest changes in attitude to make life more bearable. When outsiders were surprised about some practitioners' lack of sophistication, sophisticated clients were not because the beneficial effects they were experiencing were on the physical, emotional, social, and spiritual levels. They did not need an intellectual explanation of their condition, they needed a cure. A famous Buddhist legend relates the Buddha's words about a man who had been shot by an arrow. He said, "It is of no use to ask questions, 'Where did the arrow come from?' 'What is the material the arrow is made of?' 'Who shot the arrow?' All this has happened already. We have to take the arrow out of the body of the wounded man."

Traditional healers work mainly on levels where they don't disturb other social systems. In fact, they complement and support the other social system of their society (see Part 2, Case 16). All ages and all occupational groups as well as even members of other ethnic groups and religions can be found in the social systems around shamans, mediums, and traditional healers.

At the end, nobody is free of criticism and each practitioner is judged by his or her success rate.

4.6. What Are the Implications for Other Social Systems?

Practitioners, concerned with the spiritual world, are by nature *apolitical*. They may, however, be frequented by politicians who seek reassurance or legitimacy. In the case of Pu Sawan (Part 2, Case 17), a medium used his charisma and reputation to boost nationalism in Thailand, until he made some unfortunate predictions.

There have been millenary movements in the past in China and in Thailand where, for example, monks in the northeast claimed to possess supernatural faculties (Keyes 1973:95–101). In the Thailand of the 90s, several monks have started again movements to reform. The secret societies in Singapore have kept a low profile under the strict government of the People's Action Party. Only once I watched people listening quietly to fantastic prophecies of a devotee.

In 1978/1979, mediums, shamans, and healers respected each others territory. No coordination or cooperation between different entourages could be observed other than assistance with religious duties during festival time. Beyond these brief periods, nothing indicated that social systems around individual practitioners aspired to unite in millenary efforts.

When we look at the *economic* side, social systems around practitioners do not constitute any drain on the economy of Thailand, Malaysia, and Singapore. In 1979, the majority of the practitioners were altruistic. They had day-time jobs to earn their living. Donations were voluntary and used mainly for the upkeep of the temple and the purchase of paraphernalia. The lavish display of statues, banners, and good food during festivals entertained the clients and heightened their sense of belonging.

On the *cultural* sector, practitioners supported ethnic traditions and kept them relevant. Working on a person-to-person level, they were able to reinterpret and regenerate traditional beliefs effectively and warranted continuity. Through their participation in ceremonies of other groups, members of one ethnic group even kept the ceremonies of other groups alive. This did not seem to be just a feature of our times. A softening of borderlines must have occurred wherever different ethnic groups met in the past. Even orthodox Muslims were aware of the syncretism in local practices.

Trance and Healing in Southeast Asia Today

The *therapeutic* value of the physiological, psychological, mental, social, and spiritual services of traditional practitioners has already been explained. Safety valves are offered, so frustrations and projections of anxieties can be resolved. It is essential in Southeast Asia that spiritual beings "speak" through practitioners. Clients find consolation in the belief that gods and spirits are available in complex situations. When individuals do not find attention and understanding in public institutions, they look for solutions in the spiritual world.

Over 75 per cent of the practitioners I studied in 1978–1979 began to practice within the last seven years (i.e., after 1970). Is this phenomenon a reaction to the onslaught of modernity? Talking about Chinese in Singapore, Elliott said already in 1955:

> The classical conception of the Chinese family has not been reproduced in Singapore, partly because the persons who emigrated where of the type who never subscribed to it fully in China, and partly because the kinship system was something that belonged to the ancestral soil and could not be transplanted (1955:16).

In 1979, more than 60 per cent of all Singaporeans lived in high-rise buildings, mostly in HDB (Housing Development Board) flats. This new pattern of living accelerated the breaking-up of the extended family system for all ethnic groups. Community centers were established to reduce isolation and loneliness, however, feelings of alienation persisted.

In a rapidly changing world, with increasing modernization, urbanization and industrialization in all three Southeast Asian countries discussed in this book, individuals have left familiar grounds. They had to abandon traditional affiliations. Reliable, because already tested, defense mechanisms became inoperative. The uncertainty about the future compounded the growing anxiety in transitional periods.

In the *Thai* case, farmers, for example, sold their land to buy now available consumer goods (transistor radios, motor cycles, etc.). Not essential for survival, these goods precipitated the farmers' downfall. Having become landless, farmers moved to the cities and sought different means of sustenance. They lived now in an environment which was diametrically opposed to their life in the country. They had to become familiar with the unfamiliar which required a new set of defense and coping mechanism.[5]

In the paternalistic societies of the past, the differences between rich and poor were less aggravating. Security was found in the traditional patron-client system

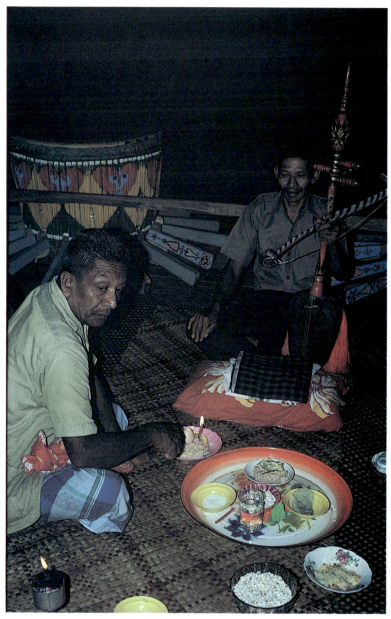

Fig. 33 *Malay bomoh, preparing for a main puteri, Kelantan, Malaysia*

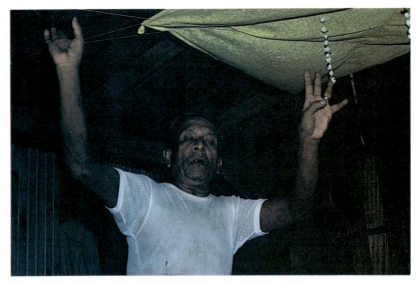

Fig. 34 *Bomoh in trance, during a main puteri, Kelantan, Malaysia*

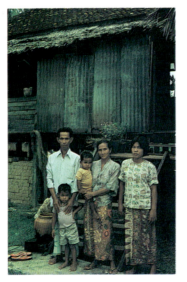

Fig. 35 *Female bomoh, Pattani, southern Thailand*

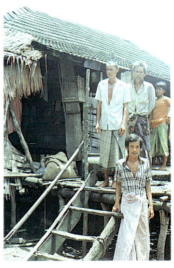

Fig. 36 *Sixty-year-old bomoh, Pattani, southern Thailand*

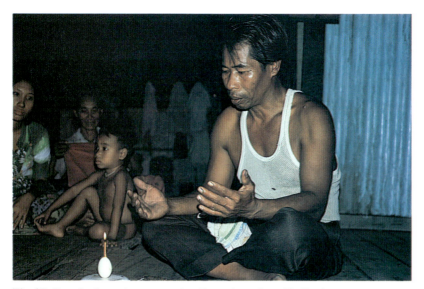

Fig. 37 *Bomoh after a tiger possession, Pattani, southern Thailand*

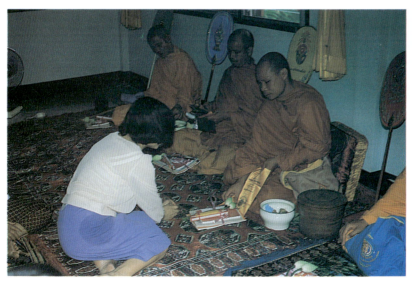

Fig. 38 *Monks performing a first-hair-cutting ceremony, Bangkok, Thailand*

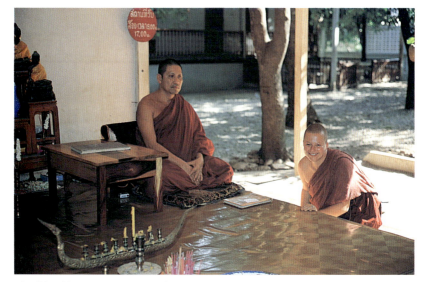

Fig. 39 *Abbot of Wat Tham Krabod, Saraburi, Thailand*

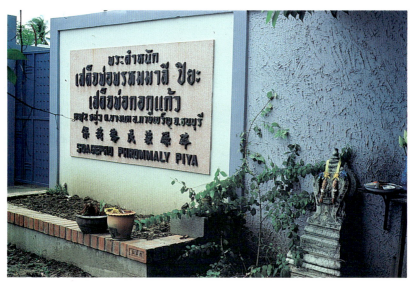

Fig. 40 *Entrance to Phrom Mali's compound, Petchkasem Road, Bangkok, Thailand*

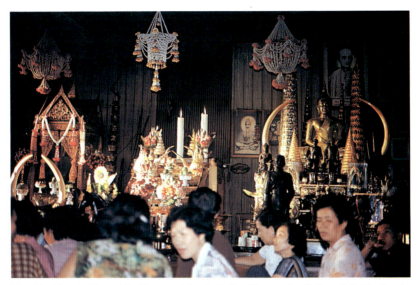

Fig. 41 *Altar in Phrom Mali's practicing hall, Petchkasem Road, Bangkok, Thailand*

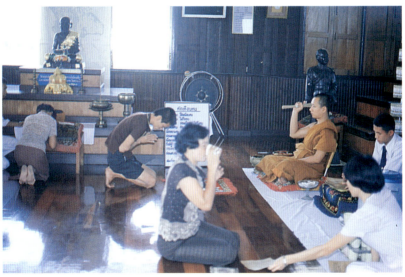

Fig. 42 *Monk blessing medicine, Pu Sawan, Petchkasem Road, Bangkok, Thailand*

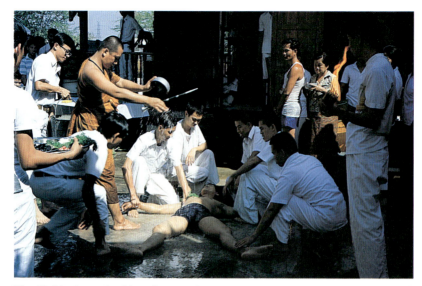

Fig. 43 *Monk pouring blessed water after an exorcism, Pu Sawan, Petchkasem Road, Bangkok, Thailand*

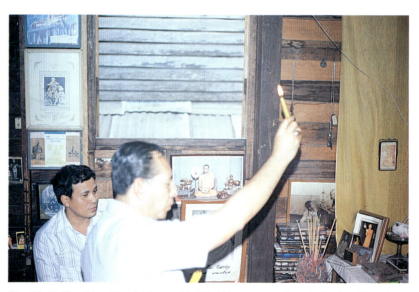

Fig. 44 *Calling Phra Narai (photo of the Thai king as a monk on the back wall), private residence, Bangkok, Thailand*

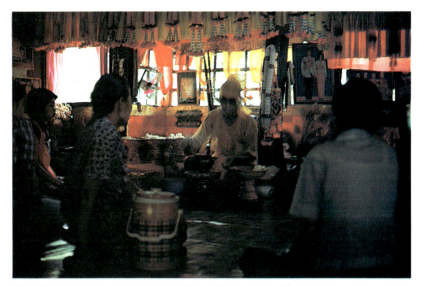

Fig. 45 *Spirit dance, Wat Chet Yot, Chiang Mai, northern Thailand*

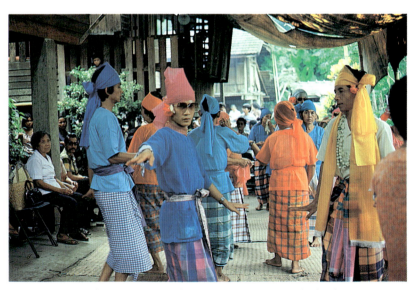

Fig. 46 *Spirit medium, Sansei, outside Chiang Mai, northern Thailand*

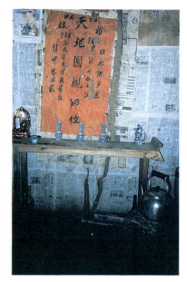

Fig. 47 *Hill tribe altar, near Chiang Mai, northern Thailand*

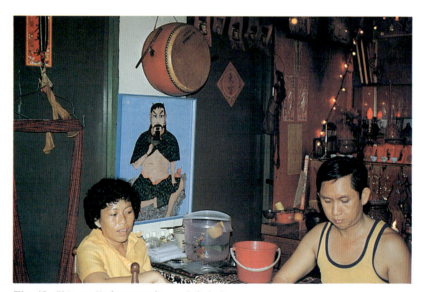

Fig. 48 *Chinese-Kadazan mediums, Sabah, Borneo*

Socio-Psychological Considerations

In democratizing societies, the number of bureaucrats grew in proportion to the increase in population. The focus and reliance on one nurturing head of state shifted to not so well-known democratic providers. Bureaucrats seemed to manipulate individuals in very impersonal ways, leaving the King of Thailand as the only remaining focus of attention. However, in a constitutional monarchy, the king has no direct influence on the policies of his country and it takes time to develop trust in new institutions. And what is worse, where new sets of ethics and values are pronounced, individuals feel their rights and needs infringed upon.

Dependency needs arise in times of social stress. When individuals look for reassurance and meaning in their lives, these efforts are not necessarily a sign for civil disobedience. The efforts, in fact, aim at going with the times.

My field data confirmed that shamans, mediums, and healers are instrumental in activating their clients' self-healing powers and in restoring their inner balance. Does this sufficiently justify the role these practitioners play in the complex social systems of Singapore, Malaysia, and Thailand? The biggest hurdle seems to be the legalization of traditional practices. To achieve this ideal solution, Western-trained scientists have first to admit the limitations of their knowledge.

Part 2

Shamanic Practices:
A Case History Approach

The following twenty-one cases have been selected from my field notes to illustrate the statements in Part 1. The cases stand by themselves, future monographs will provided more details.

Case I describes how a modern-educated, free-thinking housewife became a shaman.

Case 1 - A 39-year-old Housewife Becomes Possessed By a Deified General From the Three Kingdoms (Singapore Chinese)

In 1973, while the family was sitting around the dinner table, a 39-year-old Chinese housewife, mother of five children, became possessed by a deified general from the Three Kingdoms (220–265 A.D.). Everybody seemed to be unprepared for this event. The woman had been British educated at Raffles Girls School and had been working as a fashion model and salesgirl. She converted to Catholicism and, after some disappointments, became a free thinker.

How unexpected was this possession? The family of seven (parents and five children) were living in close quarters with in-laws. There had been health problems and difficulties with her husband's and her jobs. The future of the children caused additional concern. Year's ago, she had consulted mediums herself and had also gone to various Chinese and Indian temples as well as Christian churches, until she became resigned to the fact that she would have to cope with her situation as best as she could.

All the while she had been taking care of a house altar her father-in-law had brought from China. (Her father-in-law was Hokkien, her parents were both Straits Chinese). Her father-in-law was also a devout worshipper of the deity but after his death the altar had been left neglected. Because the altar stood in her family's room, she had taken it on herself to clean it and to put occasionally some flowers in front of the picture of the deity.

Why did a deified general, in the services of Kuan Yin (considered by Buddhists to be the *bodhisattva* of Amitābha Buddha and by Taoists the Goddess of Mercy), select a modern-educated, non-believing housewife and mother to help others, promising protection and assistance for her family, too? Her husband told me that his wife had been chosen because she was the purest in the family.

The deity was first evasive about his identity, but finally disclosed his name, *Kam T'ien Siong Teh*. He began to advise the family in their personal affairs and also instructed the medium about the services expected from her, how to meditate and how to call him.

The wife's position within the extended family changed with her being visited by a deity. The nuclear family considered her mediumship to be an act of divine grace. Their lives had come to a dead end, but now they were the first to benefit from the "salvation work."

The medium's sisters-in-law, who had scorned her in the past, brought the first clients. Because the advice, protection, and assistance of the deity (through the medium) proved to be effective, the word spread fast among relatives, friends, and colleagues. The number of clients kept growing. Some came from the nearby Malaysian city Johore Bahru, some even flew in from Jakarta, Indonesia. Within a year the family could move into a house of their own and, after four more years, into an even larger house.

The altar (see Fig.12) stands now on a raised area and occupies, together with a large waiting area below, most of the downstairs quarters. In separate rooms behind the altar, there are the kitchen, a small dining area, and a storage closet. The children live on the second floor. Husband and wife sleep downstairs, next to the altar, separated by the stairs. (Since she is serving the deity, the medium claims to have become celibate.)

The first member of the medium's entourage was her husband. He became her assistant. Because the deity speaks medieval Hokkien,[1] the husband has to translate the deity's words. Some clients may also come from other dialect and language groups, but most clients are too awed to understand what is going on anyway.

The other members of the entourage were recruited from regular devotees. They do not only relieve the husband from translating and wiping the altar clean during sessions, their duties include

1. to give out numbers to establish the waiting order;
2. to explain
   a. how joss papers have to be used (burned and the ashes mixed with water for drinking and/or bathing;
   b. how the deity has to be evoked; and
   c. how many joss sticks have to be lit when entering and leaving the temple and where they have to be put in which sequence (see Fig.11);
3. to sell joss sticks;
4. to accept offerings, e.g., *ang pows* (red envelopes with money), oil, and fruit, etc.

No musicians are needed for playing drums and gongs to induce the medium's trance, neither are singers required to chant evocations. The medium simply meditates in front of the altar until the deity "arrives."

All members of the entourage are male. They clean after each session and when there has been a large crowd on festival days. Women are only permitted to sell joss sticks and to cook the meal on special occasions (see Fig.10). The committee of approximately sixteen men stay loosely organized. They meet on the eve of a festival to put up different altars outside the temple and set up a stage for the lion dance or a bridge to cross. They agree, therefore, among themselves when their services are required.

The entourage maintain they have been appointed by the deity to help with the "salvation work." According to the length of time each member has been "serving the deity," their position is fixed in the developing hierarchy.

Another point should be mentioned here. It was the entourage who began to codify rituals. The process started when they had to coordinate their answers about the worship of the deity.

The medium's family were her first clients. They brought friends and colleagues. Those grateful for assistance, protection, and advice became regular devotees. That means, they visit the temple on the first and fifteenth day of each lunar month, on Kuan Yin's three birthdays (19th day of the 2nd, 6th, and 9th lunar month), on the deity's birthday (12th day of the 12th lunar month) and the day of the temple's inauguration (6th day of the 6th lunar month).

The medium practices each week night and on Saturday and Sundays twice, but clients may drop in anytime. They feel "at home" in the deity's presence and they participate in meals offered not only on festival days but frequently after sessions, too.

Mediums, entourage, and most of the clients belong to the lower-middle and working classes. However, representatives of other socio-economic groups, e.g., lawyers, physicians, come for advice, too. As soon as they have been accepted into the ranks of the entourage, all "serve" the deity on an equal basis. Everybody enters the state of "liminality" and enjoys the *communitas* of which Turner (1960) spoke.

The medium plays a double role. While the deity, speaking through her, is the sole authority during sessions, the medium remains a good housewife and mother, cooking and caring for husband and children in daily life. Her only change in life style was becoming a vegetarian and observing celibacy.

Her husband also plays two roles. He assists his wife and may kneel in front of her when she sits on the dragon throne, but he asserts his rights as head of household during the day.

The medium's children do not participate in the sessions. One son falls easily into trance but is discouraged from doing so. The five children (in 1979 three sons and two daughters, between the ages of seventeen and twenty-three) are well taken care of. They receive blessings and are given jewels (jade pearls or other semi-precious stones) which the deity "materializes" on special days. The future of the family appears to be secure.

The entourage experienced a rise in spiritual status, outside of the positions they hold in other social systems. More intimately related to a deity, they gained authority through their services. In fact, they support and reinforce the authority of the deity.

The clients, having accepted the authority of the deity, respect the medium even when she is not in trance. Nobody knows whether the deity is still present or not. Though many of the clients and the entourage have established themselves in life, working effectively in their professions, they become voluntarily dependent on the deity at the moment they enter the temple.

Devotees come with questions about health or problems inside their families or with their jobs. Some psychological problems may require an exorcism. Over time, the medium developed, indeed, the reputation of being an effective exorcist. She defeated mischievous spirits, went on "spirit hunts," exorcised haunted houses, and fought demons with her sword. During these battles, bloody spots would appear on her garments.

After clients had experienced relief from their frustrations, they showed their gratitude through donations. Some began to "serve the deity" and some simply come frequently to be in the presence of the deity.

[At the Third International Conference of the International Society of Shamanistic Research in Nara, Japan, November 1995, I met a Japanese colleague who told me that the medium has died of kidney failure and that her son, who had shown predisposition to trance already when he was a child, is now continuing the services dedicated to *Kam T'ien Siong Teh*.]

In the following case, I will report on a simple dock worker from a different ethnic group (Tamil, southern India). He was called in quite a different way and is using different paraphernalia but underlying concepts are quite similar. The structure of the social system around this practitioner also follows the general patterns mentioned above.

Case 2 - An Altar in Search of a Shaman and a Shaman in Search of an Altar (Singapore Indian)

When the extension of Sembawang Shipyard required clearing of brushwork in adjoining areas, a truck suddenly broke down, as it turned out, in front of a small altar (*The Malay Mail*, February 18, 1970). The altar had been built on a small hill, where snakes lived, by Indian troops in the British Army after World War II. After the troops had left, Indian workers, living nearby, had been taking care of the altar. Thus we find an entourage developing before the appearance of a shaman.

Two years later, a Tamil worker had a vision. His parents had abandoned him when he was still very young because they thought he was dying, but a *brahmin* found and raised him. Many years later, the young man wandered around and worked on odd jobs, until a vision told him to look for an altar in the area of Sembawang Shipyard. First he did not find the altar, but another vision urged him to try again.

He finally discovered the altar and voices told him to stay there, everything would be taken care of. He waited for weeks, but nothing happened. In desperation he kicked the altar and seriously injured his right foot which remained crippled from that time on.

Hindu gods began to manifest in his body and (in 1978, for the sixth year) Hanuman, Rāma, Murgam, and Mahākālī spoke through the medium to a growing community of Tamils, Bengals, Sikhs, and Chinese every Tuesday and Friday night.

Nobody dared to address the deity. It was the deity who called devotees forward. He knew their questions already and answered their problems without having listened to them. This differs from the approach used in Chinese temples, where clients ask the deity through the medium or through the interpreter.

Staying advised by "his" deities, the Tamil medium was available for consultations at other times during the week and on weekends.

Some years ago, a British colonel donated a raised platform which was built on top of the small hill so that its roof protects the altars and up to 200 devotees from rain. The medium lived in a tiny shed next to the platform. During and after the sessions, he shared the food offerings with the devotees. He served full-course Indian meals to those who come for consultation on other days.

The medium was supported by an entourage of approximately six men from lower income groups. At least three of them were present during the nights he went into trance. They helped with the *pūjā* (worship) at the five altars. Three altars, dedicated to Ganeśa, Murgam, and Murgam's *vel* (spear), were on the ground floor and stairs were leading to the three altars on the platform. On the south side was a snake altar and on the north side an altar dedicated to Bhadra Kālī. Slightly lower, on the east side, was a small altar for living snakes.

The sessions had, over time, become highly ritualized with the entourage following the *brahmin* tradition without being *brahmins* themselves. A session started with

1. ringing of the bells;
2. waiving of lights (*arati*) and
3. offering of flowers (*puṣpapūjā*);
4. sprinkling of blessed water on each altar, followed by
5. pouring milk down a hole next to the main altar for the living snakes. Each devotee brought a pint of milk. His or her name was called when the milk was poured, in this way, the deity's attention was drawn to the donor;
6. whipping of the medium to induce trance or, as was said, to show how the deity takes on the suffering of his devotees.
7. During the "appearance" of the "deity" (usually two or three manifested, one after the other), the crowd listened spellbound and enjoyed the blessings.
8. Burning camphor was put on the medium's tongue at the end of his trance to protect the departing deity from pollution.
9. The assistants collected the donations, e.g., fruit, oil. Dimes or one-dollar notes were left on the plate with *vibhuti* (cow dung ash) or in the donation box in front of the altar. The money was used for the upkeep of the temple. Donations were voluntary and nobody watched whether or not something was given at all.
10. The donated food was distributed and consumed by all present.

The six assistants of this medium alternated in their services. They all wore white *dhotis* and amulets on gold chains. Occasionally, they borrowed money from the donation box.

The medium, a humble and unassuming man, led the life of an ascetic. He distinguished himself from his entourage through his charisma and his boundless kindness. The entourage who formed before the medium appeared, respected him when a god spoke through him, however, between sessions, they treated him rather roughly. Once a "deity" predicted a lottery number. The winner shared his fortune with the medium who used the money to visit India. On his return he was physically tied up by his entourage, because they found he was enjoying himself too much.

Approximately thirty devotees came regularly twice a week to witness the manifestations of gods. They washed their feet at a well downstairs before they climbed the ladder to the platform. Together with members of the entourage, they chanted devotional songs (*bhajans*) to "invite the Gods" and to stimulate the medium's transformation. When a god manifested, devotees were called forward to be blessed with *vibhuti*. *Vibhuti* is used to mark their forehead and to cure external or internal illnesses. I myself put once some *vibhuti* on my tongue, knowing it was cow dung ash. It was silky smooth and tasted quite well, like powdered sugar. It settled, indeed, my upset stomach.

Limes were used during exorcism and were also given to devotees for protection. Weeks or months later the medium would diagnoses the fate of a devotee by checking the process of discoloration on the lime. Black spots indicated danger. White or pink colorations indicated success, prosperity, and a better future.

The clients belonged predominantly to the lower-middle and working classes. They were concerned about their health, business, job, or they had problems with their family. Women asked what to do with an unfaithful husband. Mothers wanted to know how to treat a vagrant son. Some devotees brought their business accounts to be blessed, especially when they were embarking on a new enterprise. Those whose wishes had been fulfilled, entered their names into the book for donors, i.e., they committed themselves to bring, on a certain day, *prasad* (rice cooked with milk, honey, raisins and nuts) which will be distributed after the blessings. Offered fruit were also shared by all. Although Indians do not eat left-overs, it is considered to be a sign of humility to partake of the left-overs of a deity. Like in Cases 1 and 3, the idea of a communal meal was maintained and it was said, "You bring something and you take something home."

The social system around this and most other mediums fits Turner's *communitas* (1966). Arriving at a temple, all entered the *liminal* state and their relationships to other social systems were suspended. The manifestation of deities was celebrated, the offerings distributed and, after the meal and after the deities had left, all emerged refreshed to face their daily tasks.

[Ten years later, in 1989, I tried to find the temple but the whole area near Sembawang Shipyard had been leveled. On further inquiry, I learned that the temple had been torn down by city planners and the medium had died. It was not possible to get more information about what actually transpired]

Case 3 - How Contacts to Mediums Develop (Singapore Chinese)

On October 16, 1978, I was invited to participate in the celebration of the third birthday of a shrine which had been built inside a ball-bearing factory in Jurong. This rapidly developing suburb of Singapore was home to shipyards and large factories. Because it was also the 1105th birthday of the shrine spirit, two mediums had been invited. One after the other fell into trance and offered joss sticks and fruit to the spirit in the presence of the factory workers.

Three years ago, when the factory was under construction, neighbors had warned the management not to touch a tree. At its roots, a spirit was believed to reside in an old shrine. Excavations progressed. While the area around the tree had already been leveled, the tree on the earth mound was not touched.

To solve the dilemma, the sales manager introduced the designing engineer to a group of mediums. So, for three days, mediums talked with the spirit and, with the help of the monkey god, an answer was obtained. The spirit accepted the invitation to move into better quarters, e.g., a new shrine to be built near the gate of the factory.

The construction plans were discussed with the spirit and the supervising engineer was advised to talk to the spirit, too. He did not object to spend some minutes each on three consecutive days on the hill. He told me afterwards that, when he once stood quietly on the hill, something moved in the bushes. The moving object, however, turned out to be a dog.

While the shrine was still in the planning stage, a story inside this story developed. The engineer wanted to buy a motorboat and had taken the boat out for a trial run. Unexpectedly, the engine of the boat exploded and the engineer was severely burned to a degree where he required skin transplants.

Unable to walk, he directed the construction of the factory and the shrine from his hospital bed. When the main medium came to discuss the plans for the shrine, he touched in passing the engineer's feet. The next morning, the engineer found, to his own and the hospital staff's surprise, that he was able to use his feet again. The physical effects of a traumatic experience had been removed through the soothing influence of a medium.

At the factory, construction workers, bricklayers, metalworkers, and painters contributed to the building of the shrine (*The Straits Time*, 1st of October 1975). The tree was cut down ceremoniously and some earth from its roots transferred to an urn donated by the designing engineer. The urn was then ritually placed in the new shrine.

Factory workers prayed daily at the shrine. This attracted the attention of people living and working nearby. One night the urn, allegedly containing the spirit, disappeared. The mediums were called again and they found out that another shrine had been built behind a wall just across the street. One night, a charwoman, working for the other factory, had stolen the urn. The main medium talked with the woman who had fallen ill and had already second thoughts about the kidnapping of a spirit. She was easily persuaded to return the urn and to restore the spirit to his rightful shrine. She agreed to ask the spirit for forgiveness and her immediate recuperation was no surprise. The story does not require further comment, because the woman who stole the urn was aware of her wrongdoings. She knew she would get well after righting the wrong. This leaves us with the mediums who provided the information for solving the theft and who acted as mediators for restoring the peace of mind of all involved..

The factory workers were entourage and clients of the shrine. They had taken it on themselves to care for it, by praying daily and offering flowers and fruit. Only once a year, on the shrine's and the spirit's birthday, they would again invite the mediums.

I told the story in the sequence I learned about the events to demonstrate how contacts to mediums develop.

The main medium is a Straits Chinese who, in 1978, was in his early forties. His grandparents came from Canton. Twenty years ago he converted to Catholicism. In 1978/79 he was working during the day in a clerical position. He separated from his wife, because, he told me, his mother-in-law had charmed him into this marriage. His 6-year-old son spent Sundays with his father who, although ethnic Chinese, spoke only Malay or English with his child.

Already early in life this medium recognized his gift for helping others. After he had discovered he had "good hands," he began to massage and to experiment with herbal lotions. In his search for knowledge, he apprenticed himself to a Taoist priest, but when the priest asked him to commercialize, he refused and left. He then studied with Buddhist monks at Sion Lim Temple[2] where he found spiritual guidance through meditation. In 1971, he began to practice regularly every week night and on Sundays.

On Saturdays, he went to a mental hospital where patients came to him on a voluntary basis. He brought them fruit, cookies, and cigarettes and blessed them afterwards by chanting mantras while he was putting his hand on their head. At the end, he gave them a cup of blessed water to drink.

I went twice with him to the mental hospital and observed how faces lit up when he came. Some patients prayed while they were blessed and hope showed up on their faces. (Many of them had been abandoned by their families.) The medium took recuperating patients home, so they could adjust to the life outside a mental institution. Then he found them jobs. One of his former patients drove a truck, others worked in factories or in the harbor. He practically operated a half-way house and did what public health workers did not have the time and the money to do.

The medium was also called to assist with cases of "mass hysteria" in Singapore factories and schools (see Fig.17, Chapter 4 and Kok 1975).

The main room of his small house had been converted into a temple. Left of the main room were a tiny bedroom and a sitting room. Behind the temple was a large kitchen in which he cooked every evening and on Sundays a several course vegetarian meal for his mediums and clients.

This case, like the two previous ones, is a perfect example for Turner's *communitas* (1966).

On the altar, Buddha statues of different periods (*Mahāyāna* and *Theravāda*), Thai Buddhas (Chiang Saen and Sukkhothai), Amitābha Buddha, Kuan Yin stood next to Taoist and Hindu deities, the monkey god, and a crucifix. On the walls, there were pictures of Christ, the Last Supper, Our Lady of Lourdes, Murgam, and Krishna.

The medium was, in 1978/79, training several young men who came regularly to meditate. Some went into trance under his supervision. When in trance, some of them were permitted to chant blessings, some channelled certain spirits who advised those who expected a personal encounter with the spiritual world.

Individuals or entire families, mainly from lower-middle and working classes, but also teachers, engineers and other professionals, came to the temple. They became clients for reasons similar to those mentioned before: poor health, problems within the family or with their jobs. When necessary, they received massages and herbal treatment from the main medium. They were blessed afterwards by student mediums who had developed sufficient control of their trance. (The main medium did not go into trance anymore.)

Clients drank water over which blessings had been chanted. They took blessed flowers home to mix them with their bathing water. Eggs were rolled around the heads of clients to remove evil. It was believed that eggs would absorb evil influences. When the shell was broken afterwards, it was said that the spell had been broken, too. Statues and amulets were also brought for blessings. When the influence of an evil charm was diagnosed, a coconut was left at the entrance of the house temple. When the coconut broke open on its own, they believed, the evil charm had "gone back" to the person who "sent" it.

Shamanic Practices: A Case History Approach

The entourage of this medium differed considerably from that of other temples. Many of them could go into trance and bless clients which relieved the main medium and gave him more time to use his healing hands. The social system of this temple had a strong patriarchal character. The main medium exercised his authority and was called to assist with the trances of others. Those who could go into trance on demand were one level below him, and those who assisted mediums in trance were one further level below. All showed their gratitude for having been helped in the past. Some were still in training and hoped to achieve full trance one day themselves.

The medium's motives were strictly altruistic. Whatever small donations (*ang pows*, joss sticks, flowers, fruit) were left on the altar, the money would be used for the temple and for the work with mental patients. What remained was returned to visitors in hospitality.

The following two cases describe in more detail how two Singapore Chinese became mediums.

Case 4 - How I Became a Medium (Singapore Chinese)

The writer of this report was (in 1978) a 31-year-old Singapore Chinese. His grandparents were Teochew and had come from China. He had one brother and four sisters between the ages of 24 and 36. In daily life he was a successful businessman.

The report has not been edited. It has been kept verbatim to retain the flavor of his self-assessment:

"I was educated at St.Joseph Institution and attended Sunday School at the Presbyterian Church. My parents are ancestor worshippers, but they are understanding enough to leave it to me to make my own choice of religion. All along I was a freethinker, although my sisters and brothers are Christian."

"After completing my secondary education, I was involved in the Chinese Y.M.C.A. My association with this centre was very fruitful in my general outlook of life. As a layman I did a lot of community service work and gained many friends."

"I married in 1972 and had a son a year later. After setting up a home for my family, I realized the need for a religion. That was the time when I started visiting many temples. After some time, I realized that I was drawn toward the Buddhist way of life. I developed a liking and a deep interest in Buddhism and spent many hours talking to monks in temples. From there on I had my own circle of Buddhist friends. I also realized that in Buddhism the realization of the inner self is through meditation. Meditation came to me naturally. I meditated at home daily for a few months and through a close friend of mine I came to know the Namoputaya Temple.[3] Meditating at home alone was not enough. I had to learn more and somehow I had the feeling that this was the right place for me to go."

"I had been at the temple for less than a month when I felt my body trembling. I was able to go into trance after that. Later I learned from Maison [the master medium of Case 3] that my first master was Paso-no-kota, one of the eighteen immortals. [He was unclear himself whether he was referring to one of the eighteen Buddhist lohans or whether he meant Taoist immortals or immortals in general, and he did not know either why he used the number eighteen.] In my state of trance I was taught martial arts by my master and I did my practice when in trance at the temple."

"After one year going to the temple, one night, while meditating at home, Master Osenanto [Amitābha Buddha] communicated with me through telepathy and told me that he wanted me as one of his pupils. At first I was doubtful, thinking that it was an illusion. The only way was to confirm with Maison at the temple. Maison confirmed that . . . he had been told the same thing by Lord Amitābha. I was speechless with joy that one of the Buddhas would accept me as his pupil and I resolved to serve him as best as I can by helping people who come to the temple."

Case 5 - How I Became A Medium (Singapore Chinese)

The writer of this report was (in 1978) a 39-year-old Singapore Chinese. Both of his parents were Teochew. His father, who had come from China, was working on odd jobs (e.g., shop assistant, taxi driver). He himself had been working as male nurse at Woodbridge [Mental] Hospital in Singapore for fifteen years. He was married and had a teenage son. He also had two brothers and two sisters who were in their forties.

The report has not been edited. It has been kept verbatim to retain the flavor of his self-assessment.

"On November 1, 1977, I was admitted into Ward I, Tao Payoh Hospital for compressed vertebrae, as the X-ray showed. [He had injured himself while moving and lifting furniture in his apartment.] I was paralysed from the waist downward."

"On November 5, 1977, in the early hours of the morning, at about 5 a.m., I woke up and saw a vision in which there were two high mountain peaks looming up into the clouds. In between there appeared to be a bridge hanging across. I then saw a figure walking on the bridge from the left toward the right mountain. I could not see the face clearly at first as the figure was in a profile position. On reaching the right side of the mountain, the figure turned around and I was shocked to see the face was actually mine."

"I was skeptical and troubled to visualize this picture. I asked myself how could this be? Maybe I was dreaming or was it a form of delusion or hallucination. I rubbed my eyes again and again. I also tried to erase the vision in the air with my hands but the picture persisted there in front of me. After a few minutes it vanished as mysteriously as it had appeared. I controlled myself and told myself to keep calm, but I could not explain this phenomenon. Anyway, I believed that the vision was trying to tell me that I had crossed over a certain hurdle in my life. Well! That was it. I believed that I should get out of the hospital."

"So I tried to move my toes. It worked! I was surprised. Then I turned my feet sideways. And again I did it successfully without any pain. I began to believe more strongly in my vision. Hey! Hey! My feet could be lifted up. I could move them up and down in the air. There was no pain at my backbone. My system was coming back to normal."

"At this point, I said to myself that I must try to go to the toilet which was a short distance away. I got out of bed without much difficulty but there was some pain in my lumbar region when I stood up. I moved slowly and cautiously toward the toilet and back to bed. I was very happy and told myself that I must ask for a discharge. I rested in bed and dozed off."

"When the orthopedic surgeon came around, I was awakened. I quickly requested my discharge. The surgeon was surprised but I showed him that I was able to move my legs and could stand up and walk. He was satisfied with my progress and discharged me with a twenty-five-day medical certificate and some drugs. I left the hospital on November 5, 1977, Saturday, in a taxi cab."

"On Sunday, November 6, 1977, I attended church services at Immaculate Heart of Mary. Michael Boey, my schoolmate, saw me walking in a difficult manner and told me. 'Come, let me cure your back.' I was reluctant and hesitated to impose my problem on him. Then he added, 'If I don't ask you, you'll never will ask for my help.' I was more shocked about the last remark than the first one. I knew about Mike's massage healing for several years, but I was wondering how he knew my thoughts at that moment."

"Anyway, after church services, I tagged along to Mike's place at 41C Hillside Drive. Mike massage my back and applied some medical paste."

"Later, during the week, I attended the massage sessions for three more occasions. I felt better. I could move freely without any pain. I realized that I was cured. I continued with the massage treatment only with the aim of a permanent cure. During this stage I observed that there were people in trance states, healing patients and fellow devotees with all forms of spiritual treatment and blessings. This subject of spiritual healing and trance states was new to me. I did not really bother very much with the topic, but I did respect their religious beliefs and was quite curious about the whole matter."

"On November 25, 1977, at 10 p.m., while I was sitting, waiting my turn for massage, I saw a trance devotee taking the position of somebody crucified. Suddenly I felt like something pulling my hands and pushing my back gently to kneel down. I could feel my knees glued to the floor and my body was like a stone. Only from my neck upwards, I could move my arms and hands. I felt so funny and awkward and kept wondering. I wanted to get up but could not do so. I did not know why and how. This Part is very difficult to explain. Up to today I cannot understand how and why."

"Anyway I started work the following day, November 26, 1977 [at Woodbridge Mental Hospital]. I began to be more helpful when Mike came around to help and bless the mental patients and when he distributed oranges, cookies, and cigarettes."

"My spiritual life really started seriously with this phenomenal episode. In the middle of December 1977, I arranged that a colleague of mine, another attendant, went to see Mike for treatment. This attendant had been suffering some arthritic ailment in both of his legs for three to four years and had been taking sick leave off and on when swelling and pain erupted. We arrived at Mike's place at about 8 p.m. Then, all of a sudden, I could feel my head spinning around and my temples bursting open. I felt severe pain at my left and right temporal regions as if on each side there was a long screw, about fifteen centimeters long, being driven or screwed in at a very fast speed. There were devotees and people present and the trance healing was in progress. When the devotee in trance started to chant, I felt the screwing, agonizing pain even more. I struggled with the severe pain. I put my hands over my temporal regions to stop it but it was to no avail. At last, Mike helped me and relieved my agony by praying for me, together with the devotee in trance. During this time, I screamed, shouted and struggled again in agonizing pain. I realized something abnormal and spiritual was happening to me. I prayed and cried, saying, 'My God! My God! I am only human. I am only human. I never did anything really wrong!' After Mike's prayers and help, I became well again and was back to normal, mysteriously. Excited and fearful, I stammered for an answer for this exotic behavior and these fantastic experiences, but I could not find a reasonable explanation."

"My life became more religious with all these mysterious happenings. I began to pray and to meditate more often."

"On January 6, 1978, while praying at home in the evening at 6 p.m., I suddenly felt something coming into my body and I blurted out some foreign tongue or language. I was in a trance state, I did not know and could not explain how or why, but it was a joyful feeling. This episode was short-lived, because my wife rushed into the room and shook me. - After hearing the strange sounds coming out of me, she was in fear. I told her that I did not really know the right answer, but I assured her not to be afraid, because I was going to pray and to meditate again. I wanted to find out for myself what it was all about and whether what I had experienced was true. True enough! I went into trance again. Funny and strange words which I never had known before came out of me. I realized the sensation that I was speaking in tongues. I was fine, happy and joyful. This went on for several minutes and then the spirit suddenly shot off, I was back to normal."

"At a later stage I experienced two phenomena which were of similar nature. The dates in my diary are February 16, 1978, and March 10, 1978. Peculiarly these were days off-duty from my work. I could feel that a twirling typhoon had entered my body and spun me around and around like a spinning top. I felt nauseated, cold and clammy and had a severe headache. I was turning and could not keep my balance. I crawled to vomit and to purge. I vomited and purged about six to ten times. I was surprised where all the rubbish and dirt came from. I could feel that my whole system, my body, was made of all that dirt and rubbish."

"I was fearful, scared and I pleaded for mercy. It was a horrible and terrifying experience. I was completely exhausted and slept it off."

"These two phenomena will be remembered for the rest of my life."

In 1979, the writer of this report went to the temple every Sunday morning. During the week, whenever he could take time off from his job, he would also come in the evening and, in trance, bless, heal and answer questions of patients and fellow devotees.

He said that several Nepalese Buddhas come to his body. During the Lenten season, he frequently assumed the position of Jesus on the cross. The master medium then gave him water to drink to ease his pain.

He was an example for the "cured healer" who, after purging and restructuring his life, helps others (see, e.g., Halifax 1982).

To acquaint the reader with the rationale behind exorcism, I have included the report a Chinese father wrote for me in 1978.

Case 6- Testimony of a Father about the Possession and Exorcism of His Son (Singapore Chinese)

The following account has not been edited. It has been kept verbatim to offer the reader a first-hand view of beliefs and attitudes in multi-ethnic and multi-religious Singapore. The account was, however, abbreviated to eliminate repetitions. On the request of the father also details about some belief systems have been left out to protect the identity of all involved. The boy had no recollection of the traumatic experience.

The report offers an accurate description of a medium's exorcism. It confirms also several points made in this book, showing, for example, that the borderlines between world religions are drawn only by the codifiers but, on the ritual level where universal physiological, socio-psychological, mental, and spiritual needs have to be fulfilled, dogmatic borderlines become permeable.

"It all began one week before the Lunar New Year in 1976. A teenage boy returned from school one evening and complained of unusual tiredness. After dinner, which was about 8 p.m., he retired to bed—an unusual occurrence, because his normal routine was to either do his homework or watch TV until about 11 p.m. The next morning he did not wake up at his usual time of about 9 a.m., but his family did not see anything unusual in that. However, when he was not awake at noon, his grandmother began to worry and contacted his mother at her office. The grandmother was advised to keep him under close observation. He was forced to wake up for his dinner at 7 p.m. and, pleading tiredness, he retired to bed immediately after dinner."

"The whole next day was a repeat of the previous one. The parents were by then really worried and brought him to a doctor for examination. The doctor could not find anything physically wrong with the boy and, diagnosing the problem as one of overstrain, prescribed a tonic, assuring the parents that everything would be alright the following day. This, however, proved not to be the case and, by the third morning, the grandmother began to suspect that the affliction was not completely due to physical strain. She, however, hesitated to mention her suspicions to the boy's parents, because they were of a religion which regarded any belief in the supernatural to be a superstition."

"Towards the evening of the third day, the boy awakened, but there was a marked change in his character. He sat by himself and did not appear to be able to concentrate. When spoken to, he would look beyond the person and only after words were actually shouted at him, did they seem to be able to penetrate his consciousness and register in his mind. He would then answer in the briefest of forms and lapse again into his own private world, all the time mumbling something unintelligible to himself and smiling, completely oblivious to the fact that his parents were very close to him, attempting to make out his mumbling. Only then did the grandmother voice her suspicion that the boy was probably possessed by a discarnate entity."

"Once the parents accepted that fact, they realized that spiritual help was required. However, it was only natural that the source of spiritual help thought of was that offered by their own religion. They immediately knelt down in prayer and beseeched their deity for help. The boy was also cajoled into joining in the prayers and he appeared to show slight improvement while praying. His concentration capacities were, however, very poor and he kept dozing off while praying."

"The grandmother, who is a Taoist, in desperation, contacted her relatives by telephone, telling them of her plight and enquiring whether [they] knew of any Taoist deity who was able to render help. A ray of hope finally came in the form of her daughter-in-law who informed her that there possibly was a very high-ranking Taoist deity who very probably could be of help, but, that day being the 29th day of the 12th lunar moon, the deities had all left the earth plane for Heaven and would be returning to do salvation work through mediums only on the 4th day of the Lunar New Year. Due to the urgency of the situation, however, the daughter-in-law stated that they should try to appeal to the medium for assistance on the second day of the Lunar New Year. (They did not wish to offend the medium by bringing such a case to her on the unpropitious days of New Year's Eve and New Year's Day.)"

"The next two days were truly traumatic ones for all members of the household. Doctors pronounced the child fit, but it was so clearly visible that he was not! He slept most of the time, woke up at unusual times, refused to talk to anybody, and spent his waking hours mumbling and smiling to himself. He bathed only when forced to do so and began to show disrespect to his mother and grandmother. He appeared to be fearful only of his father. The parents spent New Year's Eve and New Year's Day in prayers, forcing the child to join in the prayers, but no improvement was noticed. The mother then suddenly remembered that she had a bottle of holy water and poured out some for the child to drink, after praying over it. She was truly shocked, when the child who belonged to another dialect group and spoke only English as his mother tongue, suddenly told her in fluent Cantonese (a tongue of which he did not have a spattering knowledge of) that he knew she was giving him holy water to drink and that he was not at all fearful of it. He then took the cup from her and defiantly drank the water. Again, no positive results! By this time, the adult members of the family felt a very strong need for the companionship and consolation of close relatives and decided to stay the night with the grandmother's daughter-in-law. When they arrived at the house, the child showed no sign of recognition of his relatives and their children, the latter had been his playmates ever since they were toddlers."

"The next morning, the parents brought him to a psychiatrist of a private nursing home. The psychiatrist gave the boy a thorough examination, talked first with him and then, individually, with the parents, asking them . . . whether there was any history of madness in their ancestral lineage. (All the while, the child was told to wait in an adjacent room and he insisted on being accompanied. He said that he was afraid of 'him' who was following him around. 'He' was, of course, not visible to anybody else other than the child.) The psychiatrist finally, in a respectful tone, informed the parents that although both parents did not have any history of mental illness in their respective ancestral lines, it was his unhappy duty to tell them, he had come to the professional conclusion that the child was mentally deranged. His recommendation was that the child should be warded immediately. Though the parents had expected such a verdict, it nevertheless came as a rude shock . . . . After a quick discussion with his spouse, the father requested that the child be warded only on the following day."

"After the visit to the psychiatrist, the child became even more uncontrollable. He walked around the home without his pants, completely uncaring of the presence of ladies. His eating habits were absolutely atrocious and disgusting! At 7 p.m., when it was time to visit the temple, the child resisted and had to be forced into the car. Upon arrival, the boy refused to leave the vehicle, and finally did so only after the father threatened assault. The medium took one look at the child and, when asked to confirm whether the child was possessed, merely remarked that he looked unusual. She (the medium) then informed the parents that it was not possible to summon the deity on that day, because it was only the second day of the

Chinese New Year and that they would have to visit the temple again on the fourth day when the deity would again descend to the earth plane to do salvation work. However, in her human capacity, she would, with telepathic guidance from the deity, take stop-gap measures to arrest the condition, but she cautioned the parents not to expect too much. She then lit three joss sticks, stood in front of the altar, looked straight into the eyes of the deity's statue and, after a short while, went into meditation . . . . Shortly after, she asked for a golden needle from one of her assistants, pricked one of her fingers and drew blood with which she marked three pieces of gold-printed joss paper. She then went into further meditation, after which she dipped three fingers into a small brass urn with burning incense and made signs on the joss papers . . . . She then called for another sheaf of prayer paper on which were printed Chinese characters and a drawing of Kuanin. After marking the papers with ash from the burning incense, she asked for a sprig of pomegranate and instructed the child to stand in front of the altar with three joss sticks held in prayer. She proceeded to pass her own joss sticks, the sheaf of blessed paper and a sprig of pomegranate leaves, all held in one hand, over the child, starting from floor level behind the child, going over his head and down again to floor level in front. This process was repeated on each side of the boy, the movements being broken time and again by the medium bowing first toward the altar and then facing the open door. Finally, she instructed the child to walk across the sheaf of papers, laid on the floor in front of him. She then called for her dragon whip and lashed the air around the boy with the whip. She informed the parents that this was the best she could do for the night. She told the parents to burn one piece of blessed joss paper in a glass each day (there were three pieces in all) to add water to the ashes and to get the child to drink the water. One important aspect of the instructions was that before burning the joss paper, the deity's name had to be called (mentally) three times."

"In all candor, it must be stated that, at this point, the father was skeptical of the whole affair. Being 'educated,' he could not see how 'ash water" could accomplish what a psychiatrist could not. At the back of his mind, the word 'superstition' kept on repeating itself, but it was fortunate for everyone concerned that good sense finally prevailed and he ultimately decided that he had everything to gain and nothing to lose by agreeing to follow the medium's instruction."

"On reaching the relative's house (i.e., the house the family was 'camping' in during this period of stress), the joss paper was burnt, as instructed, and after straining the ashes, the water was offered to the child. To the surprise of everyone, unlike his defiant reaction to drinking the holy water of his own religion at his own home, fear was displayed on his face and he cowered away from the cup. He was ultimately forced to drink the water and, for the first time in six days, he slept peacefully."

"The following day, he was more subdued, though his eating habits were still disgusting. There was not much the next day (fourth day of the Chinese New Year), but when the time came to visit the temple again, he again resisted. Again, the father had to resort to a threat of force. It was the same upon arrival at the temple. When the deity came through his medium, he told the child to stand behind his chair and asked for his sword. He then brandished the sword in front of the child and demanded to know his name. The discarnate entity possessing the child was initially rebellious and, instead of replying, uttered nonsense, sang and whistled. The deity then threatened to chop of his head if he failed to respond and it was then only that the deity's threat seemed to penetrate the child's subconscious mind and, in a weak voice, he uttered his own name. The deity then returned to his chair and demanded that the child kneel before him . . . . He placed one foot on the child's shoulder and, with a flourish, he passed one hand over the child and touched his own left foot. (The parents were later told that, by this action, the deity had withdrawn the intruding entity from the child and had imprisoned it. All this sounded like a fairy tale to the father, because visually the child did not look much different after the treatment.) The deity then prepared joss paper to be burnt and mixed with seven different types of flowers plucked from the compound of worship of the child's religion. [We have to keep in mind that it was believed that the deity was acting through the medium.] He also instructed that the child should be made the godson of one of the powerful warrior deities (named by the deity) to ensure protection against future invasion by other earthbound discarnates. This was subsequently done."

"When the family returned to their temporary home, both parents were thoroughly disillusioned and disheartened. The future appeared bleak to the extreme! They resigned themselves to the fate of having to care for a mentally deranged child to the end of his days, but bravely resolved to meet this responsibility."

"Early next morning, at 6 a.m., the whole household was greeted by a pleasant surprise. They were awakened by the voice of the child who was speaking to his grandmother in normal tone. He asked her why they were staying at the relatives' house? How long had they been staying there? And when Chinese New Year would be arriving (it was then the fifth day after Chinese New Year), because he was looking forward to receiving his 'ang pows' (red packets containing money, given to children by adult visitors and relatives). The parents could not believe their ears. The joy they were experiencing and the gratitude they felt toward God were beyond words. What had happened could only be seen as a miracle for how else could a child, pronounced a mental case by a reputable psychiatrist, be *completely* cured overnight without medical treatment."

"The deity had instructed that the child was not to return to his own home until forty-nine days after the date of exorcism, but the restriction did not apply to the parents. Since they had not gone home for a full week, they decided to return that night. On reaching home, both were restless and disturbed, and although it was already after 11 p.m., both were unable to sleep. They tossed around in bed, walked around the house, turned on the lights and the sound system, but the uneasy feeling of an invisible and unwelcome presence persisted."

"The parents told themselves that the fear was psychological and the aftermath of the traumatic experience. To convince themselves, however, they visited the temple the following night . . . . the medium's assistant brushed aside the parents' suspicion of the presence of a discarnate entity in their house and attributed it to imagination. The parents, however, insisted on consulting the deity . . . . When the deity arrived, the facts were laid before him. He requested the address and held three large joss sticks away from him. After a short while, he told the parents that they had moved into their home in the seventh lunar moon (i.e., the month of the hungry ghosts). This was confirmed by the parents. No one, except the immediate family knew when they had moved into their new flat. The deity also informed them that their block of flats had been constructed on a former cemetery. This was again confirmed. He then told the parents that they had not been practicing their religion diligently, so that their flat had not been spiritually protected, thus permitting free entry by earthbound entities. He then prepared five pieces of gold-printed joss paper and instructed that, the same night, four pieces were to be burnt in the flat, one in each of the four points of the compass. Before the fifth was to be burnt at the threshold of the main entrance, the three joss sticks provided by him were to be lit and his name to be called three times."

"These instructions were followed. After the fourth joss paper had been burnt, the joss sticks were lit and the deity's name was called, Just as the main door was being opened, a glass table in the flat broke into smithereens. Everyone was dumfounded. No one had been near the table! Everyone left in a hurry, because the deity had not mentioned that this would happen."

"The deity was consulted the following night. But before the parents could mention the incident, the deity asked, 'Why are you still worried! The glass has already been broken!'"

"Peace and tranquility have since reigned at that household. Understandably, the people involved will be eternally grateful to the deity who had been big-hearted enough to help people who are not of his faith. He has never even asked them to abandon their faith to follow him. On the contrary, he has not only instructed them to continue following their faith, but has also advised them on the proper manner of honoring their deity, with the assurance that he would be ever willing to render them any assistance in times of need."

The "possession" occurred at the beginning of 1976. The father told me in 1978 that, before and after the psychotic episode, the boy did not show any sign of mental disturbance or maladjustment. I could not arrange to get a professional opinion, because the father did not want to alarm the child unnecessarily.[4] However, I observed the boy and his younger sister for ten months on numerous occasions. Both appeared to me to be as friendly and affectionate as any other well-educated Chinese children.

The following case demonstrates how religious practices relate to codified religions. The reader will be able to observe the metamorphoses of gods in Chinese popular religion. The ever growing legends were influenced also by Hindu, Mahāyāna Buddhist, and philosophical/esoteric Taoist features. During the Festival of the Nine Imperial Gods, the medium, for example, assumes the role of a water spirit, a mother goddess, a Taoist stellar deity, and a Buddhist *bodhisattva*.

Case 7 - The Nine Imperial Gods in Singapore (Singapore Chinese)

In the China of the past, on the ninth day of the ninth month[5], people would fast and climb mountains to cleanse themselves from whatever evil had gotten attached to them during the preceding year. In the Singapore of today, people of Chinese descent celebrate the Festival of the Nine Imperial Gods during the first nine days of the ninth month.

For centuries, Chinese have upheld the belief that the Nine Imperial Gods— T'ien Ying, T'ien Jen, T'ien Chu, T'ien Hsin, T'ien Ch'in, T'ien Fu, T'ien Ch'ung, T'ien Jui, and T'ien P'ong—reside in the northern heavens, each on one of the seven stars of the Big Dipper (*ursa major*) and the remaining two gods on two invisible stars nearby. Being stars of transformation, these two stars are visible only to the eyes of immortals. Four stars form the bowl (*k'uei*) of the Dipper[6] and three stars form its handle (*shuo*). When we add the two invisible stars, we reach the figure nine (Comber 1958:20).

The location of these two invisible stars has remained ambiguous. One Sung Dynasty commentator of the "Nine Songs" said that they were "Sustainer" (*Fu* or *Alcor* attached to *Mizar*) and "Far Flight" (*Chao-yao* or Boots, the tip of an extended dipper handle). The opinion of medieval Taoists, however, differ. A map

Shamanic Practices: A Case History Approach

in a canonical version shows two ancillary stars as dipper treaders, one being "Sustainer" and the other "Straightener." The former is *Alcor* and the latter is said to be attached to *Phecda*. "Straightener," though, is an invisible star and one of its names is "Void" (Schafer 1977:239). Furthermore,

> ... this arrangement of stars is surrounded by another group of nine which cast a "light that does not shine." They are inhabited by feminine divinities, consorts of the gods who reside in the first group of visible stars. The invisible divinities from the "black stars" are invoked in many of the exercises designed to confer the power of invisibility (Robinet 1979b:56, also 1979a:250–251).

Wherever patterns of seven spots in the shape of the Dipper appear, Chinese consider them to be omens. The eyebrows of Lao-tzu, for example, have been described as being shaped like the "Northern Dipper" (Schafer 1977:277).

In the past, the Northern Dipper has also been related to the Imperial Metropolis (Schafer 1977:271) and was supposed to decide the welfare of the state as well as the fate of individuals. It was believed that cosmic harmony had been restored when a ruler was in consonance with the stars of the Dipper.

The divinities who might dwell in a Taoist saint, preside over his formation and animate his subtle body, were also believed to be

> only a transformation of the nine souls of the Lord, which in the beginning, were the Nine Celestial breaths or the Nine Original Heavens. Through a series of transformations ... they became the nine divinities of the Palace of the Brain (Robinet 1979b:43).

Over time, these nine stars became part of the Taoist cabala. "Grand Supreme Perfected Men (*t'ai shang chen jen*), belonging to the most exalted class of Taoist superbeings, could summon the Polar Deity (*T'ai i*), by pacing the road of the Nine Stars" (Schafer 1977:239). The following magic square shows the positions of the Dipper stars indicating the direction of steps a practitioner should take during a ritual (Saso 1978:139–140).

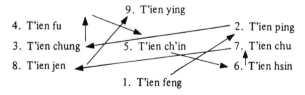

147

It is not surprising that the names of the Nine Imperial Gods correspond with the names of the stars forming the Big Dipper (the names for star 1 to 3, however, are sometimes differently transcribed).

According to legend, the ancient ruler Yu the Great used these steps to stop the floods (see Fig.26; Saso 1978:265). Dore (First Part, V, 1918:669) said that the Great Yu (2205–2197 B.C.) saw a tortoise coming from the Loh River and the animal bestowed on him a chart which showed him how to regulate the water. Schafer (1977:396), though, maintained that Yu of the Chia Dynasty (1994–1523 B.C.) was taught these steps by the "Realized Person" of Mount Chung. Yu later divided China into nine provinces and had nine *ding* ("cauldrons") cast to represent each of them. The nine *ding* then became symbols of power and prestige.

Pang (1977:113) talked about the *p'u-tu* ritual during which the souls progress through the nine courts of hell in a dance using the steps of Yu. Pang reported that Taoists used a "secret left-handed mudrā, tracing the nine steps on the palm of the left hand with the thumb."

Schafer also spoke of the

> study of methods of comprehending the esoteric meaning of the Dipper and its components, of learning to project one's secret self into it, of realizing it within one's innermost anatomical chambers, of conjuring it to inspire, to protect, to outlaw, to perform miracles. It is an active agent; its bowl will cover your head like an apotropaic shield, proof against the plague (1977:49).

In Mao Shan tradition, an adept was supposed to

> repose himself at night on a diagram of the dipper laid out on his bed, with its bowl like a canopy over his head and feet pointed to major stars. He is to recite the names of its stars, picture them in his imagination, recite prayers, and in the end bring their sublime embryonic essences into his body where they build up, in the course of time, an immortal body which will ascend to heaven in broad daylight (Schafer 1977:241).

Each of the nine stars has a secret name, each corresponds to a trigram of the *I-Ching*. A Taoist ritualist must learn which of the five cosmic elements—wood, fire, metal, water or earth—corresponds to each of the nine stars of the Big Dipper so that all their spiritual forces can be tapped.

Star	Secret Name	Trigram	Position	Element
T'ien feng	Tzu ch'in	k'an	1	water
T'ien jen	Tzu ch'ang	ken	8	earth
T'ien chung	Tzu ch'iao	chen	3	wood
T'ien fu	Tzu hsiang	hsun	4	wood
T'ien ying	Tzu ch'eng	li	9	fire
T'ien ping	Tzu hsu	k'un	2	earth
T'ien chu	Tzu chung	tui	7	metal
T'ien hsin	Tzu hsiang	ch'ien	6	metal
T'ien ch'in	Tzu chin	k'un	5	earth

Discovering further associations, Schafer (1977:50) found that stars 1, 2, and 7 are associated with cloud-soul/actualizing spirit (*hun shen*) and stars 3, 4, 5, and 6 with white-soul/embryonic essence (*p'o ching*).

In China's earliest recorded myths, the Nine Imperial Gods are the Nine Human Sovereigns who reigned a total of 45,6000 years (Comber 1958:20). There are, however, many versions which report about later events. Harada (1979), for example, spoke of nine heroes who helped the people at the end of the Ch'ing Dynasty (1644–1912).

The mother of the Nine Imperial Gods is *Tou Mu*. She was born as *Mo-li-che* in the Western Realm, *T'ien-chuh-kwoh* (i.e., in India). Having attained deep insights into heavenly mysteries, she began to radiate light. She roamed over the seas and travelled to the sun and the moon. Showing great compassion for human beings, she finally married *Ch'en-tsu-ts'ung*, King of Cheu-yu, in the northern regions of the universe and instructed her nine sons in transcendental knowledge. Because there were not many people in the north, she went with her family to an area south of Mt. Che Siu where the population believed they were genie and proclaimed the eldest son king. Later the Jade Emperor came down and took the family up to heaven where Tou Mu lives in the palace of the Polar Star near the heavenly palaces of her sons (Dore, Second Part, IX:107–108).

Schafer (1977:50) mentioned a divine mother, "Female Pivot" (*Nu Shu*) who seems to be a female version of the Polar Star. *Nu Shu* conceived the prehistorical king or demigod *Chuan-hsu* when she saw the seventh star of the Dipper, "Gemmy Light," piercing the moon like a rainbow. Similarly, Dore (Second Part, IX:20) mentioned that the Jade Emperor was considered to be a reincarnation of Yuah-shi t'ien-tsun who entered the womb of *Shan-sheng*, Queen of the Kingdom of Tsing-loh, on a ray of light.

In Taoism, Tou Mu has also been called *T'ien Hou* (Queen of Heaven) and has been compared with Kuan Yin, the female form of Avalokitesvara, the *bodhisattva* of Amitābha Buddha. Like Kuan Yin, T'ien Hou is of Indian origin. In India, she was the Goddess of Dawn, Marīcī ("Ray of Light").[7] The Tibetans called her *Semding* and the abbesses, succeeding her, were considered to be reincarnations of Marīcī.

The Chinese knew her as the god *Chun-ti*.[8] At the end of the Shang Dynasty (12th century B.C.), Chun-ti allegedly fought many wars in which gods, immortals and all kinds of spirits were involved. When in the 7th century A.D. Buddhists were persecuted in China, the Taoists adopted Chun-ti and transformed him into a goddess, retaining, however, the warlike attributes of Chun-ti. At this time, they gave her a husband and nine children.

The Queen of Heaven is also called *Ma Chu P'oh* ("Respected Grandaunt"), *Ma Tsu Ch'iung* ("Respected Mother of Hainanese") and, among others, *Su Yu Niang Niang* ("Jade Empress Who Relieves the Suffering of the People"). One Singaporean legend says she was the daughter of a Hokkien sailor. The Chinese encyclopedia *Tzu'u Yuan* (1915:377) listed her as the sixth daughter of a Fukien sailor named Lin Yuan who, at the time of the Sung Dynasty (960–1179 A.D.), lived in P'u-t'ien. Comber said,

> One day, she had a vision in which she saw her father's junk caught in a storm and in peril of capsizing. She transformed herself into a water spirit and went to his assistance. She died at the early age of twenty, but her apparition has been seen skimming the waves many times since then by sailors, In the time of Emperor Yung Lo of the Ming Dynasty (1403–1426 A.D.), she was deified as T'ien Fei (Lady-in-Waiting-to-Heaven), and not long afterwards a temple was built in her honour in the capital. Her style was subsequently changed to T'ien Hou (Queen of Heaven; 1958:27–28).

Comber also told us why the Queen of Heaven is often confused with Kuan Yin and frequently is called the Goddess of Mercy. Both have, indeed, many attributes in common. "Both are merciful and kind and offer special protection to seafarers. But the Queen of Heaven is undoubtedly a Water Spirit and her origin differs considerably from that of the Goddess of Mercy" (1958:26–28).

Furthermore, the only feature T'ien Hou, the Queen of Heaven, has in common with Tou Mu, the mother of the Nine Imperial Gods, is the indication that both have been water spirits in the past. However, Singaporeans have come to view the water spirits who have been elevated to the Taoist pantheon and Kuan Yin who is the female form of Avalokitesvara, the *bodhisattva* of Amitābha Buddha, as aspects of one and the same deity and they will name this deity according to their individual preference, another example for the tendency of moving from polytheism to monotheism.

Keeping these points in mind, let us now move to a discussion of the ceremonies in honor of the Nine Imperial Gods as they have been practiced in Singapore during the last decades.

Ong Yew Kee, whose family owns the Tou Mu Kong Temple on Upper Serangoon Road in Singapore, was (in 1978) an accountant in his forties. He maintained that the Festival of the Nine Imperial Gods was introduced to Singapore by his grandfather Choo Kee who, in 1910, had made a vow at a temple on the Malaysian Island of Penang. After a business deal had been closed successfully, the grandfather bought the statue of one of the Nine Imperial Gods to represent all Nine Venerable Sovereigns and installed it in a small temple near his home in Singapore. However, an inscription on a tablet above the main entrance of the present, much larger, temple tells us that the first temple was dedicated to Tou Mu, the mother of the Nine Imperial Gods, and was built on this site in the eighth month of 1881, that means, twenty-nine years before Mr. Ong's grandfather brought the statue of one of the Nine Imperial Gods to Singapore.

At the beginning of the 20th century, other Kau Wong Yeh temples were built in Singapore, e.g., the Hong San Temple at Lorong Tai Seng and the (Hokkien) Leong Nan ("Dragon South") Buddhist Temple at Geylang Serai. The committees of each of these temples also claim that their sponsors introduced the Festival of the Nine Imperial Gods to Singapore. All agree, however, that the festival originated on Penang and all believe the gods bestow wealth and longevity on their devotees.

Belief in the Nine Imperial Gods continues to flourish. On the third and sixth day of each lunar month, large numbers of devotees come to worship the Nine Imperial Gods in their temples. In 1978, the crowds were largest on Sundays when devotees from all walks of life brought flowers, fruit and joss sticks.

It has been said that mainly women and older people worship deities and spirits. The presence of more younger than older people and of more men than women in the temples, both during the year and at festival times in 1979, contradicted this opinion. One reason for the large number of men—especially younger men—who came to worship may be that modern life had become more competitive. Young men, in particular, experienced difficulties in "finding their way."

Representing a wide range of different age and sex groups, the devotees also came from different socio-economic sectors of Singapore society. Mr. Ong, from the Upper Serangoon temple, stressed that his "regulars" include physicians and a prominent lawyer who was imprisoned during the Japanese occupation.

Listening to the languages used in the temples of the Nine Imperial Gods, I found that most of the mediums spoke the "language of the gods" (in Singapore usually an old form of Hokkien). Some of the devotees maintained they were Cantonese, but English was used more commonly than any Chinese dialect, English is, indeed, the first language in multi-ethnic Singapore (see Chapter 2.3.). English supports the vitality of the five religions—Folk Taoism, Buddhism, Hinduism, Islam, Christianity—not to count the philosophy of Confucius, practiced in Singapore. The multi-ethnic and multi-religious environment fosters the syncretism of customs and beliefs and leads to more additions, as we will see below.

The main focus of activities around the Nine Imperial Gods is the festival during the first nine days of the ninth lunar month. As sign of their devotion, followers keep a vegetarian diet for one up to twelve days, depending on the depth of their involvement and the degree of their piety

The first day of the festival is marked by a procession to a river or the sea, whatever is closest to the temple. The Nine Imperial Gods have to be fetched from the water (we remember that their mother originally was a water spirit.) When asked why the gods have to be fetched from a river, devotees may tell the following story:

> During the Ch'ing Dynasty (1644–1912 A.D.), a rich man, head of a gentry family, invited many noblemen and wealthy people for dinner to celebrate his birthday. When a leprous beggar appeared, the guests showed their disgust and wanted to leave. The beggar advised to let the guests go, he would stay with the host overnight. The next morning it was discovered that the dikes had burst and that all those who had left during the night, had drowned in the ensuing flood. The host, his family, and his property, however, remained untouched by the raging waters. The beggar then revealed that he was one of the Nine Imperial Gods who have power over rivers and seas and who control life and death.

Harada (1979) mentioned two sources for this tale—Liu Kou Win and Chu Chin T'ao. The authors thought the Nine Imperial Gods were either *avatāras* ("incarnations") of Tou Mu or transformations of the Northern and the Southern Dipper, one representing life, one representing death, both determining the fate of people.

When the procession has reached the sea or the river, a Taoist priest invokes the spirits of the Nine Imperial Gods and invites them to descend into an urn with burning benzoin. When the sacred ashes start to burn vigorously, it is believed the spirits have entered the flames. The urn is then put on a sedan chair and ceremoniously carried to the temple where it is kept at a secret place, away from public view. The temple committee of the Tou Mu Kong Temple, Upper Serangoon Road, though, place the urn at the entrance of the central hall, so that all worshippers can pay homage to the deities when they enter the enclosure. Secrecy is retained by keeping another urn with the real ashes in a small pagoda behind the temple which can only be entered by Taoist priests and Buddhist monks.

Mr. Ong recalled that, in the past, devotees, making the pilgrimage on foot, walked for miles. The procession would wind its way in and out of traffic from the temple to the Wampon River and back. Since 1974, processions are no longer permitted to use main roads. Devotees, therefore, either board buses or drive cars or travel on foot in small groups with large distances between groups.

The number of sedan chairs used in the procession differ. Depending on the decision of the temple committee organizing the procession, two, four or nine sedan chairs seem to be in order. One of these chairs usually carries the sacred urn. One or more statues of the Nine Imperial Gods and one or two of accompanying gods may be placed on other chairs and it happens that bearers of sedan chairs may become possessed by the invisible deity they carry.

A professional medium will also accompany the procession so that messages of the gods can be related. During a procession, it is improper to ask the deity (through the medium) any question.

When the deity points to spots where fatal accidents or killings occurred, the procession comes to a halt and a Taoist priest will purify the "unclean" site with blessed water and prayers to prevent mischievous spirits from interfering with the festival and attaching themselves to participants who walk too close to the scene of the accident.

After the ritual fetching of the gods from the river, devotees start to crowd through the temple gates which have been opened already at dawn. A bamboo pole with a yellow flag on top has been erected in front of the temple. Nine oil lamps,[9] each representing one of the Nine Imperial Gods, are hung from another bamboo pole, tied crosswise to the first pole, just below the yellow flag. Every morning and every afternoon at 5 o'clock, blessed water is sprinkled on the ground directly below these lamps to purify the site. Gongs are sounded to summon the gods and a temple committee member lowers the lamps to hoist them again when the gods are supposed to have arrived. Mr. Sou Huat San (in his end twenties in 1978), serving the Hong San Temple, told me that, if one of the lights should suddenly flare up or explode, this would indicate impending disaster. He was quickly interrupted by other temple committee members who told him, in Hokkien and in Teochew, to keep quiet and hastened to explain that such things rarely happen.

A bridge is put up on the grounds for the festival. Devotees cross this bridge (see Blacker 1975) before they enter the temple. This "rite of passage" (Van Gennep 1960) symbolizes the belief that the evils of the past are left behind and that worshippers enter a better future. Midway, on the bridge, a temple committee member stamps the devotees' blouses or shirts just below the neck with a crimson stamp, bearing the insignia of the deities. The red stamp seals the promise of the deities to protect their devotees and is thought to ward off evil. At the end of the bridge, the devotees receive yellow charm papers for more protection.

The medium of the temple draws divinely inspired characters on the papers which then are burned and the ashes are mixed with water and drunk to internalize the blessings. The charm papers may also be folded and worn as amulets or they may be fixed to the outside walls of the devotees' houses. In addition, yellow threads may be tied to the wrists of devotees[10] to avert evil. The threads prevent also the *ch'i* ("life force") of the devotees from escaping and, like the red stamp, confirm the blessings and promises of the deities.

In return, devotees leave donations in red envelopes (*ang pows*), wax candles (some of these candles are up to 9 feet tall), and thick incense sticks, made out of sandalwood dust. Candles and incense sticks are frequently decorated with dragons and phoenixes. The altars are filled with fruit, rice, and other food offerings which will be distributed among the devotees after the ceremonies. During the year, they will add some of the blessed rice to their daily meals.

Wayang (i.e., Chinese operas) may be performed in the temples during the nine days of the Festival of the Nine Imperial Gods. The plot of such operas unfolds for two up to nine nights. Lion dancers and athletes may also be asked to make appearances. These shows are meant to entertain the deities while they are present in the temple, worshippers come and go. They use the opportunity to chat with other devotees they have not seen for a long time. Only a few settle down to enjoy the *wayang* for any appreciable period of time.

On the sixth day, temple compounds or the space where the festival is being celebrated are once again ritually purified with blessed water. For the Tou Mu Kong Temple, this water is drawn from the Kangkat River at the end of Upper

Serangoon Road. At the Leong Nan Buddhist Temple, this ritual is omitted but the festival is still celebrated for the whole nine days.

The requirements for participants and assistants differ. The manager of the Leong Nan Temple, who, in 1978, was in his late forties, explained to me that ceremonies have to be carried out with reverence. The people taking part in them should be dressed in white as sign of their purity. Mr. Ong of the Tou Mu Kong Temple, however, found that outward display of piety is not necessary. All depends on the sincerity of the individual devotee. The celebrations at the Tou Mu Kong Temple, therefore, are kept as simple as possible. No well-known religious leaders deliver speeches. No invitations are sent out and no dinner is prepared for a large crowd. In the past, the committee of the Tou Mu Kong Temple had requested the devotees to dress in white and had asked them to neither wear silver nor gold ornaments nor to use leather belts. Display of worldly wealth in front of the Nine Imperial Gods was regarded to be improper. When asking for wealth and prosperity, any display of what they already have would, indeed, be unwise. The present temple committee is less rigid. Devotees are asked only to abstain from eating meat during festival time and are admonished to lead a "pure life," at least during these nine days. White clothes are required only for temple assistants.

Assistants at festival time do not necessarily belong to the permanent entourage of the temple. With large crowds arriving, more volunteers are needed to keep the temple compound clean and to move the crowd through the different stages of worship. There are joss sticks, joss paper, candles, and amulets to sell. The altar lamps have to be kept supplied with oil. Joss sticks have to be removed from urns to make room for the joss sticks of the incoming devotees. The stoves have to be kept under control because joss papers are continuously burned to appease the judges in hell and to furnish the soldiers of deified generals as well as the spirits of one's own ancestors with spending money. Bridges to cross have to be manned and there are other important tasks. Most of the helpers are regular worshippers but some are total strangers. Nobody asks them for their reason to volunteer, they are only requested to abstain from eating meat during festival time.

With lion dancers, stilt walkers, and musicians playing drums, cymbals, and gongs, the festival builds up to a climax on the ninth day. The committee of the Leong Nan Buddhist Temple invites at least forty monks to conduct the ceremonial chanting which does not stop. When the monks take a brief rest, tape-recorded chanting is piped through the loudspeakers.

At the Tou Mu Kong Temple, a procession starts from the Upper Serangoon-Yio Chu Kang Junction to Kangkar at night. The procession is preceded by forty

Trance and Healing in Southeast Asia Today

boys, each holding a colorful banner. The devotees, carrying joss sticks, board trucks, buses, cars, and taxis to follow the gods. The sacred urn with the burning ashes, in which the Nine Imperial Gods are supposed to reside, is brought out of the temple and put on one of the sedan chairs. Other chairs carry statues of the deities.

As soon as they leave the temple, the chairs begin to sway and to rock. Their bearers charge into the crowd, running back and forth. Devotees bathe themselves in the smoke coming from the joss sticks and women wave the smoke into their handbags. Each devotee in the crowd is carrying at least three incense sticks. Then the chairs are put on trucks and everybody moves to a vacant lot at Kangkar where an altar has been erected and a Taoist priest is waiting.

A *chai koo* (vegetarian nun) steps in front of the priest and performs a slow ritual dance, bending back and all around, rolling her hands ever so slowly one above the other. The movements remind of *Tai Chi Chuan* (a combination of martial art and meditation). The Nine Imperial Gods are sent off. The nun bids them farewell and wishes them a pleasant journey back to their stellar thrones.

The ritual lasts about one hour. During this time the assembly remains kneeling. Then the urn is carried to the Serangoon River. The Taoist priest, holding a yellow tablet, leads the way. When the procession reaches the fishing village at Kangkar, the people living there are already asleep because they have to get up at 3 p.m. to prepare the fish they caught for the daily auction. Their boats line the bank two or three deep. The jetty is decorated with burning candles down to the water. The flaming urn is put on a small boat (see Fig.22), and the Taoist priest launches the boat on which the gods will sail home. The crowd silently waits for the boat to move, indicating the gods' departure. When, after some time, the boat still has not moved and the priest as well as the boys with their banners have left, some of the fishermen may leap into their boats and turn on their engines. The water begins to churn and the gods are on their way.

I will now report on the community of Geylang Serai who sponsor the Leong Nan Temple. From the 1st to the 10th of October, 1978, they celebrated the Festival of the Nine Imperial Gods at Katong, Mountbatten Road. Permission to use this park site had been granted by the Singapore Bus Administration and the Physical Education Office.

On one side of the huge area, a temple tent had been put up. Large crowds came daily to pay respect to the statues of Amitābha Buddha, Kuan Yin, Kuan Kong, three of the Nine Imperial Gods (the second being the most important for this community), and the nine sedan chairs for the deities. Devotees entered the tents to place their joss sticks, candles, and fruit on the different altars and to consult mediums who were available for consultation.

On the eighth day, the temple committee served a ceremonial dinner for ten thousand of their community. Ten huge tents had been put up, each sheltering ten rows of ten tables, of which each was surrounded by ten chairs. While everybody was waiting for the vegetarian meal of many courses, prepared by fifteen caterers, the ceremony started with the chanted blessings of *Theravāda* monks from local Sri Lanka and Thai temples. After thirty minutes of chanted blessings from the Pāli Canon, the interest of the crowd diminished and dragons, held up by fifteen or more young men, began to dance in the aisles, breathing fire when the dragon "tamer" threw a substance on the fire ball he was carrying on a stick. The fire ball was also used to lead the way for the dragon. Athletes somersaulted and lions danced on the stage opposite the monks' platform. A Chinese opera was performed on the stage to the right, while worshippers prayed in the temple tent at the left end of the huge area.

When the main medium, an elderly, stately woman, clad as Kuan Yin (see Fig.21), appeared, the *Theravāda* monks left in a hurry. The medium, waving swords and banners, began to consecrate the site. Considering the size of the area, it was an admirable task which took almost one hour. She symbolically fought with a lion and subdued the animal, whirling a large pole with fire balls on each end.

During the dinner, representatives of the city, members of other communities, and guest of honor delivered seemingly endless speeches. Afterwards, the nine illuminated sedan chairs danced through the aisles, making the presence of the gods felt. At the end of the long program, the medium signed a paper scroll with 108 panels (one each for the 108 different forms of Avalokitesvara, the *bodhisattva* of Amitābha Buddha). While members of the community sang Buddhist chants, she painted with a brush, divinely inspired red symbols which did not necessarily resemble any known Chinese characters. The scroll with the 108 panels was then carried to the Leong Nan Temple and it was believed that it will protect the community during the coming year.

Before sending the deities off, on the last day, the medium, again clad as Kuan Yin and wielding banners and swords, led a procession of over 10,000 devotees around the festival site. Preceded by a group of banner carriers, each of the devotees behind her was holding three joss sticks and a candle. For two hours, the crowd meandered slowly, in a very orderly way, across the huge space, while four women and three men, among them a Taoist priest and a *Mahāyāna* monk, chanted the name of Amitābha Buddha. The singers took turns, the *Mahāyāna* monk being the first to wear out and the four lay women being the most enduring chanters. Singers, sedan chair carriers, and the crowd of devotees chanted themselves into different kind of trances. The modern music, played on the stage on the far right of the area, did not disturb anybody. The musicians only stopped when the main medium, leading the procession, came close to their stage. Other mediums, who took the opportunity to offer their services, also fled when the main medium came in sight.

To illustrate the rationale behind the Festival of the Nine Imperial Gods as it was celebrated in Singapore in October 1978, I will now cite excerpts from a speech delivered at the beginning of the ceremonial dinner by Mr. Cheng Mu-Jung, Chairman of the General Administration Committee of the Leong Nan Temple.[11]

> Good believers, both male and female, honored guests, with this ceremony today, the Lung Nan (Dragon South) Temple honors the birthday of the second of the Nine Imperial Gods and also pays homage to the other Eight Imperial Gods. We are favored with the participation of high government officials and honored guests from all regions. There are senior monks conducting the ceremony and male and female believers who enthusiastically came to participate. There are certainly mountains and seas of people. All have come to accumulate good karma. We all feel honored by your presence.
>
> ... We received aid from all government departments to develop this vast site. They not only loaned the equipment but also took care of traffic and transportation problems. The enlightened government of our nation has the policy of looking at all religions equally. It has carried out this policy in a praiseworthy manner.
>
> ... The worship of the Nine Imperial Gods in our community has become more and more elaborate every year and the people who express their belief in carrying out the purifying services and in keeping the precepts[12] are also greatly increasing in number. The second eldest Lord of the Nine Imperial Gods is the Star Lord of the nine luminaries.[13] He propounds propriety and filial piety. He urges mankind to give up killing and to practice goodness. This is a wonderful law to save the world. It is also directed toward the ills of the modern world and corresponds precisely to the law of the man-god vehicle."[14]

In the preceding paragraphs, the mentioning of the "Star Lord" supports Confucian, Buddhist and Taoist ideas. Before we examine which religion prevails, let us look at the further arguments of this speech.

Shamanic Practices: A Case History Approach

Many people have a wrong conception of the dharma meeting of the Nine Imperial Gods. They take it for ordinary spiritual teaching because they don't know the complexities of Buddhist teaching. In fact, the dharma of the Buddha is divided into five vehicles. The first is the man-god vehicle, the second is that of the śravakas [disciples, "those who listen," hence "monks"], the third that of the Pratyeka Buddhas [who found enlightenment on their own but cannot teach it], the fourth that of the bodhisattvas, and the fifth and highest that of the Buddhas.[15] The man-god vehicle stresses and propagates the correct ways of behavior for people living in our times. It expounds the ethics which should be followed. The śravaka vehicle, the Hīnayāna [see Glossary], is the basic law of the Buddha. It emphasizes the observance of the precepts and encourages spiritual cultivation. At the time of the Buddha, those who truly understood the twelve nidānas [causes, underlying factors] pronounced by the Buddha, became enlightened. After the nirvāṇa of the Buddha, people were left without master. They had to find the way on their own. Through intense cultivation and one-pointed meditation they achieved the Great Release. They are called the sages of solitary enlightenment or Pratyeka Buddhas. The bodhisattva vehicle goes one step further. Those who practice this vehicle have opened their hearts and practice the six degrees and the ten thousand ways. They have foregone their own enlightenment and work for the salvation of all sentient beings, like, for example, the Bodhisattva Kuan Yin who works for the salvation of all those who suffer, and the Bodhisattva Kṣitigarbha[16] who made a vow to help all sentient beings who suffer in the hells. Having given such great examples, we can truly call them bodhisattvas. The highest vehicle is that of the Buddhas. It can only be reached by those who cultivate the way of the bodhisattvas, attain the level of highest virtue and austerity and thus achieve enlightenment. Through their virtues they reap the fruits of supreme enlightenment[17] and can be called Buddhas. You can see that, in Buddhist practices, you advance step by step and cannot attain the highest, most perfect level in one stride.

The thoughts expressed in this paragraph have been assimilated from Mahāyāna Buddhism, although the Bodhisattva Kṣitigarbha may appear in Taoist hells as well. The speaker then changed his style and preached a sermon.

The world in which we now live goes through the last stages of this kalpa ["a day of Brahmā," or 4,320 million earthly years, see Basham 1959:320]. Our thinking is extremely complex and there are all sorts of diverging and confusing conflicts in this world, people fight, commit acts of hatred, and constantly go to extremes. All this has contributed to the tragedy of the current world crisis. If we look at the causes, we

> see that basic principles have been violated. Mankind pays only attention to material happiness and no attention to the spiritual enlightenment of the masses. Human society has to be held together and peace and security have to be maintained. The goal of calling a dharma meeting of the Nine Imperial Gods is to propagate the principles of the man-god vehicle of Buddhism, that means, we promote the moral concepts of our superior Eastern tradition and make it possible for all men to carry out these principles effortless and with a heart devoted to abstaining from killing and promoting vegetarianism. We can foster benevolence to suppress violent thought and action. Once our hearts are devoted to benevolence, the virtue of forgiveness will become widespread and we will be able to coexist in peace with all nations. We also wish to promote filial piety for our father and mother and foster recognition of what others have done for us in repaying them. Doing this we truly earn the place we occupy in society and will be good citizens. When we do not think of supporting our father and mother and cast off this duty, how then can we think of the welfare of our society and make true and loyal contributions to our nation? It is clear. It has been said "to climb high, you must humble yourself; in going far, you must make the first step yourself."

The speaker used again Confucian as well as Buddhist and Taoist principles. Then he turned to the main topic of his speech—the Nine Imperial Gods.

> Why do we say that the dharma meeting of the Nine Imperial Gods follows the law of the man-god vehicle? According to the Buddhist scriptures, when the Buddha, in the Heaven of Purity, taught the essentials of the dharma to the assembled lords, Indra and Brahmā,[18] gods, yakṣas [trees spirits, giants], nāgas [mythical serpents], bhikṣus [monks], bhik unỸs [nuns], upāsakas [laymen], and upāsikās [lay women], at that time, Manjusri stood up from his seat and asked the Buddha to speak to the assembled heavenly beings about the seven primal star lords of the Northern Dipper. They were all Buddhas of the past who manifested to save and be of benefit to all sentient beings. Buddha said, "the eldest and first of the Northern Dipper is grand k'uei, luminosity of yang, the veracious wolf, the great star lord. He is the harbinger of the one who comes to the eastern world and who is called jina [conqueror], peerless."

These words imply the messianic mission of the first star lord who is compared with Maitreya, the Buddha-to-come. But let us follow the train of thought of the speaker.

Shamanic Practices: A Case History Approach

And that what Buddha mentioned appeared. "The second eldest lord of the Northern Dipper, the primal star lord, grand k'uei, essence of yin, vast gate, comes from the eastern world and is called 'wondrous treasure.'" And that what Buddha said appeared.

This quotation proves that the dharma meeting of the Nine Imperial Gods was supposed to conform with the doctrines of Buddhism.

The scriptures say, the officials and the laymen of this world, monks and nuns, those within the Tao and those without, both in high and in low positions, insofar as they have an understanding and feeling, all are under the sovereignty of the Northern Dipper. When they are capable of sincerely cultivating and keeping the precepts according to the dharma, not only will their position be raised and their lives lengthened, they will also gain salvation from being reborn or being reborn in one of the heavens, they will live beyond suffering . . . . So it is my hope that all of you listening will be able to adopt the benevolent heart of the Buddha, will abstain from killing and will release life.[19] At the time of weddings or at the time of death of a loved one, it is best to accumulate blessings by releasing life and giving alms to practice benevolence . . . . On the other hand, whoever continues to kill during this time, will reap only harm and won't get any benefit. And so I humbly and respectfully urge you to spread these teachings . . . so everyone will be happy and every home will prosper."

[The speech ended with quoting a paragraph from the *Wondrous Scripture of the Northern Dipper for the Prolongation of Life*.]

In conclusion, the worship of the Nine Imperial Gods in Singapore may occur in a Buddhist context and be reenforced by the philosophies of Lao-tzu and Confucius. The rituals during the festivals have retained elements of earlier developments.

Fetching the gods from a water way reminds us of water spirits being accepted in the Taoist pantheon where they, later, were elevated to become star gods. (We note that the Nine Imperial Gods are allegedly called by Buddha to become star gods.) When the Nine Imperial Gods then are said to reside on the stars of the Northern Dipper, we realize that the North is associated with the element of water, the principle of life and death or fate. Schafer (1977:221) told us that star worship was already firmly established in Han times (202 B.C. to A.D. 221), this means, that the Nine Imperial Gods became star lords before religious Taoism developed in the second century A.D.

Religious Taoism then absorbed Buddhist elements and the dipper gods became Buddhas who would appropriately manifest in *bodhisattvas*. The medium of the Nine Imperial Gods of the Leong Nan Temple appeared, indeed, clad as Kuan Yin (see Fig.21), the *bodhisattva* of Amitābha Buddha, and the festival of this temple in Singapore culminated appropriately with the chanting of Amitābha Buddha's name. Furthermore, Buddhist precepts calling for benevolent action and abstention from killing, are close to tenets of philosophical Taoism, too. Together with the Confucian call for filial piety and loyalty to the state, concepts blend without difficulty. Thus we find three world religions applied to Chinese religious practices.

When we talk about the Festival of the Nine Imperial Gods, we are basically talking about Folk Taoism. Esoteric Taoism is upholding the view that

> the stars were not gods but the chosen tokens and guises of cosmic beings, who might assume other guises and reveal themselves in other symbols. They were deities whose location was nowhere, who existed simultaneously in the brain and in outer space, and could exhibit their numinous presence in any manner or place that seemed desirable. It would be demeaning to suggest that the adept could invoke or command their presence—rather he could, by patient study and years of discipline, create wholesome mental and physiological conditions within his person which made it possible for the gods to reach him, or, what amounted to the same thing, made it possible for him to perceive the divine presences (Schafer 1977:224).

The practitioners of Folk Taoism seek more immediate and material rewards—longevity and wealth.

Harada (1979) reviewed some of the numerous works on dipper lore.[20] According to him, Singaporeans think the Festival of the Nine Imperial Gods came from Penang. Others point to a youth named Lin Yin who brought, at the time of an epidemic, scrolls about the Nine Imperial Gods from China to Malaysia. The scrolls are shown at the temple of the Nine Imperial Gods at Ampang near Kuala Lumpur and the master of ceremonies there still claims to be related to Lin Yin. The devotees of the Ampang Temple believe that nine retainers during the Ming Dynasty (1368–1644) were beheaded. They manifested later as spirits and became the protectors of the country. Remembered for many centuries, statues of them were commissioned and these objects of worship were, finally, called the Nine Imperial Gods.

Harada also suggested that the belief in the Nine Imperial Gods may have originated in Fukien. He was not certain how many Imperial Gods were worshipped in China and whether images existed of them or not. The belief in the Nine Imperial Gods, though, seemed to have spread to Yunnan, from where it entered Thailand and then was brought to Malaysia.

Harada added that the worship of Tou Mu, the mother of the Nine Imperial Gods, was widespread in northern as well as in southern China. Temples dedicated to her were found in Peking, Soochow, and Hainan.

The stages of the festival at Ampang are similar to those in Singapore:

1. The gods have to be summoned and brought in from a waterway.
2. Lamps and banners are hoisted in the temple compound.
3. The festival site has to be purified and all participants have to vow to lead a pure life at least for the ten days of celebration. It is generally expected that they wear white clothes when participating in the ceremonies.
4. Buckets with rice and other food are placed on the altar to be blessed by the gods. After the final ceremony, devotees take the food home and, during the year, add part of the blessed rice to their daily meals.
5. Pious devotees will walk unharmed on fire as proof of their faith. This phase was dropped in Singapore in the seventies because it was too difficult to control a crowd of over ten thousand during the fire walking. Onlookers had been in danger of being pushed into the fire. (It seems that the element of fire counteracts the effect of water. So when water prevails over fire, it symbolizes the victory of life over death.)
6. The gods are ceremonially sent off on a waterway.

The ceremonies for the Nine Imperial Gods are apparently quite similar wherever they are performed in our times.

The worship of the Nine Imperial Gods and the rationale behind it are certainly syncretistic. It is this syncretism which makes the celebrations so relevant for practitioners living in multi-ethnic and multi-religious countries.

More legends about the Nine Imperial Gods will, no doubt, be discovered in the future. They will help to analyze the underlying motifs which led to the formation of such beliefs. We can also expect that new legends will be created to keep the belief in the Nine Imperial Gods and their mother alive. The study of socio-psychological dynamics of cultural beliefs and customs has just begun. In the next case, I will discuss automatic writing in Singapore. It is important to note that the "actors" are not the men who are holding the writing stick but it is believed that the stick is moved by spirits of a higher order.

Case 8 - Automatic Writing In Singapore (Singapore Chinese)

Honegger considered automatic phenomena to be

> any phenomena experienced or produced by a subject involuntarily, for which he denies actual or potential control. These include *de novo* thoughts and images which, if veridical relative to a distant space-time event about which the subject could have acquired no normal knowledge, are referred to as clairvoyant or telepathic; automatic speech, also referred to as automatic talking or mediumship; and automatic writing, also sometimes referred to as mediumship (1980).

I studied automatic writing with professors at the University of the Philippines in Quezon City and with Javanese mystics and artists in Jakarta, Indonesia. Dr. Jaime T. Licauco, president of the Inner Mind Development Institute, Manila, also gave me a film he had produced on parapsychological phenomena. In one scene, he showed a statue of a saint, placed under a glass container, answering various questions by allegedly moving on its own.

In Singapore, I was told that spiritual forces either

1. manifest themselves unexpectedly through writing because they have messages to convey or
2. are called by those
   a. who keep channels for divine inspiration open or those
   b. who have been trained to act as relay stations for spiritual energy.

Automatic writing has been documented already over two thousand years ago in ancient China. De Groot (VI, 1910:1187–1322) cited references from the Chou Dynasty (i.e., before the second century B.C.). Tracing the development of automatic writing, Overmyer found a 5th century A.D. source reporting that

> people made an image of Tzu-ku on the fifteenth of the first lunar month, the anniversary of her death as a human being. She was invited to descend into the image, which grew heavy when she arrived. The image was then asked simple questions about the future, with "yes" or "no" answers. When the answer was "yes" the image

danced; when it was "no," it lay down as if to sleep. Most of the early devotees of this cult were women and girls, who inquired among other things about the prospects for the silk-worm season.

Simple divination with a Tzu-ku image continued through the T'ang dynasty (618–907), though evidently it was still not associated with writing. However, there are T'ang references to written predictions of personal fate composed by spirit-possessed pens or chopsticks (1981:6).

Having conducted fieldwork on Taiwan, Overmyer thought the present form of automatic writing among Chinese is "a modern manifestation of a tradition of spirit-writing in China which took form during the Sung Dynasty (960–1279 A.D.)." He suggested it began "in part as a form of non-verbal divination by common folk, but by the eleventh century was centered on written messages from immortals and deified culture heroes" (1981:3).

I found another reference in the *Standard History of the House of Ming* where it is reported that Shi Tsung who reigned from 1522 to 1567

> had erected in the private Palace a terrace for the consultation of an Immortal by means of the *ki*, and regulated the punishments and rewards (of his officers) in accordance with the oracles which that spirit gave (De Groot, VI, 1910:1314).

During the 19th and early 20th centuries, a medium sitting in front of a planchette tray had become a familiar scene at gatherings, for example, of Confucian scholars. Spirits were asked to predict success or failure at examinations, advancements in officialdom, and outcome of other career-related events. Furthermore, poems were written and collected by spirit mediums on the planchette tray. The *Pei-shan Shih T'sun*, edited by the Confucian scholar Lin Kuang-yun, is one of these collections where most of the poems have been composed through automatic writing (see, among others, Yang, 1961:259–260).

Let us look at the writing utensils. The divining pencil, *ki* or *ki pit*, had to be cut at an auspicious hour from the natural fork on the southeast side of a tree, i.e., the side where it had been exposed to the rising and the midday sun. Ideally, the pencil should be from a peach tree because this tree, according to legends, bears the fruit of immortality. A Chinese medium on the Malaysian Island on Penang, with whom I discussed Chinese symbolism, confirmed this belief (see Wan Hoi Poh 1979:38). The stick should be painted red to increase its ghost (*k'uei*) repelling capacity. The general consensus was that only the guidance of a *shen* (spirit from a higher realm) was acceptable. A prong, about 18 inches long, projects at point of bifurcation at almost right angle to the arms of the holding stick (see Figs 28 and 29). The prong serves to write on some sand or incense ashes poured out on a table or wooden platter, *ki poan*. The man who is holding the right arm of the stick with his right hand is called, *kiah tsian ki e lang* or *khan tsing ki*, bearer or holder of the right. The bearer or holder of the left arm with his left hand, *khan to ki e lang* or *kian to ki e*, is called *hu ki*, secondary or auxiliary diviner. This second holder behaves passively and just supports the stick. This form of writing has been called in China *kiah ki ch'ut ji* or *khan ch'ut ji*, "to produce characters by bearing or holding the *ki*."

Through incantations, spirits are "invited to descend" into the *ki kang ki* or "go into" the *ki tsiung ki* or "adhere to it," *hu ki*, or "contact it," *koan ki*. The movements of the *ki* holder are slow and spasmodic

> as if he is wrestling the *ki* out of the assistant's hand. All this tends to prove that the *ki* has become extremely heavy in consequence of its occupancy by the god. Suddenly the tip comes down upon the writing-table; like a hammer it jumps up and down, two, three, even more times, its violence being tempered by the automatic resistance of the other holder. But almost instantly it scrawls something, and the interpreter reads . . . (De Groot, VI, 1910:1298).

In our times, automatic writing is practiced, for example, by members of the World Red Swastika Society. The caretaker of the Society's building in Singapore told me that in 1916, Colonel Liu Shao-chi, Mr. Wu Fu-sung (District Magistrate), Jung Shih-tao (Secretary to the Magistrate) and Chow Teh Hsi (Secretary to the Colonel) met in Pin Hsien, Shantung Province, because they believed that communication could be established between living and departed spirits. They decided to use a sand box and a wooden pen. Professor Wolfram Eberhard told me (on April 30, 1980) that some Chinese dictionaries maintain Chieh-k'ung and Liu Fu-lu compiled the *T'ai ai-i pei-chi chen-chiao* ("True Teachings of the T'ai-i of the North Pole") and began to conduct religious meetings in Chi-nan in 1920. The latter names show similarities to the above-mentioned ones. However, they are religious names, *Hung* meaning "one who understands emptiness" and *Liu* "one who has luck."

In 1916, the group of sandbox writers in Pin Hsien went in their free time to a temple in the magistrate and prayed for the presence of a spirit. They were most often visited by Shang Chen-jen, the spirit of a man who had lived in the 14th century A.D. or during the latter part of the Sung Dynasty (13th century A.D.). Residing in the Feng District of Shansi Province, his earthly name had been Shang Cheng-ho. On account of his refined character, he had been a man of great learning, proficient in poetry, literature, philosophy, and painting, and for his benevolent deeds, he was deified after his death and duly canonized later on.

A publication of the World Red Swastika Society reported that, in the course of time, God Himself came to reveal words of eternal truth. Other spirits delivered messages in the name or by order of God to the society's sandboxes. According to Overmyer (1976:256, footnote 108), the chief deity is Chih-sheng hsien-t'ien lao-tsu ("Most Holy Venerable Patriarch of Primordial Times"). It is the same spirit who appeared to Taoist sages in the 4th century A.D., produced the revelations at Mt.Mao Shan, and introduced the era of religious Taoism.

In 1918, the activities of the World Red Swastika Society were moved to Tsinan, the capital of Shantung Province, and thirty-six men were appointed to build a temple and form a society. Tientsin, Peking, and Tsinin were the first three cities in which the movement took a firm root and from where it began to spread rapidly.

In 1922, the World Red Swastika Society was founded officially and duly registered. The word "world" means that the goals of the society concern the whole world, without boundaries and without discrimination of any kind. The word "red" stands for purity and innocence, like the heart of a newborn baby. Red also indicates brightness in appearance and cheerfulness in manners. The word "swastika" (*wan tzu*) symbolizes universal benevolence, extending into all directions and indicating incessant activities. The publications of the society stressed over and over again that the swastika is a "token of blessing" for their work "toward universal peace." In sum, the main goals of the society were promoting world peace and providing relief in times of need.

Professional relief squads were organized during military conflicts and assistance was rendered during and after floods and droughts in various Chinese provinces. Relief to foreign countries, e.g., was sent after an earthquake in Japan in 1923 and again in 1927. In the same year, 200 British, American, French, Norwegian and Japanese residents were saved in Nanking and, in 1929, a Frontier Relief Squad was sent out during the Sino-Russian War.

By the end of 1928, over 200 branches had been founded in nineteen Chinese provinces and one branch in Kobe, Japan. Nine years later, in 1937, before the war between China and Japan, one could find over 500 branches in China and several branches in Japan and Hong Kong. There are now branches in Singapore, Bangkok

(Thailand), Malakka (Malaysia), Taiwan (Taipei), Seoul (Korea) and in the United States (New York). The first international meetings were, in fact, held in New York in 1971 and 1973. Presently, only the headquarters in Hong Kong and in Taipei are using the sandbox for automatic writing.

Overmyer observed automatic writing in the temple of the Red Swastika Society in Taipei during September 1969 (1981:1). The ritual was called *fu-chi* ("to support a winnowing basket") or *fu-luan* ("to support a phoenix"), because a winnowing basked was used for this form of divination in earlier times. The word *luan* ("phoenix") reminds of the phoenix-drawn carriage in which the gods are believed to descend (De Groot, VI, 1910:1314). In Taipei, the ritual

> began with burning incense, ceremonial bowing and offering prayers of petition .... The officiant on stage right, wearing a long scholar's robe, in an apparently relaxed state began to move the stick over the table in long, slow circles, with the other end held up by his assistant on stage left. After a few moments the stick seemed to leap of its own accord and smashed resoundingly on the table several times .... a god had taken possession of the stick. The vertical tip began to scrawl characters in the sand in a very cursive style ... First the god announced his name and title, to verify that the coming revelation was from an orthodox spirit, and not some trouble-making demon. As each character was completed, a gentlemen beside the table called it out in a loud voice. A bit behind this "chanter" was a scribe who wrote the oracle on paper with a brush pen, in neat vertical rows. Next to the chanter was another participant who occasionally corrected his readings (Overmyer 1981:1–2).

Having studied over one hundred books "received" in this way, Overmyer found that "*fu-chi* books seem to have emerged out of the coming together of the spirit technique with the sectarian tradition of religious texts produced by lay societies" (1982:40).

When I lived in Singapore 1978–1979, the local branch of the World Red Swastika Society was located at 75 Keng Lee Road, Singapore 8.

Its sandbox is a wooden tray of 26 inches square and 2-1/4 inches high (see Fig.28). When in use, a layer of sand, 2 inches deep, will be put into the box. For writing, a wooden pen, 9 inches long, straight at the top and slightly curved at the end, is attached to a pole which is 36 inches long. Two individuals, one at each end, will hold the pole over the sandbox, the one at the left holding it with his left hand and the one on the right with his right hand.

Shamanic Practices: A Case History Approach

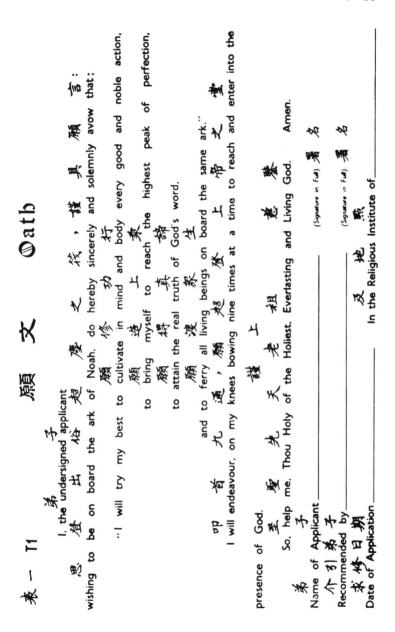

表一 T1　　　願　文　Oath

弟　　　子
I, the undersigned applicant

思　遽　出　苦　產　之　筏，　誓　具　願　言：
wishing to be on board the ark of Noah, do hereby sincerely and solemnly avow that:

願　修　功　行
"I will try my best to cultivate in mind and body every good and noble action,

願　造　上　乘
to bring myself to reach the highest peak of perfection,

願　得　真　諦
to attain the real truth of God's word,

願　渡　眾　生
and to ferry all living beings on board the same ark."

叩　首　九　通，願　起　凌　霄　上　帝　之　壇
I will endeavour, on my knees bowing nine times at a time to reach and enter into the

presence of God.

護　佑　天　老　祖
So, help me, Thou Holy of the Holiest, Everlasting and Living God. Amen.

聖　光　慈　鑒
　　　　　　　　　　　　　　　　　　　　(Signature in Full) 署　名
Name of Applicant _____

弟　　　子
介　引　弟　子
　　　　　　　　　　　　　　　　　　　　(Signature in Full) 署　名
Recommended by _____

求　修　日　期　　　　　　　　及　地　點
Date of Application _____　　In the Religious Institute of _____

I was told that when a spirit arrives, the two individuals feel pressure on the pole and will then hold the pen over the sand box so that words appear on the sand. A third person, stationed at a proper distance, calls out the words he sees written on the sand and a fourth person writes down on paper what has been called. The words are often written in rapid succession, one over the other. The third person, who is calling each word, has therefore to undergo special training to recognize a word quickly, as soon as it is completed.

When one group of sandbox writers retired in 1976, four Singaporeans began their training. In modern times, I was told by the custodian, it takes, however, longer to develop the necessary purity and sensitivity. Inquiries, from Singapore, are, therefore, sent to Hong Kong where they are answered by the sandbox writing group at their branch of the World Red Swastika Society.

What I observed in Singapore was confirmed by what Overmyer had found on Taiwan. The World Red Swastika Society is basing its activities on a collection of messages received through sandbox writing. Its "Holy Arctic Canon" (*Thai I Cheng Ching Wu*) explains in twelve chapters the universe and the meaning of life. It also contains instructions about initiating members into the subtler aspects of the infinite truth. All five religions—Christianity, Islam, Confucianism, Buddhism, and Taoism—for example, are believed to have the same origin in God. The supplementary volume (*Tao Yuan*, "moral institutions of the society") spells out the original principles for the cultivation of mind and body. It is considered to be merely the first step towards the practice of keeping a calm mind and is divided into six sections:

the *Tung Yuan*, for general purposes,
the *Tso Yuan*, for meditation,
the *T'an Yuan*, for holding seances,
the *Ching Yuan*, for keeping sūtras (scriptures, sermons),
the *Tzu Yuan*, for doing charitable work, and
the *Hsuan Yuan*, for publicity.

The first chapter, *Tung Yuan*, is supposed to exercise control over the other *Tao Yuan*. The instructions about proper behavior in the temple, and especially about spirit writing are detailed and explicit (see also Overmyer 1981:37).

Although the society fosters universal brotherhood and welcomes all people, irrespective of race, color or creed, all members in Singapore were Chinese and male. Whoever wants to be accepted into the society has to be recommended by a member. His name will then be posted at the society's bulletin board to find out whether there are any objections to his admission. Each application is also submitted to the sandbox to be answered by automatic writing, i.e., each prospective member has also to be accepted by the spirit. A brief initiation completes the process of becoming a full member. With signing the application form, each candidate already vowed to cultivate himself (see p.).

All 25 officials of the Singapore society had been appointed by the sandbox. They divided their duties into five areas: (1) headquarters and sections, (2) sandbox writing, (3) Holy Arctic Canon, (4) charity, and (5) meditation.

Free medical services were offered on weekdays. The general services, mentioned in the prospectus, were founding of hospitals and schools, conducting workshops for the poor, offering asylum for the disabled and for the elderly, collecting waste-paper, and lending money. Alms were given in form of medicine to the sick and grain, clothes, and coffins to the needy. In countries where it gets cold in winter, kitchens were opened, but this did not apply to Singapore with its tropical climate.

The downstairs hall of the three-story headquarters in Singapore was used for general meetings. Portraits of donors were displayed on the entrance wall. One donor gave 100,000 Singapore dollars, two donors gave each 50,000 Singapore dollars, and ten donors each 10,000 Singapore dollars ($50,000, 25,000, and 5,000 US dollars respectively).

The meditation hall where members meet every Sunday and where regular readings of the Canon take place, was on the second floor. Ceremonies were conducted on the third floor on the 1st and 15th day of each month. Of the five altars, the altar in the middle was devoted to the highest god, the altar to the right to the headquarters and the one to the far right to the sandbox, the altar to the left was reserved for messages and the altar to the far left was dedicated to charity. When approaching the altars, each member bows nine times to the highest god and five times to the founder of each of the five other religions.

The sandbox receiving messages from the highest god was kept in a small pavilion on the flat roof of the building (see Fig.27). The custodian remembered how, in the past, he had stood with others respectfully in front of this pavilion to wait for the descent of the highest God.

The daily practice expected from each member is called "waiting upon the Lord." Each member is supposed to sit upright on a square stool without any back rest. The stool should be 13 inches high and 14 inches square, with a soft cushion on the seat. Feet should rest squarely on the floor, with the palms of the hands touching the knees. Each sitter should abandon any thought of himself and wait in silence so that he may get into direct contact with the Lord. The room should be darkened and the sitter should not be disturbed by any noise. Aside from the joint sittings and the regular readings of the Holy Canon in the temple, members are free to attend the temples of their own religion, whether these are churches, synagogues or mosques.

The custodian mentioned especially that Singapore headquarters keeps a picture of God behind a curtain. It was said that on November 21, 1921, God permitted a photograph to be taken of Himself. Special instructions were received through the sandbox. Aimed at the clouds on top of the Mountain of a Thousand Buddhas near Tsinan and witnessed by 28 devotees, the lens was left open for a few seconds and when the film was developed, the shape of an old, dignified man appeared on it. Copies of this picture are shown in the mother temple and several other branch temples.[21]

One Singapore member told me that automatic writing is also possible with pen, ink, and paper. It still requires two writers but the presence of readers or announcers and recorders is no longer necessary. He maintained that the writing often resembles the actual handwriting of discarnate spirits when they were still in their body. Another devotee mentioned that he possesses a painting which was spiritually conceived.

Automatic writing is practiced at least at three other temples in Singapore, for example, at the Keng Yeon Taoist Association, 86-A Jurong Road. This association has been founded (in 1979) 47 years ago in Medan, Indonesia. Every 1st and 15th day of the lunar month and also every Friday the writing stick can be consulted.

The temple is perched on a hillside. The statue of a protective deity stands in a glass case on a raised platform in front of the temple. The main deity in the center hall is Lu Yen Tzu. There are smaller altars on both sides and a separate smaller hall to the right. The hall outside to the left is dedicated to Kuan Kong and his two sworn brothers.

Each ceremony starts at 8:15 p.m. with prayers. By circling the stick in front of the statues, the two holders of the writing stick pay first respect to the deities on the inside altars. Paper money is blessed by the stick and then "sent to heaven" by burning it to ashes in the oven outside the temple. Blessed rice will be thrown into the four directions. Some food is also left on the provisional outside altar.

Back in the main hall, clients approach a small wooden table with their questions. The red stick, topped by a dragon head, is held by two school teachers (see Fig.29). One of them is British educated. The temple committee has two substitutes in reserve in case one or both teachers are prevented from coming. It is said that nobody else but these four individuals can hold the writing stick with impunity. Moral qualities of the writing stick holders are of the highest importance. Overmyer said that the chief pen wielder "is supposed to be an educated and morally upright man who has purified himself before the ritual. His desires and personal opinions should be suppressed, that the spirits may better use him" (1981:3).

When I visited the Jurong temple in 1979, both pen holders appeared to be very relaxed and did not seem to go into trance at all. As soon as a question was asked, the stick kept circling over the table. Although both holders were clasping the stick firmly, it seemed to have a life of its own when it knocked the answer on the table. Sometimes, the stick drew Chinese characters on the table. They had to be read in following the movements of the stick. At other times, a brush filled with red ink was attached to the stick so that characters could be painted on joss paper. The papers were either burned and the ashes, mixed with water, internalized (drunk) or externalized (used for bathing) or they were affixed to the outside of a house for protection or folded up and worn as amulets.

As in other cases, where spirit mediumship was involved, the clients were (1) concerned about their own and their family's health or (2) had problems with members of their family or (3) needed advice in their career, job or business. Additional questions concerned (4) longevity or (5) fertility. In brief, the writing stick is considered to be as important for receiving direct answers from the world of spirits as the consultation of mediums, though the holders of the stick are not directly involved in the communication process.

When we compare Chinese records on automatic writing with the field data I collected among Singapore Chinese in 1978/79, we find the belief in spirits continues to be the basis for automatic writing.

Why automatic writing? I got the following answers:

1. Some individuals want to get in touch with the spirits of dead relatives or friends because
    a. they experienced some misfortune and want to find out how and why a spirit has been offended. Thus, on one hand, they attribute their bad luck to the dissatisfaction of a discarnate soul. On the other hand, in expecting and having faith in a moralistic answer, they allow the spirit to play the role of their own conscience, or

b. they seek the consolation and blessings of a deceased relative. Or
2. they believe that only spirits from higher realms can answer their questions. Or
3. artists, especially writers, seek divine inspiration.

The structural-symbolic dimensions have not changed, but socio-cultural circumstances are different. Modernization has changed the face of Singapore considerably. Its multi-ethnic and multi-religious society attempts to develop a Singaporean identity. However, without neglecting their loyalty to their nation-state, individuals keep channels to their own ethnic background open and continue to seek "divine guidance."

Before I comment on the psycho-dynamic dimensions of automatic writing, a comparison with occurrences in the West may be helpful.

Automatic writing has occupied the minds of eminent writers from the Swedish scientist and philosopher Emanuel Swedenborg (1688–1772) to Sir Arthur Conan Doyle (1959–1930), the author of the Sherlock Holmes novels. Automatic writing was widely practiced from the middle of the 19th century to the beginning of the 20th century. I will mention only two famous cases:

1. *Fox-Taylor*: For 23 years the Taylors were consoled by alleged messages from their dead relatives who spoke through the medium Katie Fox. From 1869 to 1873, the seances were held in a house at the corner of 6th Avenue and 38th Street and from 1873 to 1892, the year when the medium died, in the old Madison Avenue Hotel, Madison Avenue and 58th Street in New York.

2. *Patience Worth*: For 24 years, from July 8, 1913 to December 3, 1937, the spirit of a 17th century woman from Dorset, England, wrote seven full-length books, thousands of poems and carried on dialogues with the living, among them renown writers and scientists. The spirit communicated through the ouija board,[22] with the help of a St.Louis housewife.

Observers[23] agreed that

Mrs. Curran is an intelligent woman, but her mind is much inferior to that of Patience Worth. In short, here is a subconscious self far outstripping in power and range the primary consciousness (Litvag 1972:281).

Litvag suggested that

> Either our concept of what we call the subconscious must be radically altered, so as to include potencies of which we hitherto had no knowledge, or else some cause operating through but not originating in the subconscious of Mrs. Curran must be acknowledged (Litvag 1972:279).

In his essay, "The Case of Patience Worth: A Theory" in the *Journal of the American Society for Psychical Research* in 1949, Charles Waldron explained that a person's brain cells at birth

> contain a record previously made by some progenitor, and which if subsequently agitated by the functioning of the brain will cause the child or later the adult, to recall the information or knowledge acquired by its ancestor (quoted in Litvag 1972:285).

Among Western theories about automatic writing

1. the work of Myers (1897, 1903) indicated the transition between the "purely mediumistic use of automatic writing associated with spiritualism and its later more clinical and more experimental use" (Honegger 1980, Hilgard 1977:134).
2. The ideomotor theory sees automatic behavior to be "the result of involuntary motor movements resulting from thoughts of actions, thoughts of objects associated with actions, occurring in muscles which would have executed the contemplated behavior" (Honegger 1980).
3. Janet (1889) proposed the dissociation theory which maintains that automatisms are manifestations of the "personal subconscious" of an individual and Prince (1906, 1925) found a dissociated "subconscious" functionally co-conscious with the normal waking consciousness.
4. Honegger mentioned the psychoanalytic theory which

    > conceives of automated material as the "return" of actively repressed memories endogenous to the personal unconscious of the subject who produces it. Central to psychoanalytic theory is the distinction between the conscious, preconscious and unconscious mind, and the concept of repression—a much stronger concept than the amnesia of dissociation theory. In repression an active barrier is held to prevent otherwise retrievable memories from reaching awareness. Hilgard (1977)

distinguishes between repressed and dissociated information by noting that whereas dissociated memories are retrievable through non-normal means such as with the use of hypnosis, repressed memories are truly unconscious ... unavailable to the primary or any secondary awareness (1980).

5. The most extensive and comprehensive study of automatic writing has been conducted by the psychiatrist Anita Muehl (1963). Using automatic writing in her treatments, she reported that patients expressed joy and satisfaction when they realized the messages they thought coming from discarnate spirits originated in their own unconscious. Muehl made the important statement that "everything we sense (hear, see, feel, taste, touch), whether we are aware of it or not is recorded and *can be recalled* under proper conditions." Our brain processes only a very small amount of the incoming information. Though in at least two of her cases a psychoanalytic explanation for automated behavior could not be obtained, Muehl preferred not to consider supernatural explanations.

6. Hilgard (1977) was the author of the neo-dissociation theory which introduced new evidence together with the data which served as basis for Janet's original model. He mentioned, among others, Messerschmidt's study (1927–1928) where automatic writing was carried on simultaneously with a conscious task. The dissociation between the subconscious and the conscious task seemed to reduce the normal interference between them (1977:139). Hilgard maintained that amnesia is at the heart of the formation of multiple personalities. He agreed with Prince that "hidden observers" are genuinely co-conscious with primary ego observers. The best summary of the historical development of the concept of independent conscious states of non-ego consciousness, in his opinion, was Th. Wright's case history of automatic writing (1970).

7. Honegger (1980) discussed the interhemispheric communication theory where the inferior temporal lobule of the right hemisphere of the human brain in normal right-handed language users is considered to be the neurophysiological substrata of a verbal system independent of the classical left-hemisphere verbal system which is normally inhibited in its expression.

8. Obviously psycho-dynamic investigations do not attempt to account for any supernatural aspects. Krippner conducted many experiments and accumulated a wide knowledge of the field. He found that the closest he came to an answer was a medium's own description.

> When I do automatic writing, I simply relax my control over my conscious thoughts and let the thoughts from another source come into my brain and through my handwriting. It took a year before I was able to accomplish this. Other than a fraction of a second's warning, I am not aware until I am writing what I'm going to write. It is as if the conscious brain only watches while it relinquishes control of my writing mechanisms. I am able to switch back and forth to my own conscious writing during the sessions in order to write down questions for later reference. However, I am also able to ask the questions mentally and have them answered in writing (Krippner 1977:74).

9. Honegger found

   > it is also possible that psi fields associated with deceased or other living personalities may selectively trigger memory traces in the right IPL[24] of a medium around which her extra-ego consciousness may construct hybrid *persona* personalities similar to those proposed by Hart (1958).

This hypothesis was reinforced by Hilgard referring to "the automatic writing of Mrs. Verrall, reflecting communication with many departed persons" (1977:133). Detailed examinations recently suggested "that the dead person can communicate directly only for about seven years after death" (Lambert 1971).

10. Whether we consider Jung's collective unconscious" or Tyrell's suggestion that the mid-levels of human mind can make direct contact with corresponding levels of other minds, the age-old riddle remains unsolved.

In the 12th century, the Muslim mystic Averroes spoke of a "common mind around us of which we all partake." The 20th century psychologist Gardner Murphy talked of "an interpersonal mental field possessing properties which cannot be expressed in terms of any individual mind" (Litvag 1972:288).

Investigations are still in progress. On April 14, 1970, the program "60 minutes" of the television station CBS in the United States showed a London medium who composes music which, she claims, is written by the spirits of Liszt, Chopin, Brahms, Rachmaninoff and others. Though the music does not appear to be of first quality, it requires a great deal of technique to master all these different styles. The medium has been examined by psychiatrists from the University of London and was found to be neither schizophrenic nor neurotic.

I do not have an answer to the question whether automatic writing in Singapore or elsewhere is a product of the subconscious mind of a medium or the function of some spiritual entity or both, but I hope to have contributed at least some observations for consideration.

In previous cases, it was believed that deities either speak through mediums or manifest in a writing stick. Whether the phenomenon of glossolalia is another aspect of spirit mediumship will be discussed in the next case.

Case 9 - Glossolalia in Singapore (Singapore Chinese and Malay)

The term *glossolalia* is derived from the Greek words *glossa* ("tongue") and *lalein* ("to talk"). Webster called "speaking in tongues" a form of ecstatic speech that is usually unintelligible to listeners and may be accompanied by religious excitation (1990:1242) The unabridged Random House Dictionary defined glossolalia as "a prayer characterized chiefly by incomprehensible speech."

Utterance differ, indeed, from individual to individual and leave the impression that they are meaningful only to the speaker. Glossolalia has been compared with "infantile babble" similar "to the second or parataxic phase of an infant's attempt to communicate. During this period the toddler repeats sounds which are meaningless to the listener but satisfying to the child" (Kildahl 1972:31).

Those speaking in tongues usually "received the gift" during a church service. Later they speak in tongues at will. They may use this gift during meditation when they are alone. However, speaking in tongues seems to be most reassuring in a community setting where all "experience the living Christ."

Glossolalia occurrences have first been mentioned in the Bible.

> There appeared in them tongues like flames of fire, dispersed among them and resting on each one. And they are all filled with the Holy Spirit and begin to talk in other tongues as the Spirit gave them power of utterances (Acts 2:3. 4).[25]

Pentecostalism became an religious movement at the beginning of the 20th century. In the United States it was practiced in mainline Protestant churches, but also in Episcopal, Lutheran, and Presbyterian congregations. Kildahl noted that until the later 1950s in America "the practice of glossolalia . . . was confined to a few extreme theological conservative religious sects. The atmosphere in which it occurred was generally ecstatic, even hysteric" (1972:ix).

Glossolalia was supported in particular by Wesleyan Methodists who stressed "the need for a growth in sanctification beyond initial conversion" (Winthrop 1981). Sanctification was expected to manifest in outward supernatural signs.

> Such a phenomenon usually occurs at a time when prayer is more intense and seems to be poised between silence and speech. The ordinary words of shared thanksgiving—*Amen* or *Alleluja*—are no longer adequate, and one or another of those present begins to utter, half-aloud sounds that are more or less articulated and fall into a chant pattern; others gradually pick it up, always calmly and in a moderate tone. Nothing is pre-arranged, and each individual expresses himself as he wishes. You would expect cacophony, but what you hear is a soothing, attractive melody that soon stops after a short decrescendo (Laurentin 1978:73).

Catholicism adopted glossolalia in the later 1960s (Winthrop 1981:285–287). In 1972, Pope Paul VI proclaimed that the Church

> needs the Holy Spirit . . . who is the source of her charisma and her songs . . . . the Church needs to experience the praying voice of the Holy Spirit rising, like tears, out of her inmost being. For the Holy Spirit acts in our stead, praying in us and for us, "with groanings which cannot be expressed in speech," and St. Paul teaches us. The Spirit expresses what we ought to say, for, when left to ourselves, we do not know how to pray as we ought (Laurentin 1978:27

Nobody could tell me when glossolalia first occurred in Singapore. In 1978/79, one meeting place for those who spoke in tongues was the Catholic Church, Our Lady of Lourdes.

Benches were put up in front of the church for a crowd of several hundred. The priest and some members of the community sat opposite the church on a raised platform under a canvas shelter.

Every Tuesday night, people from near and far came to experience the descent of the Holy Spirit. They were predominantly converted Chinese, but there were also Singaporeans of Malay or Indian descent. They differed in socio-economic status and education, however, common to all was the search for *communitas* (Turner 1966). They were looking for a "sacred space" away from daily life, where they could unburden their minds and open their hearts.

At the beginning, the priest invited all to shake hands with the people sitting around them "to set the giving and receiving of love in motion." Then hymns were sung to invite the descent of the Holy Ghost. The singing was interrupted by testimonials. Somebody stood up and walked to the microphone to talk about his encounter with God and how he experienced the presence of God in a crisis situation.

I seldom heard a woman testifying. Neither of the three major ethnic groups represented in Singapore—Chinese, Malay and Indian—encourage women to speak up in a religious context. Women cannot be Muslim leaders, nor can they perform *brahmin* rituals or take over the duties of a Taoist priest. There are, however, female shamans, mediums, and healers, but they would not speak up in public either.

Let us go back to Our Lady of Lourdes. As the intensity of the chanting began to grow, its volume turned almost into a whisper. First one and then others of the community began to speak in tongues, very subdued, unlike the ecstatic and erratic behavior found in some Pentecostal churches in America. The community listened spellbound and experienced the presence of the Holy Spirit. After a while the phenomenon faded away and the service ended with thanksgiving hymns.

Does the glossolalia state differ considerably from alternate states of consciousness experienced by shamans and mediums? Are there similarities to the ecstasy of Indian devotees when they enter the temple? Glossolalia appears to me one step away from any professional, mediumistic "possession trance," because it does not answer any questions or needs of others, it resembles, however, the ecstasy of Indian devotees when they are in the presence of the Divine.

What have Western scholars to say about glossolalia? Is glossolalia a gift of the Holy Spirit or a trap of the devil or simply an abnormal psychological condition?

Kildahl (1972:2, 36) confirmed that practitioners do not make "a deliberate or conscious effort to control the movements" of their tongue. Thought does not seem to be involved. On the other hand, the glossolalia state is not a full trance. The senses of the practitioners continue to operate during the experience. Kildahl posed an interesting question which arose for him during his research. "How can a tongue-speaker call upon his unconscious so that he can fluently produce unintelligible speech and still maintain enough ego control to drive a truck on an interstate highway?" Maybe we should ask researchers who speak of "multiminds" (e.g., Ornstein, 1986)?

Kildahl discussed seven theories, among them the views of Laurence Christenson who did not employ psychological categories but considered glossolalia to be "a supernatural manifestation of the Holy Spirit which is clearly spoken of in the Bible."

I mentioned in Part 1 that each discipline is developing a terminology of its own. But can we apply psychological terms to theological issues? We have first to agree on universal methods and terminologies which satisfy more than one discipline. This dilemma became obvious when some psychologists considered glossolalia to be a manifestation of schizophrenia because speakers allow themselves to be possessed—or dispossessed—by the contents of their unconscious.

Cutten (in Kildahl 1972:25), offering some psychological explanations, assumed that a person speaking in tongues must be experiencing a state of personal disintegration in which the verbo-motive centers are obedient to subconscious impulses. Cutten found certain requisites for the successful inducement of the hypnotic state also being present in glossolalia, e.g., rapport between subject and leader, uniformity of perception, fixation of the subjects' attention, and suggestion.

Cutten also distinguished between various degrees of glossolalia,

1. inarticulate sounds,
2. articulate sounds which simulate words, and
3. fabricated or coined words.

Linguistic research conducted by scholars in several countries has proven that glossolalia does not seem to belong to any known language. The sounds appear to be meaningful to the speaker but not to the listener. However, most speakers don't recall what they have said during their glossolalia experience.

Kildahl (1972:27) differentiated glossolalia both in kind and quality from either hysterical or ecstatic experiences or an innocuous release of strong religious emotions. In pointing to the similarity of glossolalia to visions, he realized that in both phenomena the individual comes in contact with psychic reality (1972:29).

In the Singapore as well as the Kildahl sample, individuals seem to have a deepfelt need expressing their emotions in a safe environment. Whether they have a weak ego structure and suffer from identity problems, whether they have high anxiety levels and are somewhat unstable, more submissive, suggestible and dependent on the presence of an authority figure (Kildahl 1972:32, 50), this will differ from case to case. So called automatisms are considered to provide an escape valve for deep-seated conflicts within an individual. In glossolalia, feelings are expressed without ambivalence so that overwhelming sensations of joy and release can be felt.

Wayne E. Oats stated that "Intellectualization, institutionalization, and sophistication all result in repression of deep religious feelings" (in Kildahl 1972:31), so we may find occurrences of glosolalia in any modern country.

Can we compare glossolalia with hysteria? Hysteria is a condition in which an individual is extremely susceptible to suggestions. Any sensation s/he feels is exaggerated. Hysteria is an illness which harms the mind and sometimes the body. Glossolalia, on the other hand, increases the ability to cope with reality, both in the material and in the spiritual sense (Kildahl 1972:28).

Among psychoanalysts, Jung was willing to recognize the value of genuine religious experiences. He spoke of the numinous which seizes and controls. An individual has the impression of being acted upon rather than being the creator of the experience. Not having the scientific means to understand this phenomenon, we have to accept glossolalia as part of a belief system firmly upheld by individuals and groups wherever it occurs in the world.

From my field data, I can confirm Kildahl's findings that, after having spoken in tongues for years, individuals still experience a sense of well-being and are no more or less depressed than before. "Feeling supremely confident because of his experience of divine approval, the glossolalist is willing to risk more in life. He is bolder in his work, more active in bed" (Kildahl 1972:46).

It will require more research to understand the psychological and sociological aspects of glossolalia. Kildahl asked whether it is "harmful rather than helpful when measured by the criterion of edifying the whole group" (1972:74)? "Does it help to build up the community" (1. Corinthians 14.5)? The hypothesis, half proven already by the present research, is that glossolalia offers a safety-valve to individuals who find emotional release in a community setting. The experience gives individuals strength which has beneficial consequences for themselves as well as for the other social systems in which they operate.

Although speaking in tongues is mainly practiced in a community setting and is of benefit for other social systems, it cannot be considered to be a form of spirit mediumship. No divine messages are transmitted to others. It raises, however, the question whether the occurrences of some spirit mediums speaking an unintelligible language are not actually cases of glossolalia?

The next case illustrates an alternate state of consciousness unknown to the West. Horse possession, practiced by Malay and Indonesian Muslims, has beneficial effects for the "possessed" because it offers a culturally sanctioned safe structure for strong emotional release. It has also protective and entertaining aspects for the audience and reinforces folk beliefs.

Case 10 - *Kuda Kepang*: Horse Possession (Singapore Malay)

During the Kuda Kepang, widespread in Indonesia, dancers become possessed by horse spirits. On Bali, the dance is called *Sangkhyang Djaran* (De Zoete

1938:70–80), because "reverend divinities" (*sangkhyang*) are evoked to protect the dancers and the community from evil forces.

Performers of the Kuda Kepang in Singapore told me the following legend:

> Once a beautiful princess, Chandra Kumara, lived in the State of Kediri in South Java. Having heard about her beauty, the Raja of Gerensong sent a delegation to ask for her hand. Her father, the Sultan of Kediri, rejected the proposal because he found the Raja was too ugly for his daughter. Infuriated, the Raja of Gerensong vowed revenge and prepared to destroy Kediri and its people. When the warriors of Kediri saw themselves outnumbered by the Raja of Gerensong's army, they made the first Kuda Kepang, i.e., bamboo horses, and, after having charged these horses with spirit power, the soldiers riding on them behaved like horses themselves and defeated the Raja of Gerensong.

On May 19 and 26, 1979, I observed the Kuda Kepang performed at Rasa Singapura, the tourist center of Singapore. The 55 members of this group were mainly young men and women between the ages of 14 and 26. Nobody under 12 years of age was allowed to perform the Kuda Kepang. Furthermore, originally only young men would perform this dance, but no explanation was given why in Singapore young women are permitted to join.

The group, located in Changi at the southeast Coast of Singapore, is trained by two *pawangs* (see Fig.32). They rehearse regularly every Sunday from 2 to 5 p.m. and perform on invitation at weddings, circumcisions, and trade fairs. In 1979, they charged 200 Singapore dollars (approx. US$100) for a performance which will last from 10 a.m. to 5 p.m. When they are asked to perform until 11 p.m., there will be an extra charge. Lunch and dinner have to be provided by the patron. The income is shared by all, whether a member actually became possessed, joined the musicians or just assisted the possessed dancers.

The leader of this Kuda Kepang group is a *haji*, i.e., has made a pilgrimage to Mecca. He is married and has a son who will continue the tradition his grandfather has brought from Kendal, Central Java, to Singapore in 1948.

New members are recruited from those who approach the group after public performances. They are selected for the ease they fall into trance and for their moral conduct. All are devout Muslims who do not drink intoxicating beverages and do not eat pork. Only one member of the group is a Eurasian Christian.

Regulations differ from group to group. On Bali, for example, dancers have to remain chaste. They should not creep under beds and should not eat left-over food. They should also neither quarrel nor use bad language. On Bali, trance is still part of the culture, so dancers need not undergo any special training. Whenever needed, they fall into trance naturally (De Zoete 1938:70–80).

During the training in Singapore, while everybody is slowly moving along in a circle, the teachers shows the steps of the dance. Muslim prayers and the cyclical music of xylophones, gongs, and drums then induces the trance. Some trainees successfully fall into trance after only three rehearsals, while others need more time to build up their faculty; however, not everybody may be able to trance.

Each dancer has to be given permission by the trainer who whispers a verse from the Koran in Javanese or Arabic when he deems the dancer ready for full possession and each phase of the performance is connected with a special *mentera* (Sanskrit, *mantra*, magic formula).

The Kuda Kepang is a flat, mat-like image of a horse, made out of strips of bamboo. To charge it, it will be buried for 44 days near a cemetery. Prayers continue while it is painted and tested. Only then a rider is permitted to mount it. The Changi group bought their horses in Johore Bahru (Malaysia) for about 12 Singapore dollars (appr. US$6) each and painted the horses themselves. They are the only group in Singapore who uses bamboo poles, the other seven groups[26] use plywood. On Java, Kuda Kepang groups use either rattan or wooden horses. Sometimes, a simple rod is used to which a head and a tail is affixed.

At the beginning of each performance, the *pawang* recites appropriate *menteras* and sacrifices raw hen eggs, flowers, and grain. Then the performers start to move slowly to a monotonous tune, one standing behind the other in two rows. A main dancer leads each row. After twenty or more minutes, the orchestra of several large drums (*gedang*), gongs, and *sarons* (Javanese xylophones) starts to play more lively tunes. The dancers then move around more freely and behave like horses, prancing and rubbing their heads against their trainer's chest. They pick up a whip with their mouth and ask the trainer for a hearty whipping. They slurp water from a bucket like horses, dance with their bare feet on broken glass (see Fig.30), and eat wine glasses. The trainer told me that dancers have been X-rayed and no trace of glass could be found in their bodies. Watching closely, I did not see any performer spit out glass he or she had chewed for quite a while. The eating of glass, the licking of burning charcoal, the opening of coconuts with their head or teeth, the somersaulting over several chairs is considered to be proof of the depth of their trance. The performers have become vehicles of protective spiritual power.

Once in a while a dancer would collapse and assistants carry the individual off the floor (see Fig.31). The trainer then massages the dancer's diaphragm while

Shamanic Practices: A Case History Approach

praying appropriate *menteras*, until the dancer returns to a conscious state, somewhat exhausted but visibly elated by the experience.

The members of the Changi group have a wide range of day-time professions—from manual worker to student, from fashion model to clerk and secretary. All function well in their respective social system and claim they perform the Kuda Kepang to entertain themselves and others. None displayed any pathological symptoms.

One member, a clerk and a part-time model, was, in 1979, 21 years old. She had been recruited when she was ten years old and attended Kampong Jagoh Primary School. In Secondary Two, she fell into trance for the first time at a wedding in Sembawang. "Accidents can happen," she said. Once, at a performance in Sembawang, one of the dancers jumped into a tree and could not be persuaded to come down. The trainer added that this incident happened because the *pawang* had omitted to offer raw chicken eggs at the beginning of his prayers. The spirits could be appeased and they "released" the dancer who finally climbed down from the tree.

The alternate state of consciousness entered by Kuda Kepang dancers does not have any obvious shamanic, mediumistic or priestly functions, at least not in the form it is practiced today. The Kuda Kepang is not used to heal, to advice or to make any predictions. However, the *pawang* is a shaman instrumental in inducing the Kuda Kepang state which is beneficial to the dancers and protective and entertaining for the audience. The *pawang's* sacrifices and prayers are also important to appease and placate spirits and to drive negative influences away.

Controlling the alternate states of consciousness of his dancers, the *pawang* may use hypnosis and we can assume that the dancers are also using forms of autosuggestion. In any case, the Kuda Kepang catharsis offers the dancers relief from tension accumulated during everyday life. For them the dance is a coping mechanism while the audience feels not only entertained but protected by the present of "spiritual power."

The Javanese legend about the origin of the Kuda Kepang explains the use of bamboo horses, but we should also not forget that horses have been employed by shamans

> in various contexts, as a means of achieving ecstasy that is the "coming out of oneself" that makes the mystical journey possible. This mystical journey ... is not necessarily in the infernal direction. The "horse" enables the shaman to fly through the air, to reach the heavens. The dominant aspect of the mythology of the horse is not

infernal but funerary; the horse is a mythical image of death and hence incorporated into the ideologies and techniques of ecstasy . . . it produces the "breakthrough in plane . . . " (Eliade 1974:467).

Eliade mentioned that the horse played a role in some male initiation rites. A horse-headed stick is also used by the Buryat shamans and the horse is, for example, part of the harvest ritual of the Garo in Bangladesh.

The body of the horse is made from banana stems, its head and hoofs from bamboo. The head is mounted on a stick, held so that it reaches the height of the chest. With shuffling steps the man performs a wild dance while, facing him, the priest dances, pretending to beckon the "horse" (Eliade 1974:468).

Furthermore, in the Europe of the Middle Ages, it was believed that, at Walpurgis Night, witches ride on broomsticks to meet the Devil on the Brocken (peak in the Harz Mountains of Germany). These are examples from ethnic groups outside the Malay-Muslim world.

The Kuda Kepang, if ever, is neither a part of a male initiation ritual, nor is it connected with any harvest ritual. We may get closer to the original meaning when we consider that a new bamboo horse has to be buried near a cemetery for a certain amount of time (i.e., 44 days and nights). This proximity to the "essence of bones" activated the powers which enable the dancers to enter different states of consciousness.

With the following four cases, we will continue to explore the world of Malay-Muslim shamans, mediums, and healers.

Case 11 - A Male Muslim Bomoh in Singapore (Malay)

At several occasions, I observed a *bomoh* in Singapore who was, in 1979, in his sixties. At the age of 18 he had come from the island of Madura near Surabaya, East Java. He worked first, for 9 years, for the Sultan of Johore and then enlisted in the British Army. When the Japanese occupied Southeast Asia during World War II, he left the army and began to work as a truck driver, an occupation he was earning his living with ever since. He married and had 5 sons and 2 daughters.

He became a *bomoh* when he was in his forties, i.e., in 1979, he had already practiced for 20 years. Being the 7th son of a 7th son, he inherited the "power"

Shamanic Practices: A Case History Approach

from his grandmother. He was not certain whether his 7th child (a son) would take over after he has died. It will depend on the deity's decision.

He lived with his family in two rooms which were part of a long, one-story house in one of Singapore's back lanes. Other families lived in adjoining rooms. In the hallway from which all rooms branched off, there were a sleeping platform as well as chairs for clients who came either alone or in small groups, i.e., with their families and friends.

Every time, when I arrived, some of the other tenants sat around a table at the other end of the hallway, consuming their evening meal. Children were reciting verses from the Koran in one of the *bomoh*'s rooms. In the room in front of his bedroom, there were comfortable armchairs, a television set, a stereo as well as school trophies and presents in glass cases along the walls. The *bomoh* was relaxing in one of the armchairs, watching *Candid Camera* with the sound turned off. In front of the large bed in the back room, a mat and a pillow were lying on the floor.

At 7:40 p.m., the *bomoh* began to yawn. He went into his bedroom and lay down on the bed, meditating quietly. Then his right arm went limp and fell from his chest. He stood up and lay down on the mat spread out on the floor. After some more minutes, he turned to lie on his stomach. His eyes were closed, but his face did not show any sign of trance. He smiled mildly and began to speak in a very low voice. His older brother told us that the *bomoh* was now "possessed" by an Indonesian earth goddess. (The *bomoh* had said before that he does not remember what occurs during trance.) During the sessions, he had to be assisted either by his older brother or his youngest daughter. They translated when clients could not understand the spirit voice. They handed the *bomoh* the objects for blessing. They were also the ones who asked the questions of the clients. That means, the spirit (through the *bomoh* in trance) addressed the clients, the clients were not permitted to talk to the spirit themselves (see, Case 2, where Indian devotees had to wait until the god addressed them).

This *bomoh* was mainly consulted in health problems. He also developed the reputation of being a good diviner. He spoke *jampis* (magic words) over water brought in bottles and he cut lemons into water brought in pails, adding flower petals and stirring the water with a knife to strengthen its protective power. The water was then used for bathing. I saw a girl enter the communal bathroom to use the blessed water. She returned dripping wet (Malay girls bathe fully dressed, i.e., wearing a blouse and a *sarong*). He blessed the girl again, blowing gently on her head and she was told not to change her clothes but discard them after wearing them for one more day. Such sympathetic actions seemed to be very effective.

A mother brought an 8-month-old baby who could not sleep at night. The *bomoh* massaged the baby and blew on his head.

An old man, suffering from arthritis, brought a bottle with water to be blessed. He was also given a glass of the "magic" water to drink.

The clients come predominantly from lower socio-economic groups but there are also some middle-class women who seek reassurance and protection to handle their everyday anxieties. They come for blessings and take blessed water home.

The *bomoh* practices only on Wednesday and Thursday nights, starting at 8 p.m. and going on as long as there are clients. He told me that he feels a strong compulsion to go into trance every Wednesday and Thursday night. One Thursday night his return home was delayed, because he had to take his truck a different route. At 8 p.m., he felt onsetting trance, while he was still driving. He just managed to get home before the spirit took over.

Serving the earth goddess in helping those in need has filled his life with purpose. He is interconnected inside and outside of trance.

Case 12 - A Female Muslim *Bomoh* in Singapore (Malay)

On November 6, 1978, I went with a Chinese physician and a Malay student to a *bomoh* who lived in a modern HDB flat in Woodland New Town, near Admiralty Road, in Singapore. The woman was in her forties and claimed to be a faithful Muslim. One of her daughters was living with her and she mentioned that she had already several grandchildren.

Her living room was the receiving area. There were armchairs around a glass-top table, a color T.V., and glass cases along two walls, in which, among others, seven different headdresses she had worn at her wedding were displayed.

The *bomoh* practiced in a side room, where she was sitting crosslegged on the floor, facing the client who sat opposite her also on the floor. She preferred to see her clients alone. When requested to divine, she cut lemons into four pieces. When the majority of pieces fell cut-side up (*buka*), the answer was yes. When the majority of pieces fell cut-side down (*tutup*), the answer was no.

One client requested a lottery number but was told that it was not the right time. When the client asked why, it was explained to her that her hands were "dirty." (It turned out that the client was working in a hospital delivery room and blood shed

Shamanic Practices: A Case History Approach

during childbirth is considered to be the most impure substance. Although this blood can be used to attract lovers, it also attracts mischievous spirits.)

A student asked about her prospects for getting a job and received an encouraging answer.

When an elderly woman asked about her health, the *bomoh* used a wooden knife to diagnose the problem. She put a 4-inch-long knife between the second and third toe of the client's right foot and pressed the toes together. This test allows to find out whether a spirit caused the illness. It is assumed that the spirit, feeling the knife, will cry in pain. The obesity of the woman was diagnosed to be the result of too much "wind" (see also Case 13).

The woman went on inquiring about her job prospects. When the *bomoh* cut lemon pieces, all fell cut-side up. She was delighted and explained at length why the client would have a good future.

The maid of the Chinese physician with whom I had visited the *bomoh* told me, that she had been helped with her divorce. She had been encouraged and given a charm and the judge had, indeed, decided in favor of her and her five children.

Case 13 - Main Puteri Performed by a Muslim Shaman in Kelantan (Malay)

On September 11, 1978, I attended a *main puteri* near Kota Bahru, Kelantan, in the most northern part of the east coast of Mainland Malaysia. The ceremony was conducted by Che Abdullah bin Che Mamate, an experienced *bomoh* who, in 1979, was in his early fifties. His fee had been negotiated with the owner of the house in which he performed the ritual. (The owner himself was a famous *dalang*, i.e., shadow puppet player. This is of significance because shadow puppet players function as ritualists in Asia.) The fee of 60 Malay dollars (less than US$30) covered the *bomoh's* travel and the expenses for the seven musicians he brought with him. There were one player of the spike fiddle (*rebab*), as well as three drummers and three gong players.

A *bomoh puteri* is expected to evoke spirits for the benefit of clients (Benjamin 1979:19). The custom predates the arrival of Islam in Malaysia. The present Malaysian government does not encourage the performance of *main puteri*, however, the demand for "calling the spirits" persists. According to Gimlette (1975:77–94), *main puteris* are not only performed to cure but also to punish, to discover stolen property, to avert epidemic diseases, to establish proof for the infidelity of a wife, and to win the love of somebody.

On September 11, 1978, the *main puteri* was performed to cure the *sakit berangin* (sickness from wind) of a young man.

> The pressure of angin building up in the body destroys the balance of the four elements from which the world is made. The spirits must be sent back to their place of origin so that the universal divisions between darkness and light, the spiritual and human realms are clear once more. Excess balance must be allowed to escape from the body so that balance can be restored (Laderman 1980:39).

Malays are not supposed to express emotions. The client, having repressed his anger about an incident at his job, was now suffering from excess *angin* (wind).

The *bomoh* proceeded by hanging a canopy of yellow cloth (*langit*) over the area selected for healing. He fastened garlands of jasmine flowers at the four ends. A lighted candle on top of an egg was also hung from the ceiling. Then the first invocational song was directed to the *guru* (teacher). The *bomoh* blessed the instruments with uncooked rice and waved the smoke of burning incense toward the players. Offerings were made of five kinds of rice, areca nut, betel leaves, tobacco, and lime (see Fig.33). "To open the stage," he sang *buka panggung* which was followed by *lagu setayu*. The *bomoh* wound a red and white patterned scarf around his waist and blessed again the space and himself with sacred water and incense.

To diagnose the illness and to find out which of the four humors was in excess, the *bomoh* counted kernels of rice—two kernels each for earth, fire, water, and air. Bartlett reported in his "Directions for the Ceremonies":

> When there is sickness, there is requested medicine of the datoe. Coming, he says, the datoe, let us bestir ourselves, there is labor to be done. There are to be taken one egg, of rice one cupful, of palm-leaf stalks seven, bound up with thread of three colors, with one ring, of the things needful for sirih chewing, one leaf come. Of sirih, four mouthful are to be offered at the path. To be invited is the soul of the sick person. This having been done, there is to be taken with thumb and two fingers rice, an even number (of grains). If it is the right amount, it will be an even number. If it is uneven, not divisible by two, it is to be taken a second time, and wrapped up, the rice of even number. This accomplished, return to the house. To be boiled by him without salt . . . . That done, there is to be held between thumb and two fingers the rice at the head of the

sick person. By this time cooked, the egg is to be given to the datoe. To be examined by the datoe is this egg (1931).

After counting rice kernels, the *bomoh puteri* in Kota Bahru confirmed his findings by reading the flame of a wax candle. This checks with Eliade who said, "The arrival of the spirit is manifested by the quivering of a candle flame . . . and hence the shaman keeps his eyes fixed on the flame for a long time, hoping thus to discover the cause of the illness" (1974:345).

The *bomoh* continued to sing long evocations directed at a number of nature spirits as well as spirits of Muslim saints (see Fig.34). The chanting was interrupted by dialogues with the *rebab* (spike fiddle) player, commonly called *mindok*. The highly stylized invocations were very similar to those recorded by Cuisinier in 1936. The music attracted neighbors and the audience grew during the evening. The community obviously wanted to participate in this auspicious event which was also the only available entertainment in this distant area.

The fiddle player, sitting opposite the *bomoh*, was facing west, while the *bomoh* faced east. The *mindok* furnished cues and supported the continuity of the *main puteri* with exclamations like "ah, yeah," "tell us!," etc. When the *bomoh* signaled the musicians, they sped up their tune, so that he could work himself into trance and, with quick rotations of his head, deepen it. He grabbed the big toes of the patient and tried to pull and suck out the excess "wind." He went on calling spirits and sucking until he was satisfied with his results. (A traditional *main puteri* may go on for three days and nights.)

The *bomohs* in Malaysia all claim to be good Muslims. Though it is said that a *dalang* will loss his skill when he goes to Mecca, it is also reported that one *bomoh* received his "call" on a pilgrimage to the most venerated site of Islamic belief (personal communication, Carol Laderman, March 1980).

Asked why the belief in spirits survived in a Muslim country, I agree with Carol Laderman who said

> The shamanistic healer opens the floodgates of emotion and exorcises the demons of disease. His cures, rather than merely byproducts of a magical ceremony, are the result of conscious psychotherapy. The concept of angin, in the hands of the Malay shamans, becomes a powerful therapeutic tool, perhaps as useful in the context of Malay culture as the Freudian concepts of id, ego, and superego have proven to be in

the West. The healing role of the shaman is not likely to be filled by someone trained in another medical tradition in the foreseeable future. He remains an important resource for the people of the east coast of Malaysia (1980:39).

Though Carol Laderman and I mainly conducted research on the east coast of Mainland Malaysia, reports from other Malaysian states confirm that *bomohs* continue to be consulted throughout Malaysia.

The following cases illustrate the work of seven *bomohs* at the east coast of the Malaysian Peninsula in southern Thailand, north of the Malay state of Kelantan. The population on both sides of the border are predominantly Thai-Malay who are Muslims and speak a mutually intelligible language.

Case 14 - One Female and Six Male Muslim *Bomohs* in Pattani, Thailand (Thai-Malay)

Having prepared the ground during previous field trips in 1972 and 1975, I worked in September 1978 with seven *bomohs* in and near the city of Pattani in southern Thailand. Six of them were men and one a woman. They were between 40 and 80 years old. All of them claimed to be devout Muslims. They never saw clients on Fridays between 10 a.m. and sundown and all stressed that they perform their daily prayers.

None of them appeared to be wealthy. They owned a minimum in household equipment. In the houses, either on stilts in Thai style or simple wooden structures, there were neither tables nor chairs but a few mats on the floor to sit and some others rolled up against the wall to be used at night for sleeping. There were also charcoal braziers and a few utensils for cooking. If anything was on the walls, there would be either a metal or wooden plate or a scroll with verses from the Koran.

Two *bomohs*, though, showed some signs of prosperity in owning a refrigerator and an electric fan, and in displaying presents in glass cases. One of the two *bomohs* was a *haji* (had gone on a pilgrimage to Mecca). It was also said that he was of royal ancestry. The other was the assistant of an American anthropologist.

The *first bomoh*, a 50-year-old housewife (see Fig.35), told me that the grandfather from her father's side appeared to her in a dream when she was 20 years old and in good health. The dream was completely unexpected. She did not know why the spirit had selected her, but he taught her how to heal. She married afterwards and had children (in 1978, four boys and three girls). Her husband worked as a fisherman to support the family. She herself had no fee schedule. The voluntary donations seldom amounted to more than 20 baht (US$1).

At the beginning, she called her grandfather's spirit when she needed help for her family. Step by step, the spirit taught her how to help other people, too. Within three years, she was able to call her grandfather's spirit whenever help was needed. In 1979, more spirits came and spoke to her in Malay or in Thai. Her clients came mainly to be healed from various kinds of illnesses.

Her trances, if any, were light and controllable and, as personal and as individual, as her relationships were with her clients, were also her relationships with her helping spirits. She called the spirits directly, in her own way, that means, she did not use any incantations. The spirits never failed to come. Ritualization of her healing had not yet set in and did not seem to be expected by the people who consult her. She also did not require any entourage, in fact, nobody assisted when she was healing.

Her family life as a Muslim wife and mother did not appear to suffer serious interruptions from her healing work.

The *second bomoh* was a construction worker who, in 1978, was 50 years of age. He was married to a wife ten years younger and had with her ten children, five boys and five girls between the ages of 3 and 22. He became *bomoh* when he was 34 years old. The father of his father appeared to him in a dream and told him that he will, from now on, advise him how to help others.

Many people came to him. He also went to the houses of those who needed help. Aside from healing, he was sometimes asked to reconcile husbands and wives. He explained to me the "scientific" methods he was utilizing for diagnosis, e.g., taking a patient's pulse. He had read some medical books and had looked for other opportunities to increase his knowledge. Obviously, he was endeavored to reconcile traditional and Western medicine.

The *third bomoh* was, in 1978, in his sixties. He had forty-five children from nine wives whom he had married in succession. From his present wife he had three children, all girls. His decrepit wooden house on poles did not show any sign of his fame. Walls and poles badly needed repair. He and his family, though, looked quite content (see Fig.36). Their pride and dignity was in tact.

Like most other *bomohs*, this *bomoh* had his first dream when he was 20 years of age. The spirit of the father of his father came to him in a vision. He could not see the spirit, but a bowl with a lighted candle came flying and disappeared in his body. Then he lost consciousness.

He was mainly consulted for curing stomach ailments and headaches. A demented woman lived near the entrance of his house under a wooden roof propped up with four poles. He controlled her insanity with his presence.

He spoke at length about spirits in big trees of which some can assume human shape. When put to test, their skin will change and their claws will come out. A patient's skin also will show some reddish hue where a spirit has entered. The spirit of his grandfather can remove intruding spirits. He himself had no recall of what takes place when a spirit uses his body, mainly for curing.

The *fourth bomoh* was, in 1978, 80 years old and lived in a village outside of Pattani. He was treated with great respect because he was a *haji* and, as a client told me, of royal blood. He had been an only child and had inherited the office of a *bomoh* in direct line. Having had his initial dream at the age of 20, since then he had been practicing for sixty years.

He owned a large house in which he lived with three children and three grandchildren. Leather armchairs stood around a glass table in the living room and receiving area. There were curtains at the windows and curtains separated the large room from its back part. A rug in one corner apparently served for daily prayers. While I was there, one of his daughters changed into a simple white dress and knelt down in the corner to pray.

When a young man came to complain about the loss of his motorcycle, the *bomoh* asked him how it had happened. As it turned out, the young man had lent his motorcycle to an acquaintance who had driven off with it. The *bomoh* suggested the young man should be more careful with the people he trusts. Then he took a glass of water and silently recited some *jampis* over it. He told the young man to find out whether he could spot the thief in the water. The wife of the *bomoh* encouraged the young man and suggested how he should slowly turn the glass. Though the young man tried hard, he could not see anything.

The *bomoh* then tapped his own arms from the elbows to the wrists, the left arm with the second and third fingers of his right hand and his right arm with the first and third fingers of his left hand. He read the vibrations and finally announced the thief was dead and the motorcycle was used by insurgents outside of Golok near the Thai border to Malaysia. "They are taking good care of it," he added. All these statements could have been made without the consultation of spirits. The closeness of the border and the insurgents' need for motorcycles were well-known facts. To pronounce the thief dead, however, seemed to deflect the young man's anger. One cannot take revenge on the dead.

Although the results of the consultation were inconclusive and the *bomoh* had not made any suggestions how to get the motorcycle back, the young man, who had paid 100 baht (US$5) before the session, put another 100 baht on the table, urging the *bomoh* to get his motorcycle back. The theft was a great loss. He was still paying the installments, but he did not hesitate to spend even more money on the rather futile attempt to retrieve the vehicle.

This *bomoh* had the reputation to find lost objects and persons. He also treated people in absentia by reciting *jampis*. His clients were predominantly women for whom he prepared love charms to bring back their straying husbands. When he exorcised, he used lemons like other Malay and Indian shamans. He mentioned especially the profusion of spirits in the Pattani area where there were more Muslim than Thai spirits.

The *fifth bomoh* was, in 1978, in his forties. He was married and had a small boy. Following the pattern of the other *bomohs*, he had his initiatory dream when he was 20.

When I mentioned the legend of shamans turning into weretigers after they have died, he did something unexpected. He simply said, "Do you want to see it?" I quickly answered "yes" and asked whether I could use a tape recorder. He agreed, but I forgot to ask whether I could also take a photo with my flashlight camera. (In the past, some Chinese mediums had no objections when I used a flashlight, they only insisted that I waited until they were in full trance.)

He told me that tigers with a skin whiter than others are former shamans. Sometimes a neophyte has to live in the jungle for several years until a shaman tiger finds and trains him. Elephant spirits (*hantu raja*) and monkey spirits (*hantu pogu*) can become teachers, too. Then he spoke of a specialist, across the border on the Malaysian side in the Kelantan region who had met a tiger in the jungle. Mounting the tiger's back, he was taken to *Kadang baluk*, the underworld in the bush where initiations are performed. He said, however, that not all initiations would be shamanic. After having stayed for 3 years at this mythical place where tiger men lived, the man became a *bomoh belian* and did not suffer from epileptic seizures anymore (see, among others, Cuisinier 1936:5ff, 38ff, 74ff, and Eliade 1974:339 and 344–345).

When I previously had asked where weretigers could be found, the Kerinci Plateau on Sumatra had been mentioned. This *bomoh* knew a place not far from Pattani. He said also that people, who want to become a *bomoh*, go to a nearby fishing village and stay there near a *keramat* (tomb of a Muslim saint).

The *bomoh* then proceeded with calling his spirits. He lit incense and waved the curling white incense clouds toward his body, cleaning his hands and face with them. Then he asked me to put 20 baht (US$1) on a new role of incense. Producing a modern cigarette lighter, he lit a candle and lifted the burning candle into the five directions—east, west, north, south and above. Chanting for ten minutes, his voice suddenly faded away. His articulation became slurred and his hands began to shake. He fell down on his hands and knees and stalked around like a tiger. He jumped from one wall to the other with giant leaps, toppling the incense burner. Then he fell back and rolled on the floor.

Because his co-shaman had not been available, his wife joined us to act as assistant. She addressed the tiger spirit politely and inquired about his well-being. The gratified spirit made some predictions. The wife then asked whether he could call a Javanese ancestor. This was done. One spirit replaced the other. The wife thanked the spirits for coming and the *bomoh* awoke without having any recollection about what had transpired during the various stages of possession (see Fig.37).

Listening to the tape recording afterwards, a Malay expert and I found that, during his incantations, he had called twelve ancestors (some from Java, some from Pattani), also seven *walis* (Muslim saints) as well as white snake, raven, and shark spirits.

The *sixth bomoh* was, in 1978, in his forties. He was married to a woman who looked as if she were his mother. They had no children. Working as a fisherman, he would lend his boat also to others to increase his income. In 1978, he worked furthermore as an assistant to an American anthropologist. His readiness to talk was almost compulsive. It was not so much the joy of "telling stories" than the satisfaction he derived from the "exchange of professional experiences."

In 1978, he had been a *bomoh* for nine years. At the age of thirty-five, he had a dream in which an old man asked him to climb through a hole in the ground. He described how he found himself in a cave with old men who taught him various kinds of knowledge. (I was reminded of the descriptions of American Indians talking about their journey into the earth to meet their power animals or other spirits who become their teachers. I do not think there is any connection between the dream of a Thai-Muslim and the vision of an American Indian other than a substratum in the human mind which leads to similar, archetypal experiences among different ethnic groups.)

The *bomoh* showed me his large collection of herbs, different kinds of bark and minerals from which he concocted love potions and draughts to increase virility.

He offered to prepare an elixir which, put into my eyes, would make me see spirits. He also volunteered to produce a spirit helper using substances from a fresh corpse. He was obviously trying to impress me with his expertise, because he sensed that I had studied different techniques. It cannot be excluded that he wanted to test my knowledge, too.

He had written down all what his spirit teachers had taught him and had added knowledge acquired from other *bomohs*. He was especially proud of a chart which listed the auspicious hours for healing for all days of the week. He did not allow me to look closely at the chart, but he did not hesitate to read off the respective hours.

Sunday	11 a.m.	and	2 p.m.
Monday	8 a.m.	and	3 p.m.
Tuesday		12 noon	
Wednesday	9 a.m.,	4 p.m.,	4 a.m.,
Thursday	6 a.m.	and	1 p.m.
Friday	11 a.m.	and	5 p.m.
Saturday	7 a.m.	and	2 p.m.

To determine which spirit possesses a person, he suggested to put small green peppers into the ears of the patient. The owner of the spirit (i.e., the individual who sent the affliction) will cry in pain.

This *bomoh* was not available at certain hours because, he said, he was saying his prayers and studying the Koran.

When I visited the *seventh bomoh* in his small wooden house located in a side lane of Pattani City, he did not show any idiosyncracies. In fact, the features common to all Thai-Muslim *bomohs* were confirmed.

Bomohs experience a dream or a vision when they are in their beginning twenties or mid-thirties, i.e., after puberty or in mid-life. Six of the seven *bomohs* I talked to had first been called by the spirit of the father of their father, i.e., received their instructions from an ancestral spirit. It appears that certain families inherit the "duty" to become shamans, i.e., one family member has to take over and serve the community. I was told that the 7th son of the 7th son has to become a *bomoh* whether he has any talent or not. In cases, when there is no 7th son, a daughter may inherit the office. Only one of the seven *bomohs* in my sample had received his instructions from a tiger spirit. In such case, individuals had been chosen by an unrelated shaman spirit or they decided to go on a vision quest on their own.

In 1978, I had no difficulties locating *bomohs* in Pattani. They were easily accessible and part of daily life. They all had day-time jobs and they all said they were good Muslims.

Bomohs gave advice in interpersonal relationships. They were consulted in cases of theft and other losses. They provided protection, love and other charms and, most of all, they approached health problems holistically.

Having talked about an Indian shaman in Singapore in Case 2, I will now discuss a Thai shaman who follows *brahmin/animistic* customs.

Case 15 - A Brahmin Shaman in Bangkok (Thai)

The boatman of the British Naval Attache in Bangkok had invited the wife of his employer and me to attend the first-hair cutting of his one-month-old son. The boatman was a native of Central Thailand and had moved to Bangkok's twin city Thonburi shortly before the birth of his first child. His wife hailed from Chiang Mai.

After crossing the Menam River to Thonburi, the car passed several other smaller bridges and we finally managed to locate the boatman's house built out of teakwood in traditional Thai style along one of the back lanes. Flowers, some food, candles, and incense sticks had been placed on banana-leaf trays and left at the spirit house outside the building and there were other offerings on the threshold of the house.

The room on the ground floor was furnished with bare essentials. In one corner there were two tables and some chairs for Western guests, the mats on the floor were for the owners and their Thai visitors. The cupboards along one wall were reserved for clothes. Photographs of the Thai king and his queen hung on one wall next to family pictures. One of them showed the boatman in monk's robes. It had been taken at the time he had spent in a Buddhist monastery. (After having reached the age of twenty-one, Thai men are expected to spend at least one rainy season in a Buddhist monastery to become "ripe." The pattern has now changed to entering monkshood for a brief period of time after having finished education, so they may get vacation pay from their employer.)

The boatman wore an immaculately white shirt and grey trousers, his wife a yellow blouse and a full-length skirt. Both were in their end twenties. They greeted the visitors in the large downstairs room. A betel-chewing grandmother was preparing various Thai dishes on a charcoal brazier in the back room kitchen. Offerings to monks had been made already in the morning.

Shamanic Practices: A Case History Approach

The boy had been born in Siriraj Hospital, Thonburi, where he and his mother remained for one week before returning home. Wrapped in a pink blanket and sound asleep, he was briefly introduced and then returned to his cradle which had been a present of his father's Western employer.

Refreshments, i.e., tea as well as mineral water, were served. Shortly after, the local police chief and another government official in uniform dropped in and started to sample the whiskey the Western guests had brought as an appropriate present.

The invitation had been for ten a.m., but time passed with discussions about the weather and the latest rice prices. In the meantime, the wife had put on a flowered cotton tunic and dark blue trousers, blue and yellow being the colors of her native Chiang Mai. She wore discrete make-up and had pinned some flowers into her hair. The boatman had changed into a white cotton tee shirt and white shorts. Somewhat absentmindedly he went upstairs.

Suddenly we heard a loud thump, as though someone had struck the floor above with a heavy mallet. The boatman's sister appeared on the wooden staircase and gestured us to ascend. In the upper room the boatman was kneeling in front of the family altar. He wore now a white *phanung*, a *dhoti*-like piece of white cloth wrapped around his hips and he had a white scarf wrapped across his upper garment like the cord *brahmins* wear as sign of their caste. It became obvious that he emulated a *brahmin* and soon after it turned out that he was also a *khon song* (spirit medium).

A teakwood table, painted black with gold ornaments, served as an altar. Candles, incense sticks, and some flowers had been placed in front of the Buddha statue. Right and left of the statue stood small golden and silver trees. (In the past, such trees were presented by vassals to their overlord. In this case, monk had given these trees to the householder at a special occasion.) Two coconut halves were lying on the floor. Next to the photographs of the Thai king and queen, behind the main Buddha statue, was an image of Luang Po Thuad, together with a small image of the meditating Buddha to the left. The smaller statue to the right was the four-faced Hindu god Brahmā.

Luang Po Thuad had lived approximately 100 years ago near Nakhon Si Thammarath in southern Thailand. He was known for his supernatural powers, he could, for example, transform salt water into water fit for drinking. He is still well known in southern Thailand. No explanation was given why his spirit was visiting the boatman, however, there was no doubt about his assistance and advice.

The boatman's body was shaking. He managed to recite an invocation and then turned to calling the spirit of Luang Po Thuad. His wife squatted nearby and the embassy driver, a friend of the family, was holding the baby, his little hands covered with felt mittens, was gyrating his arms wildly in the air.

The boatman fell forward, hitting again the floor with his head, which explained the sound we had heard earlier. He was now deep in trance and "possessed" by the spirit of Luang Po Thuad. He seemed to sustain the possession state by inhaling incense and by occasionally taken some puffs from a cigarette his wife passed on to him. Although his speech was slurred, as if he was talking in his sleep, he still was able to communicate with her.

He took a bundle of small lighted wax candles and waved them three times around the baby's head. Then he held his hand into the flames, evidently feeling no pain. Touching different parts of the baby's head with his fingers, he transferred purity and protection to his child.

The baby, held head first, could not see what was happening, but when the smoke reached his nostrils, he became a little uneasy and started to whimper. The boatman extinguished the candles in his mouth and asked Luang Po Thuad about the child's future. His possession differed from the trance experienced by Chinese mediums. We neither heard the father's questions nor the messages of the spirit, we only saw the boatman's lips move.

A large pair of scissors was produced and the father, still in trance, cut all of the baby's hair, leaving only one lock in the middle of his son's head, the place of the fontanella, where, it was believed, the baby's soul had entered the child and would escape through if left uncovered. The hair was collected in the coconut shells and set afloat afterwards on a nearby *klong* (small waterway).

Each of the baby's wrists was tied with pieces of unspun cotton threads. The father purified these threads by holding them in the palm of his left hand while he chanted verses from the Pāli Canon, allowing the hot wax from a burning candle to fall on the threads. Again he did not seem to feel any pain.

The baby stretched out his arms as though it was inviting his father to tie his *khwan* (vital essence). This was considered to be a good sign and registered by all with a smile. Tying the threads around the right wrist, the *khwan* is invited to come. Tying the threads around the left wrist, the *khwan* is invited to stay (Heinze, 1981a:8–9).

After some more chanting, the boatman fell forward again, hitting the floor with his head for the third time. This broke his trance. He gradually returned to his normal self, seemingly exhausted but smiling. Luang Po Thuad had forecast a good future for his son.

We were told that, aside from his daily duties as boatman of the British Naval Attache in Bangkok, this man served as the medium of Luang Po Thuad. During his off-work hours, people came for advice. When something had been stolen, he might be able to tell where it could be found. In some cases, he even identified the thief. He did not accept any money, except for the *tham khwan,* the ceremony to "make the vital essence." According to the socio-economic status of the client, he charged from 5 salyng to 6 baht (a fraction of a cent to 30 cents; quoted in 1972).

The Thai shaman, described in the following case, calls herself the "wife of Brahmā." She claims to be visited by the spirit of King Chulalongkorn, the fifth king of the Chakri Dynasty, who died in 1910. The name "Brahmā" is used as a generic term for spirits of a higher order and does not necessarily indicate the creator god of the Hindu trinity.

Case 16 - The Wife of Brahma: *Phrom Mali* (Central Thai)

I don't know her real name. For decades she has called herself and is called by others "Phrom Mali." She lives in a large compound off Petchkasem Road in Bangkae outside of Bangkok (see Fig.40). When she was in her middle thirties, she became very ill. She stayed for 10 days in a hospital, but the physicians could not find the cause of her illness. When she went home, her condition worsened. Frequently she would lose consciousness. Finally, she consulted a medium and learned that she was about to be possessed by the spirit of King Chulalongkorn who wanted to help his people. As soon as she accepted the "call," her health improved. Since then she helped and healed up to three days and nights without getting up from her seat. She told me that during this time her body is taken care of by deities.

Phrom Mali did not "work" on *wan phra,* the half phases of the moon, the Buddhist equivalent to our Sunday observances (i.e., she did not practice the 1st and 15th day of the lunar month and two days before these Buddhist holidays.

Every time I went to see Phrom Mali, a large crowd had congregated in her hall. Three walls were covered with pictures of Thai kings and of herself in religious functions, e.g., laying foundation stones. (She has, among others, built a monastery, Wat Bod Phrom Mali, in the Province of Trad.) A bronze statue of King Chulalongkorn stands on the large altar and there are elephant tusks and statues of famous monks (see Fig.41). Her seat, prepared like a throne, was on the wall left of the altar. People came and sat patiently on the floor, moving up until it was their turn.

Before Phrom Mali came out of the adjoining private quarters, a moaning sound was heard, indicating that the spirit was about to descend into her body. The crowd knelt, lifting their hands to a *wai* (holding both hands, like in prayer, together in front of their faces). Then the door opened and Phrom Mali made her entrance. She was clad in brocade and silk, befitting a royal spirit of the turn of the century. Smoking five cigarettes simultaneously in one silver cigarette holder, she slowly walked to the cushioned seat and sat down crosslegged. Her attendants had prepared tea, fresh betel leaves, areca nut and lime. They also kept lighted cigarettes ready. Phrom Mali would continue chewing betel during the session, vigorously spitting out the red juice once in a while and then polishing her teeth with a small twig. Because she was meticulous in brushing, her teeth stayed white and hardly showed any of the red stains of heavy betel chewers.

At the beginning of the session, she chanted invocations to deities in Thai. Then she encouraged the first patient to speak up. During the first three hours of the session I attended, I counted 73 clients, 52 of them were women, 15 men, and 5 were children. A soldier came with one of his shoulders bandaged. A girl had a large open wound on her back which was dressed by Phrom Mali with an herbal mixture. A young man had six fingers on each hand and six toes on each foot. He said a twin brother was inside of him and had not been able to come out.

A monk came with his mother and one of his sisters who had become "possessed" when she had not been allowed to marry the man she loved. Phrom Mali did not exorcise her. She reprimanded the girl for not obeying her parents, "They have raised you and have your best in mind." Talking firmly about the behavior the society expected from her, she prepared the girl for reintegration. Phrom Mali was obviously reinforcing societal norms. The girl stopped her wailing and attempted to pull herself together. She looked subdued but no longer unhappy when she left. Whether this had any lasting effect, I could not ascertain. After the consultation, the family went to a huge earthen jug to fill blessed water into a bottle to be used later, when necessary, at home.

Phrom Mali used mainly herbal potions to drink and herbal paste for her massages. To ease headaches, she blew gently on the forehead of the patient.

She also advised in matters other than health. One man reported his grandmother left 4 million baht. Having been illiterate, she had not written a will. One nephew stole a check over a large sum and also passed bad checks to workers. Phrom Mali told this client that he will get some of his money back. "No lawyer can solve this problem, so they come to me," she remarked to me.

Quite frequently she repeated, "I can cure and I can help all those who have not committed any evil." Everything she said was accompanied by moral instructions. Though dressed like a man and speaking authoritatively, she radiated motherly love and charisma. She embraced each client and spoke kindly but sternly to all. Many of her clients experienced for the first time that somebody cared for them. They visibly cheered up and followed her words like obedient children. She was able to inspire hope which, in case of illness, triggered self-healing powers.

During her treatments and consultations, she joked with old acquaintances, sitting close by or greeted friends when they entered the large hall. After I had waited for 7 hours, moving up with the others until it was my turn, she did not mind to talk about half an hour about her work and how it related to the world of souls.

What were Phrom Mali's rewards? She enjoyed the unrestricted respect and gratitude of thousands of people. Aside from that, each client took a tray at the entrance of the hall. The trays were provided for offerings, customarily a lotus bud, a pack of Phrom Mali's brand of cigarettes, a candle and a pack of incense sticks. Some clients added fruit or other gifts. Those who wanted to become Phrom Mali's disciples put 36 baht (US$1.80) on the tray.

Near the gate behind the high concrete walls of the compound, relatives had opened a shop and sold incense, flowers, fruit, cigarettes, and candles as well as Thai dishes for those hungry from waiting seven hours or more. New buildings were in construction for Phrom Mali's relatives. She had built already a monastery and remained generous with other donations.

Her sound advice and her knowledge of herbal cures attracted thousands of people. She established her own network and operated with a small entourage (mainly her relatives). She certainly had a beneficial influence on other social systems in Thailand, but she did not enter the political arena like the shaman described in the following case.

Case 17 - The Divine Sages: Pu Sawan (Central Thai)

Peace Envoy Suchart Kosolkitiwongs was the Prime Director of Samnak Pu Sawan ("House of the Divine Sages"), 270 Soi Chaturongsonggram off Petchkasem Highway in Nakhorn Pathom. He was also the founder of the Centre of Psychical Phenomena Research at Anachak Hoop Sawan ("Valley of the Divine Paradise"), Pak Thor, Ratchaburi.

Khun Suchart was born on March 28, 1943 in Bangkok. In 1964, he was drafted into the army and served for one year in an anti-aircraft regiment. In 1966, at the age of 22, he was appointed Director of the House of the Divine Sages. What happened in the 12 months after he had left the army?

Staying at Bang Pak Thor, Khun Suchart became "possessed" by the spirit of Supreme Patriarch Luang Pu Tuad (see also Case 15) and the spirit of Somdetch Phra Phutajarn Brahma Rangsi. The Supreme Patriarch Luang Pu Tuad lived 400 years ago in Ayuthya, the former capital of Thailand. His spirit helps diagnose illnesses and prescribes herbs and lustral water for the clients who come every Sunday to the House of the Divine Sages. The second spirit, affectionately called Somdetch Toh, has been Supreme Patriarch last century during King Mongkut's reign. He preached and answered religious and other questions. The third spirit to appear was Tao Maha Brahma Jina Panara. He was a follower of Moggallana, the disciple of the Buddha, known for his supernatural faculties. Tao Maha Brahma Jina Panara is the exorcist.

These three spirits continued to appear regularly to Khun Suchart. They are present also at Pu Sawan when Khun Suchart is travelling and a monks steps in to bless and to exorcise. As has been mentioned before, each of these spirit has a special mission. One helps to diagnose and to cure the growing crowd of people, the second preaches, and the third lends his powers to fight spirit intrusion.

Khun Suchart lived in a small house in the Valley of the Divine Paradise. His lifestyle was frugal and he practiced meditation several hours each day. He encouraged his followers to observe Buddhist tenets and discouraged ritual activities. He continuously trained and purified his mind to refine his psychic powers. When speaking, Khun Suchart would elaborate on the three roots of evil—greed, hatred, and delusion. No one should trust any theory or text or word of mouth blindly. Everyone should investigate, contemplate and cultivate himself (the same was taught by the Buddha). Khun Suchart's followers said he is one "who gilds the back of the Buddha statue," that means, he works behind the scene.

Khun Suchart, however, became quite visible when he talked about the nation, religion and monarchy, encouraging people to fight against unrighteousness. He traveled through the Thai provinces and delivered speeches on morality to military units in border camps or to students in schools, colleges, and universities. Sometimes he distributed a consecrated cloth, called "national liberty," to soldiers and children (e.g., at the Juvenile Reform Center in Chiang Mai). When he visited soldiers, policemen and civil volunteers throughout Thailand, he attempted to boost their morale in fighting terrorists and saboteurs. He extolled the German dictator Hitler for building a strong army, working for the unity of his country, and solidifying the "Reich". He also mentioned Mussolini and Mao Tse-tung along similar lines. Obviously, Khun Suchart was not judging these leaders by their ethics and the consequences of their ideas.

On his trips, Khun Suchart also distributed medicine, clothes and supplies among the needy. He offered school children 5 baht notes for correct answers to questions of national or religious concern and he propagated the *Dhamma* in stressing *sīla* (moral conduct), *samādhi* (concentration) and *paññā* (wisdom).

He went on pilgrimages to Burma, Laos, Malaysia, Singapore, Indonesia, Vietnam, Sri Lanka, India, Nepal, and the United States. In 1966, the first year of his "possession," the spirit of Luang Pu Tad told Khun Suchart to go to Malaysia and collect earth from a sacred place at Alor Star. The earth was then used for making an image of Phra Sri Arya Maitreya, the Buddha-to-come. In 1969, when Khun Suchart moved to the present center, soil was collected from sacred places in other countries and put into 8,000 miniature statues of Phra Sri Arya Maitreya, to be distributed all over the world.

In May 1977, Khun Suchart met with Pope Paul VI in Rome. Afterwards he went to Israel to obtain holy soil and a stone from the mountain of crucifixion. He also visited the Mufti of Jerusalem and, in November 1977, His Holiness Sri Satguru Jagsit Singh Si Maharaj, the leader of the Sikhs, in the Punjab. He talked to Prime Minister Morarji Desai in Delhi and headed a delegation to the XXIV World Vegetarian Congress and the Asian Conference on Religion and Peace in May 1978. In November 1978, he went again to Italy (Assisi and Florence) and met in December of the same year with Pope John Paul II in Rome. He went to London, Warsaw and Cracow. On May 14, 1979, he met with Secretary General of the United Nations, Kurt Waldheim, in Bangkok and he kept writing letters to foreign ministers and heads of state. On January 16, 1975, he wrote a letter to the Russian leader Breshnew and, in February 1975, a letter to Henry Kissinger, other letters went to President Carter and the Egyptian leader Sadat.

In 1975, Khun Suchart was elected President of the International Federation of Religion. His aims are expressed in the following ten points:

1. to help relieve the physical and spiritual suffering of the people,
2. to work for the removal of senseless greed in the minds of men,
3. to encourage efforts to banish ignorance,
4. to uphold justice and righteousness in all societies,
5. to push for truly world peace as the sublime goal,

6. to promote religious work in every possible way,
7. to support the practice of concentrating the mind to finally attain *nirvāṇa*,
8. to fully cooperate with everyone working to become a *bodhisattva*,
9. to encourage and promote the upgrading of moral standards and conduct of the younger generation,
10. to firmly stress the existence of life after death so that nobody will deceive himself of being absolved of all sins.

In a publication, *The Blights and Blooms of Thailand*, distributed with the compliments of the International Federation of Religions, the Peace Envoy from the World of Divinity saw the blights of Thailand in the tolerance toward the wrongdoings of neighbors, colleagues and friends who were harmful to society. "People lack responsibility," said Khun Suchart, "They are buried in self-interest. They do not carry out what they are supposed to do. They criticize on false premises and they do not work for the sake of unity. People do not rectify unjustified opinions and do not resent disastrous acts. They neglect the cause of common people and only a few perform their duty with zest and zeal." Suchart warned of people who indulge in boasting and who refuse to rectify their mistakes.

The Religious Land Hoopha Sawan covers 10 acres. It was discovered in May of 1970 when Khun Suchart travelled with a young novice to Salika Cave and crossed the Valley of the Divine Paradise at Pak Thor, Ratchaburi, 100 km south of Bangkok. Thirty-five years before, on February 25, 1935, the cave had already been declared an archaeological site by the Minister of Education, Luang Vichit Vadakaran. According to legends, the cave served as shelter for the first Buddhist missionaries to Suvannabhumi ("Land of Gold," presumably either Lower Burma or the Thai-Malay Peninsula). It is said that the Indian Emperor Asoka, approximately 279 B.C., sent the Venerables Sona Mahathera and Uttara Mahathera to spread Buddhism in Southeast Asia. The venerables proceeded to Khu Bua, now a village 10 km northeast of the Religious Land and founded the Buddhist empire around Nakhorn Pathom where the largest and oldest *stūpa* (dome-shaped mound, topped by a relic chamber and a many-tiered umbrella) remained as a witness.

The highest peak near the Religious Land rises 185 m above sea level. A 9 m high Buddha statue has been put on its top. Statues of founders of other world religions as well as symbolic structures will be placed on neighboring peaks. On October 19, 1976, together with devotees from several world religions, the Supreme Patriarch of the Thai Sangha and Air Chief Marshal Davee Chullasap climbed the 559 concrete steps to the Peace Pagoda at 9 p.m. They spent the night, until 4 a.m., in meditation, praying for world peace. Since then services are held at the Peace Pagoda on the 19th of each month.

Other important ceremonies at the Religious Land have been

> consecration of the image of the late Supreme Patriarch of Ayuthya, Luang Pu Thuad (1582–1681), at Salika Cave, April 12, 1972;

> consecration of the image of Somdetch Phra Phutajarn Brahma Rangsi (Toh, 1788–1872), at Singh-Monkol Cave, July 16, 1973;

> laying of the foundation stone for the Jinnaputo Memorial Foundation Hall, October 12, 1973;

> Dhamma Chakra Flag Hoisting, January 24, 1974 (the "Wheel of the Law" symbolizes the Teachings of the Buddha);

> opening ceremony for the Hall of the Chief Lord Indra, January 14, 1974 (Indra is the chief god in Tusita Heaven, considered to be a protector of the Buddha and his teachings);

> consecration of Buddha images, containing Holy Soil from nine countries in the presence of the Minister of Education, the Supreme Patriarch, royalty, generals, the Deputy Prime Minister, and Air Marshall Davee Chullasap, March 31 and April 7, 1974. (The soil had been collected from 3 places of national importance in each of the participating countries: (1) the parliament, (2) the government building, and (3) the most venerated temple, church, mosque or official residence of the head of the state. - Earth is considered to be the mother, cradle, and grave of all life. The three different places of collection were compared with the three pillars of Buddhism, known as the Triple Gems—the Buddha, the *Dhamma*, and the Sangha or the Three Realms—The World of Desire, the World of Pure Form, and the World Without Form (see Heinze 1977b:215–216). Participating countries were Australia, Egypt, India, Philippines, Sweden, Sri Lanka, Turkey, with Japan and New Zealand having promised to join;

> laying of the foundation stone for the Peace Pagoda, October 19, 1974;

Songkran festivals, every April 12 to 13, since 1975;

opening of the Public Health Center, November 25, 1975;

casting of the statue of Rama I, February 15, 1976;

laying of the foundation stone for a 9-meter high Buddha image, March 28, 1976;

enshrinement of Buddhist relics in the Peace Pagoda, October 19, 1976;

opening of the exhibition of Religious Missions Work at Vatican City and Jerusalem, October 19, 1977;

laying of the foundation stone of a 9-meter high statue of Jesus Christ, December 25, 1977;

opening of the Buddhist-Sikh exhibition, February 19, 1978;

laying of the foundation stone for the World Eternal Peace Conference Hall, October 19, 1978, etc.

The House of the Divine Sages and the Religious Land Hoopa Sawan are both under the patronage of the Jinnaputo Memorial Foundation. Its president is Professor Dr. Klum Vajropala. His Royal Highness Prince Chumpakaputra Jumbal is the Vice President. Police Major General Pibul Pasawat is the Honorary Secretary General. The Branches in others parts of Thailand are coordinated by Prija Jumchai, the founding Secretary General of the World Fellowship of Buddhist Youth. The objects of the Jinnaputo Memorial Foundation are:

1. to help promote religious practice among members so that the teachings of the great founders of religions remain observed;
2. to help strengthen unity, solidarity, and brotherhood among its members;
3. to help propagate the sublime doctrines of religions;
4. to cooperate in social, educational, cultural, and other humanitarian services;
5. to promote lasting peace and harmony for all mankind and to collaborate with other organizations working toward the same goal;

6. to promote unity among men toward achieving world unity;
7. to help eliminate controversial disagreement about religious and political doctrines in order to raise the spirit of religious brotherhood and equality of all mankind;
8. to help promote human rights so that neither harm nor difficulties arise for mankind;
9. to search for ways and means to work on the convention of eternal peace in this world.

Aside from the Jinnaputo Memorial Fund, the Religious Land Hoopa Sawan was, in 1979, also the headquarters of the International Federation of Religions, the Office of the Peace Envoy of the World of Divinity, the Council of Mind Development of the Youth, the International Medical Center, the Religious Brotherhood Promotion Project, the Vegetarian Promotion Center, the Project on the World Eternal Peace Conference, the Project on Faith Healing through Meditation, and the Bodhisattva Village Project. All ten projects are headed by Khun Suchart who, when I visited Pu Sawan again in June 1979, was traveling through the USSR to promote the World Peace Conference, planned to be held in 1984 to prevent the outbreak of World War III.

Two marble tablets at the Religious Land bear the auspicious time and date when the foundation stone for the conference hall was laid. This ceremony was attended by 20,000 people, presided by the Head of the Sikhs, and in the presence of members of the diplomatic corps, royalty, representatives of all world religions (Buddhism, Christianity, Islam, Sikh, Bahai, etc.) The band of the Royal Army played Auld Lang Syne while the flags of 85 countries were hoisted. Police cadets as well as boy scouts sang the victory song. Balloons were released and Holy Soil was deposited ceremoniously by representatives of the participating 19 countries—Australia, Austria, Burma, Great Britain, Indian, Iran, Israel, Japan, Malaysia, Nepal, Philippines, Poland, Spain, Sri Lanka, Turkey, USA, USSR, Vietnam, and West Germany.

Aside from his efforts to spread world peace, the medium received messages from the "world of souls" with the help of "Our Great Father Somdetch Phra Phutajarn Brahma Rangsi" (Toh). For example, on August 8, 1968, 8:30 p.m., the spirit, speaking through Khun Suchart, announced, "the world of souls wishes it to be known among men what is the true cause of the present world crisis." An appeal was directed to all in power to promote peace. On June 16, 1968, 2 p.m., while Toh was preaching, Jesus Christ came to the Center and the spirit of the Somdetch translated Christ's words into Thai. On July 12, 1969, 7:20 p.m., Napoleon came and spoke in Cutave (?). The speech and the Thai translation by the Somdetch's spirit were tape-recorded and later translated into English by Professor Klum Vajropala. Napoleon reminded his audience to live without attachments (Buddhist words in the mouth of a French emperor). A consultation among spirits of religious leaders took place on July 19, 1969. It was followed by Mahatma Gandhi's spirit appearing on November 16, 1969, and Pandit Javaharlal Nehru's spirit on December 11, 1971. One of the Samnak Pu Sawan's publication mentions the prophesies of the Divine Sages:

1957	we are in the middle of the Buddhist era (2,500 year after the death of the historical Buddha);
1967–2007	half of all human and all animal life will perish in a massive holocaust;
1974–1984	a World War is likely to break out if no help should come from the World of the Divine Sages;
2007	the feudal and bourgeoisie classes will be destroyed and lose their power to communism and democracy;
2108–2307	communism will rule the world for 200 years;
2307	communism will fall from grace and the Ten Points of the House of the Divine Sages will become canonized;
2457	a new bodhisattva will be born and bring back Buddhism. He will reside at the House of the Divine Sages;
2947	a religious war will break out;
4457	there will be a worldwide annihilation war. Then a new world era will emerge and Phra Sri Arya Maitreya will proclaim his religion.

In 1979, every Sunday, hundreds of people came to Pu Sawan. In the morning, they received a number to establish the waiting order. At 1 p.m., the monk who was helping Khun Suchart, mounted the stairs to the consultation hall. The crowd sat on the floor to the left of the statues of the three guiding spirits, moving forward, one by one. Each draws 4 numbers out of a box in front of Luang Pu Tuad's image. A helper would call out these numbers while the monk blessed each client with sacred water (see Fig.42). Clients then moved on their knees to another group of helpers who dispensed sacred water to drink and handed out paper bags with the numbers clients had drawn. To receive herbal medicine, clients then showed the

Shamanic Practices: A Case History Approach

bag with the numbers to the dispensary downstairs. This procedure was adopted since Khun Suchart was not always available for consultation.

After all had received the number for their medicine, had been blessed and drunk the blessed water, the crowd moved downstairs to an adjoining building where those who wanted to be exorcised, had lined up. They have partially disrobed, i.e., had only a cloth wrapped around their hips, leaving the upper part of their body bare, when they were men or had slipped into old clothes when they were women. From the top of the stairs of an adjoining building, the monk would pour blessed water through a bunch of lighted candles on those who sat below him. It was amazing to watch how possession came out in the presence of a Buddhist monk. A group of helpers assisted in restraining the patient. They threw also a cloth over writhing women to keep them decent. The possessing spirit was asked to identify him- or herself and to say what he or she wanted. After having been promised that his wishes would be fulfilled, the spirit was then admonished to leave. Seven substances—charcoal, uncooked rice, onions, parsley, sulfur, salt, and small green beans—were thrown from a tray over the patient (see Fig.43). After one or two minutes of acting out, the shaking subsided and then stopped. The patient stood up and walked away as if nothing had happened.

The books of the Center recorded, among others, the case of Khun Vichai Sae Tia, who, in August 1970, had been advised to go to Samnak Pu Sawan to ask the spirit of Tao Maha Brahma Jina Panara for help. Khun Vichai was, at that time, 21 years old and a dealer in ready-made clothes. He lived at 76/24 Krung Kasem Road, Talat Bobe, Bangkok. For one year he had felt that something was wrong with him. He had frequent spells of headaches, had become bad-tempered, and began to walk through the streets aimlessly. Medical treatment brought no relief. A physician diagnosed that he was working too hard and that stress, together with lack of sleep, had caused his nervous condition.

When Khun Vichai sat down on the stairs at Samnak Pu Sawan and the blessed water was poured over his head and body, he began to howl and his arms moved like the forelegs of a dog. This caused consternation and remained unexplained, but Vichai felt relieved from his headaches and his health improved. Because the monk took ill, he was treated only once. Vichai returned to Samnak Pu Sawan later for four consecutive treatments until he was considered to be completely cured. After a few weeks, however, Vichai felt as bad as before and received blessed water for six more weeks. The spirit of Luang Pu Tuad, through the medium, finally told him that in a previous life Vichai had been a Vietnamese who had killed a dog named Tum Tah with the intention to eat it. (This custom was not uncommon in Vietnam and southern China.) In excruciating pain before his death, the dog had avenging thoughts. The spirit of the dog then began to look for his killer. He found him in Thailand where he had been reborn as Vichai Sae Tia, a Thai of Chinese descent. When the spirit dog continued to cause mental and physical suffering, Vichai was told to apologize to the dog for what he had done to him in a previous life. Vichai also donated money to Samnak Pu Sawan so that a shrine to Phra Bodhisat could be constructed. The shrine was dedicated to the dog Tum Tah. Vichai recovered completely afterwards. He received his final treatment on December 13, 1970. His case has been certified by reputable Thai officials.

Who were Khun Suchart's coworkers?

There was Professor Klum Vajropala, born on June 17, 1907. He graduated from Wat Dhebsirindra Secondary School in 1924 and completed the pre-medical courses at Chulalongkorn University in 1926. Then he was granted the King's Father Scholarship to study in England at London University in 1927. He was granted an honors degree in Biology in 1932. He finished his Ph.D. at London University in 1934 and conducted post-doctoral research at Cambridge University. In 1935, he became lecturer at Chulalongkorn University. In 1960, he was professor and chairman of the Biology Department. In 1965, he retired, but continued teaching at Mahidol University and also instructed the royal children at Chitralada Palace. He is the founder and life member of the Science Society of Thailand. His interests are Buddhism, parapsychology, meditation and spiritualism. He was ordained for three months at Wat Pak Nam, Thonburi, in 1956. During his meditations, he had four visions. In 1969, he visited Samnak Pu Sawn and became convinced of the supernatural phenomena of the spirits of Luang Pu Tuad and Luang Po Somdetch Toh entering the body of Khun Suchart.

Luang Samanvanakit (Charoen), born on December 19, 1896, in Ampoe Chaibadan, Lopburi Province, received his primary education at Wat Singaram. At the age of 16, he enrolled at the Dhebsirindra School in Bangkok and continued at Chulalongkorn University which had only 50 students at that time. After graduation, he won a government scholarship to study forestry in Burma. Returning in 1917, he entered the civil service and worked in the Department of Forestry. in 1949, he was appointed Director General of this department. During his government services he had been offered bribes for concessions in teak forests amounting to over 200 million baht (US$10 million). He recommended, however, that the concessions should be granted to Kasetsart University and the earnings accrued be used for the promotion of agricultural education so that trained personnel could help poor Thai farmers. The government followed his advice. Shortly after, a high official attempted to frame him with thirty-six false charges. Thailand's Prime Minister set up an investigation committee and the charges were proven to be groundless. The King appointed then Luang Charoen to the position of Dean of Agriculture at Kasetart University and, on recommendation of the university, Luang Charoen received the honorary doctorate in forestry from the hands of the King. Having served the government from 1917 to 1953 and, after having been Dean of Agriculture at Kasetart University from 1954 to 1958, Luang Charoen retired and was, in 1979, life member of the Science Society of Thailand, Chairman of the Association for the Conservation of Wild Life and leader of the Agricultural Project at the Religious Land Hoopha Sawan.

Major General Thawil Kasetratat, born on July 7, 1912, graduated from the Military Cadet School in 1933. Then he went to the General Staff National Defense College and took courses in supply management at Fort Lee, USA, as well as modern weapons courses at Fort Bliss. In 1957, he was temporary UN Commander in Tokyo. He is now retired from the Army Cavalry.

Mr. Bun Yong Vangvanij, born on January 24, 1923, received his primary education at Assumption College in Bangkok and St.Stephens College, Hong Kong, where he passed his final examination in 1951. In 1954, he studied at Columbia University, New York and, in 1963, he completed the International Management Course at Indiana University, USA. In 1979, he was managing director of the British Dispensary Company, the L.P. Stanford Laboratories Company, and Universal Food Company. He was, furthermore, managing partner of Vongvanij Limited Partnership and Vongvanij Investment Limited Partnership. He was also Vice President of the Young Buddhist Association of Thailand, Honorary Secretary of the Association of Thai Industries; member of the committee for the Welfare of the Crippled; member of the Sub-Committee for Industrial Development of the Private Sector of the National Economic Development Board, and member of the Community of the Druggist Association.

The prospectus of Pu Sawan in 1975 listed many prominent supporters of Khun Suchart. Among his advisors were Field Marshall Prapas Charusathiera, General Kruan Sutthanindra, and Professor Dr. Nibhon Sasithorn. Khun Suchart used to quote Gandhi, "He who says that religion has nothing to do with politics, does not understand at all the true meaning of religion."

The above record was written in 1979. Two years later, on December 18, 1981, *The National Review* (Bangkok) reported on page 3 of their local news that Police Lieutenant Chaovarin Latthasaksiri had been appointed "by lawmakers of all political parties" to submit an urgent motion to the House of Representatives to set up a commission to probe into the activities of Samnak Pu Sawan and Samnak Hoopa Sawan which were described as "two controversial semi-religious schools in Ratchaburi." The schools were accused "of being involved in scandalous rituals," "curing illness through superstitious means," and "using religion for personal gains." It was also demanded to find out whether the schools' activities were a threat to national security. Khun Suchart Kosolkittwong had allegedly proclaimed himself to be the president of the World Religious Relations Organization, affiliated to the United Nations, and Thai envoys had helped him to meet UN Secretary General Kurt Waldheim. When he sought support from international organizations, no official hesitated to defend Khun Suchart.

On December 22, 1981, Khun Suchart's name appeared again in the local news of *The National Review*. Members of the so-called "Chanuan (Igniter) Movement," led by the well-known Buddhist monk Phra Anant Senakkhan, had registered a series of charges with the Ratchaburi police on December 21, 1981. Phra Anant, a former police activist, had been dismissed from police service after having been found guilty of inciting policemen in 1976 to storm the residence of former Premier Minister M.R. Kukrit Pramoj, located in Soi Aree off Paholyothin Road. The Chanuan Movement had been active in waging a campaign against corruption among government officials from 1974 to 1976. Their controversial magazine, *Chanuan*, listed the names of individuals they found corrupt. Phra Anant, who had held the rank of police major before he was dismissed from government services, had already earlier registered a charge against Suchart because the latter had accused the Chanuan Movement of being communist oriented.

On December 21, 1981, the Minister of Interior, General Sitthi Chirarochana, declared that legal action may be taken against Samnak Hoopa Sawan for "making grim predictions about the future of Thailand." In a book, *The Doomsday of Thailand*, Suchart had said that Thailand will soon be occupied by communists. The publisher of the book was sentenced to six months in jail and all copies of the book were confiscated. The licenses of the Religious Relations Association and the Jinnaputo Memorial Foundation were revoked by the National Committee on Culture (ONCC). The schools were searched for weapons and a warrant was issued for the arrest of Khun Suchart.

There were other allegations that Khun Suchart had written a letter to the king, urging him to abdicate and that, on July 19, 1981, he had proclaimed himself to be the second king. Confusion arose about the Hoopa Sawan Center allegedly being an independent state with a peace ambassador and an Islamic monument which had been erected against Islamic principles.

The issues lingered on and on January 4, 1987, the *Bangkok Post* published on p.3, under the heading, "Reopen Hooppha Sawan for tourists":

> Suchart Kosolkittiwong, former leader of the Hooppha Sawan Religious Centre, has urged the government to reopen the controversial site as a tourist attraction. It is located in Pak Tho District of Ratchaburi Province.
> Mr. Suchart was charged with illegal renovation of the ruins at the site and illegal encroachment on public property. His cases are being forwarded to the court.
> He said that since the Government had proclaimed 1987 as "Visit Thailand Year," it should take the advantage of a large investment in the religious centre and reopen it for foreign tourists and the public.
> Mr. Suchart once spoke of his aim to establish a world government based at Hooppha Sawan and was called "world peace envoy" by his followers.
> He said that more than 30 million baht collected from his followers had been spent to construct statues of various religious figures. He said other tourist attractions there include the Salika Cave, the holy image of "Luang Poo Thuad," the 559 man-made concrete steps to the Peace Pagoda on a mountain peak, a 9-meter statue of the Buddha and another of Jesus Christ.
> Hooppha Sawan was ordered closed in 1982 by Ratchaburi authorities after an arms cache was uncovered in front of its entrance. Six charges were filed against Mr. Suchart who surrendered to police last year after five years in hiding.
> He said that before the centre was closed, he had intended to turn it over to the Government for public visits and study.
> Ratchaburi MP Pol.Lt. Chaovarin Latthasaksiri once proposed that the Education Ministry turn the site into a provincial college, but no action was taken by the Government.

Khun Suchart's role as shaman and medium of divine spirits has become overshadowed by his involvement in political affairs.

The following case describes what happens when ethnic Thai decide to acquire shamanic power.

Case 18 - Calling Phra Narai (Central Thai)

The contact to a shaman in the Ministry of Education was made through his secretary who was a classmate of my assistant at Mahidol University. The government official was quite willing to talk about his practice for the "sake of knowledge." He indicated that, in June 1978, there were about 60 to 70 shamans like him practicing in Bangkok. Many of them were holding high positions. Many more were waiting to be accepted for training.

The official considered himself to be a Buddhist who was following the four precepts. They turned out to be the four Buddhist *brahma vihara*: *metta* (loving kindness), *karuna* (compassion), *mudita* (altruistic joy) and *upekkha* (equanimity). He pulled out a necklace with several Buddhist amulets which he was wearing under his shirt. The amulets had been given to him by Buddhist monks. He told me that he can determine the quality of different spiritual entities by their temperature.

Asked how he acquired his power, the official reported that he had been searching for some time, until he finally was accepted for training by a group of prestigious shamans. He had been worthy on account of the merit he had accumulated in previous lives as well as the meditation he was practicing and the *samādhi* (concentration) he had cultivated in his present life.

His actual training consisted of seven days of intense practice which included exercises to retain his breath. During two additional days, he was taught four words for practice and four words for calling, as he said, the *winyan* (spiritual essence) of Phrom (Brahmā, see Case 16, a generic word for a "high spirit").

When people were disturbed by spirits or wanted to know where the posts for a new house should be put or where a new Buddha statue should be placed, he was asked to provide divine advice, i.e., he was expected to consult the gods.

He remembered a case when the soul of a dead baby had been thirsty and was disturbing the family. He told the family how to satisfy the spirit, and, out of gratitude, the baby spirit disclosed a lottery number which subsequently won.

The official was born in 1929 of Thai-Chinese parents. After some years in business, he became a school teacher in 1957. He was soon promoted to the position of district superintendent of education and then called to serve in the Ministry of Education. He became a shaman when he was 37 years of age.

He and his clients belonged to the middle and upper socio-economic groups and he was consulted not only by clients from Bangkok but also by people living as far as the island of Phuket in southern Thailand. He invited me to drive down with him in a police van to observe a spirit-calling ceremony.

I attended one of his sessions, held in the house of a colleague in Bangkok. Expected to become "possessed" by spirits from higher heavens, the colleague changed into white clothes and we all sat down on the floor in front of an altar with Buddha statues from different periods. Pictures of famous monks, among them the present king in monk robes[27] (see Fig.44), were hanging on the walls. The official

Shamanic Practices: A Case History Approach

lit candles and led the prayers to call the spirits. The white-clad colleague meditated to prepare himself for spirit entry.

Soon the face of the medium changed. Viṣṇu[28] began to talk through him, disclosing that he lives in the sixth heaven where a language is spoken which differs from the language in which he was communicating with us. (He spoke Central Thai, intermixed with Pāli words, known to ever Theravāda Buddhist.) The official thanked Viṣṇu for coming and asked for his forgiveness that he had been called.

Phra Narai was second in making an appearance in the medium's body. The third was Somdetch Toh[29] who ended the session in delivering a Buddhist sermon on the Four Noble Truths. He preached in Thai, using frequently Pāli terms:

The Four Noble Truths (*catvary ariyasatyani*) are:
The First Noble Truth of *dukkha* (suffering, unsatisfactoriness) tells us that birth is suffering, old age is suffering, disease is suffering, death is suffering, to be separated from the pleasant is suffering, not to be separated from the unpleasant is suffering, not to receive what one craves for is suffering.

The Second Noble Truth speaks of *samudaya* (arising) of *dukkha* through craving for sensual pleasures, for existence, and for annihilation which leads to rebirth.

The Third Noble Truth speaks of *nirodha* (annihilation) of *dukkha* which is achieved by forsaking of craving, by breaking loose, and thus being delivered.

The Fourth Noble Truth speaks of the *magga* (path) which leads to the annihilation of *dukkha*. This is the Noble Eightfold Path *(atthangikamagga).*

Why do mediums work in a Buddhist context? The Buddha has entered *parinibbana* (complete extinction) and cannot be approached any longer. Hindu gods have, therefore, become protectors of His Teachings *(Dhamma).* Together with the spirits of saintly monks, they can be consulted through mediums.

The following case introduces spirit medium lineages, still active, especially in northern Thailand.

Case 19 - Spirit Dances in Chiang Mai (Northern Thai)

In northern Thailand, we find mediums, shamans, and healers who draw their authority from certain lineages of spirit teachers. These lineages are exclusive and operate on principles similar to trade unions. The leader of each lineage will decide who can become a new member and who not.

Every year, toward the end of June, the different lineages of spirit mediums organize spirit dances in Chiang Mai City. These spirit dances are performed to *wai khru* ("pay respect to one's teachers"). The participants, in dancing themselves into possession, attempt to placate their "possessing" spirits (see Fig.45).

The lineage leader has, each time, to be asked for permission to join an annual spirit dance. To be seen dancing, therefore, has legitimatizing functions and increases the reputation of all participants. Public recognition is also connected with an invitation to join the spirit dance of another lineage.

I had already attended some spirit dances in 1972 and returned at the end of June 1978 just in time to attend a spirit dance behind Wat Chet Yot, the Monastery of the Seven Spires which had been the site of a Buddhist council in the 15th century under King Tiloka.

Spirit dances are usually performed in the compound of a lineage member. In 1978 a canvas roof had been erected in the large space between two Thai-style houses to protect the dancers from the sun. Two *piphat* bands, each consisting of one *song na* (double sided drum), one *ranad ek* (xylophone), one *khon hui* (gong), one *pi nai* (wooden wind instrument), and one set of *ching* (cymbals), alternated in providing the music. They played either traditional *ramwong* (round dance) melodies, special tunes for calling ancestral spirits or modern hit songs.

Mediums kept arriving in bicycle rikshas or small open trucks available anywhere in Chiang Mai City (in 1972 for 1, in 1978 for 2 bahts, i.e., 5 or 10 cents, respectively). Some mediums came on their bicycles or motorcycles. Not all of them hailed from Chiang Mai, some came from as far as Chiang Rai in the north, Fang in the south or Udorn in the northeast. In 1978, approximately 20 mediums were dancing at any time. During the five hours I was watching, at least 100 dancers had come and left again, after having briefly joined the dance.

First, the dancers paid respect to their leader in the back room where they got permission to join the dance. Some came already in the traditional costume, some changed in a back room or in full sight of the audience composed of friends, relatives, and clients. Whether male or female, all dancers wore a simple, long-sleeved blouse and a *phanung* (a skirt-like piece of cloth wrapped around their hips and reaching down to their ankles). Of contrasting colors, blouse and skirt were held together by a sash which matched either the skirt or the small piece of cloth wrapped around their head. All colors—yellow, blue, pink, purple, and green—matched well (see Fig.45). It was said that the mediums wore the costume of their spirits. Some of them changed their costume from two up to five times during the day, depending on the nature of the spirit who had just arrived to possess them.

Shamanic Practices: A Case History Approach

Though most of the dancers were northern Thai, their costumes showed Burmese influence. Some of the possessing spirits were, indeed, Burmese warriors who had died in this valley in battles centuries ago. (Chiang Mai Province has been an independent kingdom in the past, ruled by Thai and Laotian princes. It became vassal to Burma in 1550 and returned to Thailand as late as 1775.)

In 1978, hardly any ancestor spirits were possessing the dancers. Ancestor rituals were performed in a private setting, because the guardian spirits of families and clans in northern Thailand are inherited and cared for matrilinearly (see, among others, Turton 1972). In 1978, there were legendary princes and kings and other souls manifesting. It is believed that some dead heroes have not fulfilled their destiny during their lifetime (see Zuehlsdorf 1972:85). One of them maintained to be 8,000 years old. The woman possessed by this ancient spirit was herself 80 years of age. She told me apologetically that "he could not find anybody better." She showed, however, much vigor during possession. Her arms and fingers stiffened visibly and, at times, she had to be supported when she was overestimating her (or the spirit's) strength. Another woman in her thirties talked about the fierceness of her spirit soldier and promised to send him to my hotel room the next night. I was waiting with candle, incense and some offerings, tape recorder ready. He did not arrive, but, the next morning, I overheard a conversation at the hotel desk. A traveling salesman complained, he had been disturbed the whole night by a spirit who tried to shake him awake and wanted to communicate something to him. (Did the spirit soldier mix up hotel room numbers?) A Shan girl insisted on predicting a lottery number for me, free of charge, but the ticket did not win. I decided not to pursue both cases any further. The spirit dances are really not meant for practice. The mediums dance to entertain (*fawn len*) themselves and their spirits. During the rest of the year, mediums, as they said, study (*rian*) and cure (*raksa*) They also assisted in finding lost persons or objects and predict events.

Cold drinks and *miang* (fermented green tea leaves wrapped into small cubes) were offered to dancers and audience. Used like chewing gum, the fermented tea apparently served as a stimulant. Some hard liquor was consumed in the background, however, it was mostly drunk by the musicians and the spectators. Only some of the older and more hardy dancers allowed themselves to partake of alcohol.

The bodies of the dancers swayed when they moved around. They danced individually, using traditional Thai dance steps. The faces of the dancers did not betray any emotions. Emphasis was put on the movements of fingers and hands which were turned gracefully, like weaving flowers into a wreath. Once in a while the tune of the band would work up to a climax, dancers would move faster, uttering short cries, returning soon to quieter rhythms again.

Pausing once in a while, dancers came up and ask me about my family and what I was teaching at the University of California. Going to a university was to them as natural as they were taught by spirits. "Some people have a pleasant voice to sing, some have a good mind to study and to teach, and some have been selected by spirits 'to do salvation work.'" The answer to the question why these spirits do not incarnate themselves was that nobody can die and be reborn at will. *Karma* determines the fate not only of mediums but also of the possessing spirits (Zuehlsdorf 1972). *Karma*, however, did not seem to interfere with the benefits spirits and their mediums can confer (see also Delaney 1977:16).

The dancers either had followed the call of their own lineage or enjoyed the privilege of having been invited by another lineage. Their age ranged from 16 (i.e., after puberty) to 80 years of age. There were men and women, though in northern Thailand female mediums are in the majority. In 1972, there were only two male dancers, a 16-year-old boy and a transvestite (an entertainer from a nearby bar). In 1978, there were more male dancers but women still stayed in the majority. The dancers came from all walks of life and different regions of Thailand. There were farmers, laborers, street vendors and women from the upper classes.

When a woman changed back from her dancing clothes into an elegantly tailored suit made out of expensive foreign material, I asked her why she participated in the dance. She told me that in her teens she had begun to experience sudden headaches, vomiting, dizziness, and other inexplicable illnesses (classic symptoms for onsetting shamanism, see Eliade 1974). Bangkok physicians could not find anything wrong with her, but when her parents went to a spirit medium, she diagnosed onsetting spirit possession. The medium suggested to participate in the annual spirit dances in Chiang Mai. She reluctantly went north and found that her health improved considerably already after the first dance. Since then she had come regularly every year to dance in Chiang Mai. One year she decided not to come. The day when the others began to dance, she fell seriously ill and stayed ailing until she danced again the following year.

Thailand has been a patriarchal society for at least 700 years. Clients looked for patrons who responded to their needs as much as patrons gained power through their followership. With the political and economic developments in Thailand and traditional patron-client relationships breaking up, clients now sought patrons in the spiritual world.

Shamanic Practices: A Case History Approach

Case 20 - One Lineage of Spirit Mediums in Chiang Mai (Northern Thai)

Chiang Mai Valley appears to be especially blessed with spirits. Chiang Mai itself is the second largest city in Thailand, in 1978, with approximately one million people living inside the city boundaries and adjoining areas. How does this figure check with the spirit world? Counting the mediums, I observed during various spirit dances and considering the fact that some mediums are possessed by several spirits (one appearing when the preceding spirit fades away) and according to the mediums' own estimate, there must be hundreds of thousands spirits in Chiang Mai as well as in Lampang and up to 50,000 in Lamphun. They are either nature spirits, living in trees or mountains or spirits of dead heroes and kings and other legendary personalities. They are unrelated to the mediums they "possess." The placating of ancestor spirits occurs in a private setting and is inherited by the women of a certain family or clan (Turton 1972:217–256). None of these women become possessed.

Nature spirits are considered to be the most powerful. They rank higher than other spirits, but they are not so popular because they cannot be so easily manipulated. One mountain spirit in the Chiang Mai area is Phu Sae Ja Sae. His medium, a middle-aged woman, lived close to his open-air altar at the slopes of Doi Suthep. The altar was a plain platform around which people congregate to celebrate, for example, the spirit's birthday. Legends tell of three spirits, a couple and their son, who formerly lived on this mountain. When the Buddha visited this area, they accepted his *Dhamma* and the son became a monk.[30] His true nature as a *yakka* (giant nature spirit), however, did not allow him to stay long in monkshood. After having left the monastery, though, he continued to live like a hermit.

The lineage I mainly collected data on was the most prestigious in Chiang Mai City. Headed by a woman in her fifties, the lineage traced its origin back to Moggallana, the disciple of the Buddha who became known for his faculty to enter alternate states of consciousness and who visited regions above and below the earth. On one of such journeys, he discovered his mother in the realm of the *petas* (hungry ghosts) and became the first Buddhist to perform a spirit ceremony, in this case, to alleviate the fate of his dead mother (see, Spiro 1967, on *pereitta* ceremonies). Other spiritual teachers of this lineage are Phra Phrom, the spirit of the Brahmā statue near the Erawan Hotel in Bangkok, and legendary heroes like Chao Pho San Prakab, Chao Pho Chong Ang, and Chao Phi Saen Saeb.

In June 1978, I visited the medium who had been the *ma khi* (vehicle) of Chao Phi Saen Saeb for seven years. Born in northern Thailand, he was in 1978 a man in his thirties with a wife and two small children. Before he became a medium, he had been the owner of a noodle shop which did not strive. He tried his luck as taxi driver, also without success. Then his health began to fail and he consulted a spirit medium who diagnosed that Chao Phi Sae Saeb had selected him to be his "horse." The lineage elders recognized the taxi driver's potentials and recruited him because he added to the prestige of their group.

Without any training he began to practice. Eating only two meals a day, before and after "possession," he put in a full working schedule. That means, the spirit spoke through him from 9 o'clock in the morning until 5 o'clock in the afternoon. His health and general well-being had considerably improved and he drew great satisfaction out of being able to help many people.

When we drove to Sansei Village, a few miles outside of Chiang Mai City, a road sign pointed to the turn-off where his house stood in a compound. The largest of the Thai-style buildings on poles was devoted to his practice. Relatives and assistants lived in the other houses inside the compound.

The medium greeted us with a smile. His outgoing, self-assured way, his sense of humor, and his charisma explained his success. He was neatly dressed in white pants. Because it was a hot day, he wore only a white piece of cloth over the left shoulder. Wandering around in the compound, he gave orders in household affairs with the air of an office manager, confident about himself and what he was doing.

After a while he began to prepare flowers for the upcoming session. He lit several bundles of three incense sticks. With the first bundle he paid respect to the main Buddha statue on the altar to the right against the east wall of the practice hall. The first incense stick was lit for the Buddha, the second for the *Dhamma* (Buddha's Teachings), and the third for the *Sangha* (community of monks and novices), these three are called the Triple Gem and are evoked at every Buddhist event. There were numerous other Buddha statues as well as statues and paintings of Hindu gods, e.g., Krishna and Murgam. To the left was a second altar for Chao Pho San Prakab, and to the far left, against the same wall and in front of a window, there was an elevated seat with pillows on which he would sit during "possession." i.e., when a high-ranking spirit speaks through him. Above the two altars and the seat, there was a smaller altar devoted to Moggallana. Photos of the king, the queen, the crown prince, and famous monks were hanging on the walls. There were also posters of cats and small pieces of paper fastened to the rafters of the roof on which quotations from the Buddhist Canon were handwritten in Thai script. For example, "When there is no *Dhamma* in your heart, the world will be in flames." One poster announced the fee schedule: "Pay 138 baht (US$6.90) for consultation and 232 baht (US$11.60) when satisfied with the results." This adds up to 470 baht (US$23.50), not a small sum for the average client. Donations per day amounted to at least to 500 baht (US$25), in 1978, half the monthly salary of a school teacher.

The medium subsequently went outside and burned incense in front of the three spirit houses behind the east wall of his practice hall. Then he kept lingering around until almost 10 a.m., apparently giving his clients time to arrive.

Finally, he knelt down in front of the Buddhist altar and started to beat his chest and back with his fist. His face began to show some changes. He stood up and slipped into brocade pants of a deep red color interwoven with gold ornaments, typical for his lineage. Other mediums, whether male or female, usually wear a *pha sin* (long piece of cloth wrapped around their hips). Next came a yellow blouse and a sash. Then he draped a yellow turban around his head and put a flower behind each ear. He donned large sun glasses, another characteristic of northern Thai mediums, and put several large rings on his fingers, but he did not take off his modern wrist watch (see Fig.46).

He did not show any appreciable signs of trance other than speaking in a high-pitched, child-like voice, occasionally clearing his throat when he had fallen back into using his everyday voice. Before the session, he had already told me that Chao Phi Saen Saeb died at the age of 80. His spirit, however, comes to him as a 20-year-old man. Why a 20-year-old man would speak with the voice of a child was not explained. The high-pitched voice, though is not only a characteristics of many mediums in the Chiang Mai area, most Chinese mediums in Singapore also speak with a very high pitch.

On June 21, 1978, his first client was a young girl concerned about her health. He told her to be careful. Her *khwan* (vital essence) was weakening and a *su khwan* (ritual propitiation of her *khwan*) would extend her life. He rolled some small wax candles from raw bee wax, blowing on them and reciting *mantras* which were mainly verses from the Buddhist Pāli Canon. He also advised the girl to light some candles in a *nāga*-shaped[31] candleholder in front of his main altar.

The next client was a woman in her 80s. She could not walk and had to be carried by her son. Chao Phi Saen Saeb, through his medium, diagnosed paralysis and asked me whether we have similar cases in the United States. He gave the woman a cup of blessed water to drink. She was so awed that she swallowed the water the wrong way, started to gasp and nearly suffocated. A few pats on her back restored normal breathing. Her upper garments were removed and the medium brushed her body with pomegranate leaves, dipped in blessed water. Then he blew gently over her limbs. She smiled and looked better when her son carried her out. Some hope had been kindled and might have stimulated her self-healing power. She had been relieved of pain.

The third client was an elderly woman who was upset about her son who did not work and had taken to drinking. He also separated from his wife. The spirit of Chao Phi Saen Saeb said the son had been cursed by his wife's black magic. It was then discussed how evil influences could be removed. The main instruction being, the son should change his attitude toward his wife.

During all consultations, the spirit continued to give moral advice. Before the session, the medium had already told me that his ethics forbid him, for example, to help second wives.[32]

Faithful clients asked for permission to be adopted. They became the spirit's *luk liang* (adopted children) and would maintain their relationship with the spirit, i.e., the medium, for the rest of their lives.

People consulted the medium of Chao Phi Saen Saeb either

1. in matters of health. Contrary to other mediums who use herbal remedies, he did not prescribe any medicine other than blessed water to drink and to rub their bodies with it. Sometimes, he used pomegranate leaves to brush off pain. He also handed out candles over which he had chanted *mantras*. They had to be lit when the client would pray in front of a Buddhist altars. Or
2. they wanted to learn more about their future,
   a. when they were students, whether they would pass an exam,
   b. when they were professionals, whether they would be promoted, or
   c. when they were merchants, whether they would be successful in business and how, or
3. they sought advice with family problems (with their parents, spouses, in-laws, children and other relatives).

The clients of this medium belonged mainly to the farming and working classes of the Chiang Mai area, but he was also known on the national level and consulted by representatives of the elite. One government official, for example, came to him before the 1976 election. He was subsequently elected to represent Chiang Mai in the parliament and invited to join the cabinet. Another client, after having visited the medium, became police general in Bangkok under the Kukrit regime. And, in 1975, a professor of Chiang Mai University asked for advice because he was dissatisfied with his career. His subsequent promotion to become the head of the research department at Chiang Mai University was a definite turn for the better. His colleagues firmly believed that this promotion was connected with the medium's interference.

Between consultations, which went on until after 5 p.m., the medium chatted and joked with me, using the voice of the possessing spirit. He even suggested that a picture of him should be taken in front of the house. When I pointed out that the sun was getting into my lens, the "deity" moved willingly into the shade. The matter of fact attitude during the whole session was striking.

A "job" was done and it was done well.

For comparison, I have added the case of a Meo shamaness.

Case 21 - A Meo Shamaness (Northern Thai Hill Tribe)

In summer of 1972, we drove in a jeep to a Meo village behind the summer palace of the Thai king in Chiang Mai Province. After climbing Doi Suthep a few miles outside of Chiang Mai City, we passed the famous monastery on its top and then our jeep circled the royal summer palace and its gardens. Finally, we descended a loamy, winding road which was wet and slippery from a recent rain. It led to another valley where, on the slope of an adjoining hill we saw a Meo village.

The houses were simple wooden structures, just one room, perhaps with a partition, an open fire burning in the middle. Aside from kitchen utensils, there was hardly any furniture. Blankets, mats, clothes were rolled up and stacked against the walls. The Meo tribesmen and -women wore their traditional handwoven clothes, dyed blue and embroidered in red.

In the past, the Meo had been a nomadic tribe whose means of sustenance were hunting and slash-and-burn cultivation. They mainly grew opium poppies. The Meo said they did not cultivate opium anymore, but when we approached a house, pipes had been prepared and an elderly man lay down on the floor, propping his head up comfortably, a smile of anticipation on his face.

The Meo are encouraged to settle down. Christian missionaries, and especially the Border Police, opened trading posts to sell handwoven and embroidered Meo cloth, silver jewelry, as well as reed and bamboo instruments. We saw a pan-like flute (*kaen*), made out of five reeds and there were daggers and swords next to bows and arrows which the Meo still used for hunting birds and small animals in the jungle.

Climbing the hill, we heard chanting coming from a small house. A Meo shaman, an elderly woman, was "at work." Compared with the other shamans, mediums, and healers I worked with, she came the closest to the prototype of a shaman mentioned by Eliade (1974).

She "rode" into the spirit world. A board had been propped up between two stands and she sat on it as if riding a horse. Blindfolded with a black piece of cloth, she was holding in both hands iron objects which she shook vigorously to the rhythm of her chant.

The chant reflected her ride through the spirit world. Once in a while, she curbed her imaginary horse and called the spirit she had just encountered. Naming him, she incorporated his power into her body. Such chanting may go on for one up to two full days, depending on the seriousness of the patient's illness. After several hours of "riding" and charging her body with more spirit power, she felt prepared to cure a child who was suffering from a severe cold.

The "profession" of a Meo shaman is hereditary, though some shamans select a "talented" boy or girl themselves to transmit their knowledge of incantations and rituals.

The above event did not draw much attention from other Meo villagers. Calling a shamaness in times of need was not only socially acceptable but it was also considered to be a wise move. Shamanic performances have exorcising side effects. Positive powers are generated by the shaman and put to action. This is very reassuring because the presence of hosts of spirits hovering around houses and the fields, around trees closeby and in the forest is strongly felt and the Meo consider themselves to be blessed that there are still enough shamans to handle their various problems (see also Duerrenberger 1976:151–160).

Summary

What have we learned from these cases?

A Meo shamaness rode into the spirit world (see Case 21) and the god Rāma descended into the body of an Indian worker (see Case 2). A Thai-Malay *bomoh* transformed into a tiger (see Case 14) and Malay-Muslims behaved, during the Kuda Kepang, like horses (see Case 10). While performing a *main puteri*, another Malay *bomoh* balanced the "wind" of a client (see Case 13) and Chinese mediums removed bad luck with the help of Taoist deities (see Cases 1 and 6). It is believed that, during automatic writing (see Case 8), spiritual power moves the stick to answer urgent questions. Glossolalia (see Case 9), however, is an experience which, though occurring in a supportive social setting, still remains an individual event.

In sum, shamans, mediums, and healers in Thailand, Malaysia and Singapore still access alternate states of consciousness. Malay-Muslim *bomohs* inherit their faculties from their ancestors and may also create familiar spirits themselves. Chinese Taoists and Buddhists, Thai-Buddhists and Hindus lend their bodies to deities who want to do "salvation work," but some of them also search for spiritual power on their own. Personality profiles differ considerably, the common element, however, is availability to respond to needs of their community which otherwise are not met.

Shamans, mediums, and healers in Southeast Asia operate either in their own home or are connected with a temple where they practice on demand, at regular hours, on certain days or during festivals. Some serve their neighborhood, others are known regionally or even nationally, with one practitioner in my sample who worked globally for world peace but got caught in politics (see Case 17).

The role of shamans, mediums, and healers in Southeast Asia, to whatever ethnic group they may belong and with whatever religion they are affiliated, is determined by their personality matching the needs of a certain clientele. Strong personalities cross the borderline, not only of their social system but also geographic and ethnic borderlines (see Case 17). The majority of the shamans, mediums, and healers I studied were modest. They worked on an individual basis and gave immediate attention to whatever problem was presented to them. Clients were, for example, embraced by the Wife of Brahmā (i.e., the spirit of King Chulalongkorn, Case 16) or they felt acknowledged when the God Rāma knew their pain (see Case 2).

People go to shamans, mediums, and healers when they have entered a transitional period in their life and feel lonely and alienated. They have become vulnerable and dependent on understanding and empathy.

Modern physicians and psychiatrists are not equipped to provide spiritual help. They also do not have the time to render individualized assistance to patients belonging to lower income brackets. Similarly, priests of codified religions perform life-cycle rituals and deliver sermons, but in large communities there is not enough time left for solving individual problems. Priests "interpret the word of" God but they are not the "voice of God."

Gods and great teachers of codified religions have become inaccessible. They can be approached only through mediators. At this point, shamans, mediums, and traditional healers emerge and render the urgently sought services. They offer access to divine advice, protection, and blessings and, in doing so, activate their clients' self-healing power. They are effective as long as they can instill faith, they sink into anonymity when they don't fulfill expectations.

With a few exceptions, shamans, mediums, and healers have high ethical standards and do not accept cases they cannot solve. Therefore, as long as public health services are understaffed, lay practitioners can take a large load from the hands of representatives of Western medicine. The attempt to strike the middle way between traditional and modern approaches to healing has been made in Malaysia already. Authorities in Thailand and Singapore, though to a lesser degree, took also steps toward co-existence of different healing systems. To prove the efficacy of alternative healing systems, we need more longitudinal studies and, most of all, we need governmental recognition.

The study of shamanism, mediumship, and traditional healing has come a long way. Shamanism and mediumship have been considered a form of psychopathology by Hallowell (1941) and Belo (1960); a sanctioned form of psychological release by Mischel and Mischel (1958; a form of psychotherapy by Messing (1958) and Kennedy (1967); a social strategy of the oppressed by Hamer and Hamer (1966), Lewis (1971) and Potter (1974); a form of social control by Douglas (1970), Fischer (1971), Ludwig (1969), and Ornstein (1972). Then, Prince (1966), Bourguignon (1965, 1966, and 1978), and Tart (1969, 1986) began to study alternate states of consciousness more extensively, while, e.g., Frank (1961) and Krippner and Villoldo (1976) explored the "realms of healing." They prepared the ground for psychoneuroimmunology which recognized the "role of the mind in the onset and exacerbation of disease" (Achterberg, 1989:95). Achterberg listened to "healing stories" and found four common qualities:

1. none saw their recovery as "a matter of chance,"
2. all saw "the controlling factors in their lives . . . [as] highly intrinsic and internal,"
3. all experienced some "major change . . . insight" or personal decision "that facilitated the return of passion and creativity" into their lifestyles, and
4. the majority practiced "imagery or meditation." regularly (Achterberg, 1989:95–96.

Individuals are "tugged out of their passivity and experience of idiosyncratic symptoms" (Delaney 1977:30), so that possibilities for healing open up. Achterberg recognized the effectiveness of rituals which depend on

1. patient and healer expectancies,
2. trust between patient and healer,

3. patient's sense of urgency and spiritual quest,
4. patient's abilities to enter into the transformative process of his/her suffering (Achterberg, 1989:9–12).

Rituals encourage self-reflection and offer opportunities to reassess priorities.

1. They reduce anxiety, depression and feelings of helplessness;
2. they allow family and friends to provide support;
3. they encourage self-acceptance;
4. they evoke a higher power and "encourage deeper wisdom coming from these visionary levels";
5. they provide a "comforting rhythm of thought and activities" as well as a "structure . . . during times of change" (Achterberg, 1989:14–19).

Similar discoveries had already been made by Van Gennep (1960), Turner (1966), and more specifically Torrey (1986) and Heinze (1991).

Shamans, mediums, and healers are certainly multifunctional. They provide identity, order social relationships in a complex setting, enhance personal status, and compensate for the loss of integrative social systems. The new discipline of psychoneuroimmunology discovered what has been practiced already thousands of years ago by folk practitioners.

With the data, I presented in this book, I have attempted to provide answers to the eight questions I posed in the Introduction:

1. Faith still *is* part of the belief systems in Southeast Asia and this element of faith is essential for the success of folk practitioners.
2. *Physiological, emotional, mental, social*, and *spiritual needs continue to support traditional* as well as *create new cultural systems* around folk practitioners.
3. The reports on *twenty-one cases allowed a closer look* at those who meditate between different levels of consciousness to fulfill the needs of their community.
5. The *need* for spiritual guidance and help has *certainly not declined*, whether it increased is hard to measure.
6. The *syncretism* in contemporary belief systems is a *theoretical issue* and of no importance to practitioners and clients who participate in folk-religious rituals.

7. Shamanism, i.e., all folk practices described in this book, carry the characteristics of *elementary forms of the religious life*.
8. *Needs* have, indeed, *led to the emergence of need fulfillers*. Practitioners are successful when they are able to shift the attention of their clients out of an unhealthy (unbalanced) frame of mind onto a level where change becomes possible and harmony is restored within themselves, with their contemporaries, and their environment.

An Office for Alternative Medicine has officially been established in the United States in the last decade of the 20th century. More knowledge about health and healing is made available to the public. How our approaches to healing are changing is expressed by a certified M.D., Elliott S. Dacher, in his essay, "Old Landscapes, New Eyes, From Treatment to Healing,"

> We no longer believe that there is a single cause for each illness. We now recognize that disease, like health, is the result of a web of circumstances that involve our mind, body, spirit, and environment.
>
> We no longer believe that there is only one way to heal. We now recognize that no single approach, practice, or treatment has all of the answers.
>
> We no longer believe that the power to heal is exclusively contained in external agents or treatments. We now recognize the wealth of healing capacities that are built into our mind, body, and spirit.
>
> We no longer believe that health professionals have all the answers to our questions about health and disease. We now recognize that there are answers that we must seek ourselves (1995:11).

With this book, I attempted to contribute to the understanding of the work and success of folk practitioners who are responsible for trance and healing in Southeast Asia today. Longitudinal studies and case histories will provide more detailed information in the future.

Appendix 1
Chinese Terms Used in the Text

ang pow 紅包	red envelope (containing donations, left on an altar after consulting a spirit medium or given to children at Chinese New Year)
chai koo 齋姑	vegetarian nun
Chang Fei 張飛	sworn brother of Kuan Kong and Liu Pei (Three Kingdoms," 220-265 A.D.)
chao hun 招魂	calling back the soul
Chao-yao 昭耀	the star "Far Flight," also called Bootis (see Case 7)
chen jen 真人	perfected man, a spiritual man who has attained Tao
chi 祭	to sacrifice
chia t'ang 家堂	household shrine
chiang chun t'ou 將軍頭	five generals' heads, one for each of the five directions on top of a skewer used by mediums to be pierced through the skin of their upper left arm at special occasions
chiao 教	guiding doctrine, religion
ching 經	sacred book, *sūtra* (see Appendix III – Indian Terms Used in the Text)
Chun-ti 君帝	a male form of the Indian goddess Marici who later became the Queen of Heaven *(T'ien Hou)* in Taoism (see Case 7)
ch'e sin	to seek ghosts
Ch'eng Huang 城隍	Guardian God of City Walls and Moats
ch'i 氣	breath, air, life force
ch'i kiu 刺球	prick ball (with 108 spikes)
ch'ing ming 清明	"Cleaning the Graves," during the first week of the third lunar month
ding 鼎	cauldron (see Case 7)
Feng-shen yen-i 封神演義	"Metamorphoses of the Gods" (see Case 7)
feng shui 封水	geomancy
Fu 輔	the star "Sustainer," also called Alcor, attached to Mizar (see Case 7)

Appendix 1

fu 符	charm paper
fu chi 扶箕	to support a winnowing basket (for divination), e.g., automatic writing (see Case 8)
fu luan 扶鸞	to support a phoenix, e.g., automatic writing (see Case 8)
fu-mo che 優魔者	exorcist
Gak Teh Ia 嶽帝爺	Lord of the Underworld
hoat-su 法師	exorcist, magician
hsiao 孝	filial piety
hsien 仙	immortal, spiritual being
Hsüan-tsang 玄藏	Buddhist monk who, in 629 A.D., went to India to secure Buddhist scriptures
Huang Ti 黃帝	legendary Yellow Emperor who lived approximately around 2697 B.C.
hun 魂	soul, the spiritual part of man that ascends to heaven after death; *hun shen* 魂神 cloud-soul, actualizing spirit
I-Ching 易經	"Book of Changes," using combinations of 64 hexagrams for divination
jin shen 進身	to approach a body
ju chiao 儒教	Confucianism
Ju Lai 如來	Chinese name for Buddha
Kam T'ien Sion Teh 感天上帝	honorific title for one of Kuan Kong's sworn brothers (see Case 1)
Kau Wong Yeh 九王爺	the Nine Imperial Gods (see Case 7)
khan bong	to bring up the dead
ki pit 乩筆	divining pencil; *kiah tsian ki e lang* 攀正乩之人 or *khan tsian ki e* 攀正乩者 bearer or holder of the right branch of the writing stick; *khan to ki e lang* 攀左乩之人 or *kian to ki e* 攀左乩者 holder of the left branch of the writing stick, also called *hu ki* 輔乩, secondary or auxiliary diviner. Spirit writing is called *kiah ki ch'ut ji* 攀乩出字 or *khan ch'u ji* 攀乩出字, to produce characters by bearing or holding the *ki*. *Kang ki* 祭乩 means to descend into the *ki; tsiung ki* 開乩 to go into the *ki*; *hu ki* 輔乩 to adhere to the *ki* and *koan*

Chinese Terms Used in the Text

	ki to contact. (see Case 8)
ki poan 乩盤	wooden platter for automatic writing
Kuan Kong 關公	sworn brother of Chang Fei and Liu Pei (see above and below), also called Kuan Teh; red-faced, blackbearded God of War
Kuan Yin 關音	female *bodhisattva of* Amitābha Buddha. She can assume eighty-four different manifestations and is considered to be a form of the Bodhisattva Avalokiteśvara
kuay oon 改運	to change luck
kuei 鬼	disembodied spirit; *kuei min* 鬼民 demons; *kuei tsu* 鬼卒 demon soldiers
li 禮	propriety, rite, ceremonial
li 理	principle
li shu 理書	almanach with climatological information and instructions for activities in daily life
Liu Pei 劉備	sworn brother of Chang Fei and Kuan Kong (see above)
lung 龍	dragon; *lung wang* 龍王 dragon king; *lung wei* 龍位 dragon throne
Ma Chu P'oh 媽祖婆	"Respected Grandaunt," honorific title for the Queen of Heaven (see Case 7)
Ma Tsu Ch'iung 媽祖瓊	"Respected Mother of Hainanese," honorific title for the Queen of Heaven (see Case 7)
man seng p'oh 問醒婆	old woman who demands that a spirit should be raised
miao 廟	temple for public worship
Miao-shen 妙善	legendary princess of the Chou dynasty who later was deified by the Jade Emperor and allegedly became Kuan Yin (see Case 7)
Mi-lo-fo 彌勒佛	Chinese name for Maitreya, the Buddha-to-come
mi tsung 密宗	Tantric Buddhism
mu bei 木杯	divining blocks
mu yü 木魚	wooden fish, a skull-shaped block which is beaten while chanting

Appendix 1

Nor Cha Sam T'ai Tze	哪吒三太子	the Third Prince, represented with a magic bracelet in one hand and a magic sword in the other, having "wind-and-fire" wheels under his feet
Nü Shu	女樞	"Female Pivot," female version of the Polar Star (see Case 7)
O-mi-t'o-fo	阿彌陀佛	Chinese name for Amitābha Buddha
Ong T'ien Koon	王天君	door guardian
Pa Kua	八卦	Eight Trigrams
pai shen	拜神	to worship a deity
Pei-shan Shih Ts'un	北山詩存	collection of poems, edited by the Confucian scholar Lin Kuang-yün
pu	卜	to divine, to foretell
p'ing an ch'iao	平安橋	"Bridge of Peace"
p'o	魄	animal or inferior soul which fades away with the body after death; *p'o ching* 魄精 white-soul/embryonic essence.
p'u-tu	普度	a lengthy ritual the merits of which are thought to release all suffering souls from hell. It is also performed to integrate alienated members back into the community (see Case 7).
Shang Ti	上帝	Supreme Deity
shen	神	spirit, god, divine, soul; *shen chu* 神柱 spirit tablet
sheng-jen	聖人	sage
Shin-chia-mo-ni-fo	釋迦牟尼佛	Sakyamuni Buddha (the historical Buddha)
Shih Chieh Hungwan Tzu Hui	世界紅卍字會	the World Red Swastika Society (see Case 8)
shuo	槓	handle
Si-yiu-ki	西遊記	"A Record of Travels in the West," written by Wu Ch'eng En (1500-82 A.D.) about the Buddhist monk Hsüan-tsang who went to India to secure Buddhist scriptures.
siu to	綠兜	stomacher made of embroidered silk, fastened across the front part of a medium's body to identify the "possessing"

		shen
Su Yu Niang Niang	蘇玉娘娘	"Jade Empress Who Relieves the Suffering of People"
Sun-heu-tze	孫猴子	see *Ts'oi T'in Tai Seng Yeh*
ta t'i	大體	the essential part of human nature
Tai Chi Chuan	太極拳	certain spiritual as well as physical exercises
tang-ki	童乩	"divining youth," spirit medium (see also p. 46)
Tao	道	the "Way," eternal principle; *tao shih* 道師 Taoist master; *Tao Yuan* 道院
teng k'au	釘球	spike/prick ball
teng kio	釘轎	chair with sharp spikes on the seat, back, arm, and foot rests
Ti	帝	God, deified being
Ti Ts'ang	地藏	God of the Underworld; the Bodhisattva Kṣitigarbha (see Case 7)
to-kio	刀轎	chair with sharp swords or knives on the seat, back, arm, and foot rests
Toa Peh Kong	大伯公	Grand Old Man, depicted red-cheeked with a white beard, gold ingots in one hand and in the other a walking stick; tutelary deity of Straits Chinese
Tou Mu	斗母	Goddess of the North Star, Mother of the Nine Imperial Gods (see Case 7)
Tsao Chün	竈君	Kitchen God
tsu	祖	ancestor
Tz'u Yuan	辭源	Chinese encyclopedia
Ts'oi T'in Tai Seng Yeh	齊天大聖爺	"The Great Sage of All the Heavens," irreverently in English called the Monkey God; see *Sun-heu-tze;* the monkey who accompanied Hsüan-tsang to India.
tz'u	祠	shrine, sanctuary
T'ai i	太乙	"Polar Deity" (see Case 7)
T'ai-i-pei-chi chen-chiao	太乙北極真教	"True Teachings of the T'ai-i of the North Pole" (see Case 8)
t'ai shang chen jen	太上真人	"Grand Supreme Perfected Men" (see Case 7)
t'ang	堂	household altar, shrine

Appendix 1

T'ien 天	Heaven; *T'ien Chu* 天主 Heavenly Lord; *T'ien Hou* 天后 Queen of Heaven; *T'ien Mu Niang Niang* 天母娘娘 Heavenly Mother
t'u ti 土地	tutelary deity, earth god
t'ung shu 通書	Chinese almanach
wang 王	king
wu 巫	shaman; *wu chia* 巫家 shaman family; *wu erh* 巫兒 shaman
yang 陽	light, bright, positive, male principle
yin 陰	dark, negative, female principle
yin chen 銀針	silver needles, used to pierce cheeks and tongue
Yü 禹	legendary emperor of China who, according to some scholars, ruled either 2205-2197 B.C. or during the Chia dynasty (1994-1523 B.C.)
Yü-hung-shang-ti 玉皇上帝	Jade Emperor

Note: The above words are mainly Hokkien terms. They are transcribed as they are most frequently spelled in Singapore. It was not possible to find agreement between dialect groups nor did members of the same dialect group completely agree on one spelling.

Appendix 2
Malay Terms Used in the Text

adat	traditional, customary law
agama	religion
angin	wind, breath
angklung	frame where a number of bamboo tubes have been mounted in such a way that when the instrument is shaken, it produces a musical chord.
ayer tawar	holy water
azimat, jimat	talisman, small metal pendants containing words of the Qur'ān
bahasa pantang	taboo language
Batara Guru	Śiva
batu keras	quartz crystal used to detect the whereabouts of a soul
bekam	cupping
belajar	to study
beralin	sucking charm
berdosa	sinful
bidan	village midwife
bomoh	medicine man, somebody who practises the healing arts by utilizing the knowledge of traditional medicine. He may also foretell the future and raise spirits by reciting verses from the Qur'an, e.g., *berkat, el fateha, terang hati, sembahyang haja* (see Danaraj 1964; Gimlette 1974: 18-19; Hartog 1973:352-72; Mustapha 1977; and others).
bomoh belian	spirit-raising exorcist
bomoh gebien	spirit medium
bomoh mok peh	curer of the sick. He also discovers lost and stolen objects and divines, with a bundle of small canes. He can tell whether a witchcraft charm has been hidden under the house.

Appendix 2

bomoh patah	fracture doctor
bomoh pesaka	hereditary medicine man
bomoh puteri	raiser of the *puteri* (princess?) and other spirits for curing purposes
buah limau	lime
buah pinang	betel nut
buka	open; lime piece has fallen outside up; positive answer
bunga melur	jasmin
dargāh**	tomb of a Sūfī saint
dato	tutelary spirit, mainly identified with the soul of a Muslim saint; title
daun sireh	betel leaves
djinn**	see *jin*
engkarabun	(Iban), magic substance which makes the user invisible to spirits
gila	nervous disorder, madness
hadith**	sayings of the Prophet; traditional stories which aid in governing Islamic life and in interpreting the Qu'ran
hādjdjī,** haji	Muslim who has made a pilgrimage to Mekka; honorific title
hantu	spirit, ghost; there are hundreds of different spirits
hantu buyu	incubus, evil spirit supposed to descend on sleepers, especially seeking intercourse with women
hantu raya	Mythical Hunter, Specter, supposed to be Śiva (Rudra)
hantu penyakit	spirit who causes illness
hantu rimau	tiger spirit (soul of a dead shaman)
harans	forbidden
hukum adat	customary law
hukum sharia	law of the Prophet
ilmu	knowledge
imam**	leader of a Muslim community
jami	major mosque where official Friday services are held
jampi	spell, incantation (which can be an amal-

	gam of Muslim and Hindu prayers, secret magical words possibly of Sanskrit origin; mostly inherited from grandparents)
jin	genii, elemental (manifestation of fire)
jin hitam	black spirit
jin putih, puteh	white spirit who lives in the sun and guards the gates of the sky. His brother has seven heads and is called Maharaja Dewa (Śiva).
kampung, kampong	village
kadhi	Muslim court judge
kavacha	Indian talisman
kemenyan	benzoin resin, incense
kenduri	religious feast, offerings to the spirits
kepercayan	belief
keramat	sacred thing, place, tomb of a Muslim saint
keris, kris	Malay dagger
ketua	village headman
khalwat	"close proximity" (of men and women who are not married to each other, punishable by Muslim law)
kunci	lock to keep spirits out
latah	nervous disorder, also called "startle syndrome," kind of hysteria
lupa	forgetfulness, trance (from Sanskrit *lopa*, loss, disappearance)
Mahadewi	Kumari, Sri, Goddess of the Rice Fields, wife of Śiva
main gebiah	divining with green twigs (village custom, accompanied by drumming)
main puteri	"calling the spirits," amalgam of folk medicine and drama, performed mainly at the east coast of the Malaysian Peninsula (Kelantan). Accompanied by a seven-piece orchestra, the main performers are the *bomoh puteri* and the *minduk* (narrator), both interact with the patient and the audience. The *bomoh* mainly

Appendix 2

	calls nature spirits and deities from the Hindu Rāmāyaṇa. (see Case 13)
majlis ugama	religious council
manang	Iban shaman
manang balang	transformed Iban shaman
manang mansau	ripe Iban shaman
manang mata	raw Iban shaman
masdjid**	mosque; any place where worship is performed in groups
menurun	to descend, to go into trance
minduk, mindok	narrator, spiked-fiddle player in the main puteri (see Case 13)
mu'azzin**	one who calls the faithful to prayers
mullah	religious teacher and preacher
nasi kunyit	yellow rice
nasi semangat	ceremonial rice for the soul/spirit
orang asli	aborigine
orang halus	refined man; spirit in the shape of a man; invisible man
palu batil	musician who beats a brass bowl with two pieces of bamboo
palu redap	drummer
panas	hot (food)
pengaruh, pangaroh	influence; charm
pasang	leg stocks
pawang	another name for *bomoh;* agent between man and the spirit-controlled elements; priest-healer. He propitiates God and the spirits during rice and fish harvests. He stops rain and occasionally protects a village from epidemics. (see Case 10)
pelesit	familiar who works for the benefit of its owner. He can be sent out to weaken or to kill an enemy.
pelian	Iban ritual to safeguard the psychic welfare of clients
pelias	magic charm
penunggu	tutelary spirit
puaka	soul of an object

Malay Terms Used in the Text

qadar**	fate
Qur'ān,** Koran	sacred book of the Muslims, written in Arabic, containing the words of God as revealed to the Prophet Muhammad by the Archangel Gabriel
rebab	three-stringed spike fiddle
rimau keramat	ghost tiger, weretiger
sakit berangin	sickness from wind
sejuk	cool (food)
semangat	soul which separates from the body of its owner during sleep and at the time of death. When wandering around, it may become lost or be ensnared by a malevolent spirit.
shahada	profession of faith, "There is no God but God and Muhammad is his Messenger."
sharī'a**	the whole body of rules governing the life of a Muslim (religiously, politically, socially, and ethically; legal doctrine derived from the Qur'ān and the sunna, an indisputable source for regulating relationships with Allāh, it does not concern itself with inner consciousness.
shaitān**	Satan
shī'a**	branch of Islam whose followers hold that Ali, Muhammad's cousin and son-in-law, was Muhammad's successor; now found principally in Iran, Iraq, Yemen, Afghanistan, and Pakistan
shi'ite**	"partisan of Ali"
sinseh	Chinese medicine man
sunna**	"beaten path" or body of traditions recounting the deeds, sayings, and silent approval of the Prophet covering the details of community life
sunni	branch of Islam whose followers believe that Muhammad's successor should be elected; presently comprises about 85% of all Muslims

Appendix 2

sunn'ite*	sunn'ite follower of the tradition, "orthodox"
sūra**	chapter or division of the Qur'ān, altogether 114
tangkal	talisman
tutup	closed; lime piece has fallen outside down; negative answer
ulamā**	men learned in the law and religious studies; the class responsible for determining Muslim orthodoxy
umma**	Muslim community
yakin	faith and trust, keystone for Malaysian folk treatment
zakāt**	tithe or tax; almsgiving to the poor

* Many of these terms differ from location to location.
** Arabic and Persian words used by Muslims in Singapore, Malaysia, and Thailand.

Appendix 3
Indian Terms Used in the Text

avatāra*	descent, incarnation, a god manifesting in human form, e.g., the ten *avatāras* of Viṣṇu
bodhisattva*	in Theravāda Buddhism, a Buddha-to-be, somebody who is destined for enlightenment; in Mahāyāna Buddhism, somebody who foregoes his own entry into *nirvāṇa* (to save all sentient beings)
Brahmā*	creator god (of the Hindu trinity)
brahmin*	"possessing sacred knowledge," highest caste, priest
bhajan	devotional song
bhikṣu*	monk; *bhikṣuni**, nun
dharma*	the Universal Law; the teachings of the historical Buddha
dhoti	a loin cloth worn by Hindu men
Ganeśa*	elephant-headed son of Śiva, god who grants wealth and fertility, especially worshipped by merchants and women who want children
guru*	religious teacher, spiritual adviser
Hanumat, Hanuman*	"having large jaws," semi-divine monkey chief who helped Rāma to retrieve Sītā from the demon king Rāvaṇa
jina*	conqueror, standard epithet of a Buddha
kalpa*	aeon, a fabulous period of time
karma*	"what has been done," act or deed and its consequences; the fruit of each thought, word or action; law of causality during the successive states of human existence
Kārtikeya*	son of Śiva, also called *Murgam, Skanda* and *Subramanya*
kavadi	anything from a relatively small wooden yoke to a 60-pound steel frame, attached with 108 hooks to the body of a devotee,

Appendix 3

	symbolising Lord Murgam's steed — the peacock
Mahākāli*	wrathful form of Siva's consort
mantra*	verbal spell, ritual incantation; mystical formula used devotionally in Hinduism and Buddhism, supposed to transform the mind of those who repeatedly recite it
mokṣa*	liberation, emancipation; final release from worldly existence and transmigration
mudrā*	identifying seal, sign; a stylized symbolic gesture used in Indian dances and rituals, especially an intricate movement or positioning of the hands and fingers:
abhaya*	dispelling fear; raising the right hand with the palm turned outward
añjali*	adorative; raising both hands, palm against palm, to one's forehead
bhūmisparśa*	calling the Earth as a witness, conquering Mara (the Evil One, tempting the Buddha under the bodhi tree); touching the ground with the right hand, the left hand (palm up) resting on the crossed legs
dharmacakra*	preaching; turning the Wheel of Law; thumb and index finger of each hand held together, forming the spokes of an imaginary wheel
vajra*	thunderbolt; holding this symbol of Tantric Buddhism
vara*	dispersing favors; stretching out the right hand, palm up
vitarka*	argumentative; lifting the right hand with the palm toward the body
muni*	saint, sage, seer, ascetic, monk, hermit (especially one who has taken the vow of silence)
Murgam	son of Śiva, also called *Kārtikeya, Skanda,* and *Subramanya*
nāga*	mythical serpent, protector of the Buddha

Indian Terms Used in the Text

	and his teachings
nerthikkatan	vow
nirvāna*	"blowing out," extinction (of defilements and attachments to material things), enlightenment
Pārvati*	consort of Siva, daughter of Hima-vat, king of the snowy mountains
prasāda*	a propitiatory offering of food (after the ritual, distributed to the worshippers)
pūjā*	worship, homage; *puspapuja,* offering of flowers
Rāma*	seventh reincarnation of Visnu
Siva*	the "Auspicious One," desintegrating or destroying and reproducing deity of the Hindu trinity
Skanda*	son of Śiva, also called *Kārtikeya, Murgam,* and *Subramanya*
stūpa*	dome-shaped mound, built of earth, bricks or stones, topped by a relic chamber and a spire which usually has the shape of a many-tiered umbrella
Subramanya*	"dear to Brāhmans," son of Śiva, also called *Kārtikeya, Murgam,* and *Skanda*
sūtra*	thread; verse; discourse, one of the historical Buddha's sermons
swami	respectful address for a Hindu ascetic or religious leader
upāsaka*	male Buddhist devotee (who keeps the ten precepts)
upāsika*	female Buddhist devotee (who keeps the ten precepts)
vel	Murgam's three-pronged spear
vibhuti	cowdung ash, used for blessing to be applied externally on the forehead after the ritual, also used on wounds and put on the tongue for internal ailments
Visnu*	the protecting deity of the Hindu trinity, manifesting on earth in ten incar-

Appendix 3

                                nations (Rāma was the seventh and Buddha the ninth incarnation of Viṣṇu)

yakṣa[*]   dryad, tree spirit, giant

[*] Sanskrit; the other words are either Hindi or Tamil

Appendix 4
Thai Terms Used in the Text

akhom อาคม	Vedic speel
bap บาป	sin (accumulating bad *karma*)
bun บุญ	merit
chao khao เจ้าเขา	Lord of the Mountain
chao phi เจ้าผี	Spirit Lord; ancestor spirit
chao thi เจ้าที่	Lord of the Place
chao thung เจ้าทุ่ง	Lord of the Open Land
khao song เข้าทรง	to enter trance
khon song คนทรง	medium
khryang raeng กระยางแรง	talisman
khwan ขวัญ	vital essence
lak myang หลักเมือง	pillar of the city (inhabited by the city's guardian spirit)
len phi chan เล่นผี	to catch spirits
ma khi ม้าขี่	"horse of the spirit," spirit medium
mae ja nang แม่ย่านาง	Boat Mother
mae phosop แม่โพสพ	Rice Mother
mae thorani แม่ธรณี	Mother Earth
miang เมี่ยง	fermented tea, rolled into small cubes to be chewed as a stimulant
nai ariyaban นายอริยาบาน	chief jailer in hell, also called *phra jom phraban*
nam mon น้ำมนต์	*mantra* water, blessed water
ong องค์	sacred
phanung ผ้านุ่ง	cloth wrapped around the hips
phasin ผ้าซิ่น	"Chinese cloth," cloth wrapped around the hips (like Chinese would formerly do)
phi ผี	any kind of spirit, ghost, demon or deity
phi am ผีอำ	ghost who sits on the chest or liver of a sleeper
phi ca kla ผี	spirit in the shape of a jungle cat
phi chamob ผีชมอบ	ghost who haunts where a woman died in the jungle. It is harmless.
phi ha ผีห่า	violent spirit of a woman who died in childbirth

phi khamod ผีโขมด	spirit in the shape of a red star who misleads wanderers
phi khrut ผีครุฑ	Garuda, mythical bird; vehicle of Viṣṇu
phi king hoi ผีกิงห้อย	spirit in the shape of a vampire bat
phi kong koi ผีกองกอย	one-legged spirit
phi krahang ผีกระหัง	this ghost appears as a man with feathers and a tail like a bird. It eats filth and glows at night like the *phi krasy*. In northern and northeastern Thailand, this spirit is called *phi hoang*.
phi krasy ผีกระสือ	this spirit lives inside a witch and leaves her during sleep by her mouth, It has the color of fire, a head the size of an electric light bulb, and a half-a-meter-long bluish tail. It likes dirt and generally does not harm people, but when it consumes entrails, it can cause death. *Krasy* witches have a sleepy appearance during the day. Their eyes don't blink and they can never look anybody into the face. They also don't cast any reflection into a mirror. Before *krasy* witches can die they have to find somebody who inherits the *krasy* by eating the old *krasy*'s witches spittle.
phi kuman ผีกุมาร	spirit of an infant who died before or shortly after birth. If the infant is not properly buried, its *phi* may enter the mother's womb again. The corpse has to be put into a pot, closed with leaves and paper on which charms have been written, and set afloat on the next water course.
phi lang kluang ผีหลังกลวง	spirit through whose body one can see
phi ling lom ผีลิงลม	windborn monkey spirit
phi lok ผีหลอก	this spirit haunts certain places, misleading people. It can be seen as well as felt.
phi mahesak ผีมเหศักดิ์	*Mahasakka*, spirit of great power
phi nag ผีนาค	mythical serpent

Thai Terms Used in the Text

phi nang tai	ผีนางไต้	female tree spirit who may fill the alms-bowls of wandering monks (can reside in any wood but teak).
phi pa	ผีป่า	forest spirit; also spirit of someone who died away from home
phi phrai	ผีไพร	spirit of a woman who died in childbirth, the essence of *phi tai hong,* sometimes also called *phi phut*
phi phung tai	ผีพุ่งไต้	spirit in the shape of a shooting star
phi poang khang	ผีพ่วงข้าง	spirit in the shape of a black monkey
phi pret, peta	ผีเปรต	hungry ghost (those who have been preoccupied with attachments, e.g., with family, money, will be reborn as a *peta,* have a giant belly and a small mouth like the eye of a needle. A *peta,* may whistle at night looking for somebody to make merit for him.
phi ryan	ผีไร่อัน	guardian spirit who takes residence in a spirit house
phi sum	ผีสุ่ม	fish-trap ghost
phi ta haeg raeg	ผีตาแห้งแร้ง	spirit of the land
phi tai ha	ผีตายห่า	spirit of a woman who died of malaria. It will spread this disease.
phi tai hong	ผีตายโหง	headless spirit of one who died a violent death (e.g., in childbed, falling, being killed by a weapon or an animal)
phra phum	พระภูมิ	guardian spirit of the land (like the *chao thi*), ancestor spirit, spirit of the former owner of the land
phrai nam	พรายน้ำ	water spirit
phraya maccurat	พระยามัจจุราช	King of Death
phrom	พรหม	god from the higher heavens, one of the *Brahma* gods
su khwan	สู่ขวัญ	to propitiate the *khwan*
takrut	ตะกรุด	talisman in form of a small cylinder which contains a *mantra*
tham khwan	ทำขวัญ	to make the *khwan,* to fasten the *khwan* (to the body of its owner)
thao Wedsuwan or	ท้าวเวสสุวรรณ	*Kuween,* King of the Spirits; Guar-

Appendix 4

		dian of the Northern Direction; Kubera (in Sanskrit)
thevada	เทวดา	deity
thevada cuti	เทวดาจุติ	god who became a mortal rising from the tail of a green snake
wai khru	ไหว้ครู	to pay respect to one's teachers
wan phra	วันพระ	"monk's day"; Buddhist holiday, observed at the four phases of the moon
yak	ยักษ์	(fierce looking) giant (usually with an iron club); tree spirit; *yakṣa* (in Sanskrit)

Appendix 5
Chinese Festivals*

First month	On New Year's Eve slips of red paper are fastened slantwise on doors which should not be opened before dawn, so that happiness would not escape. Shoes are put down sole upward so that no god of epidemics can deposit germs of fatal diseases in them.
1st-15th day	Chinese New Year, Kong Hee Fatt Choy ("Wishing Prosperity")
	The 1st and 2nd day [Jan. 28-30, 1979] are celebrated with feasting and visiting relatives. Children receive their *ang pows*. Mandarin oranges are eaten as symbols of happiness. Brooms are hidden until the 5th day not to sweep luck away. The 3rd day is inauspicious, people stay home and feast.
	The 4th day, the gods return from heaven; celebration for the Kitchen God, Tsao-shen
	The 9th day [Feb. 4, 1979], celebration for the Jade Emperor, Yu Shang-ti
	The 10th day, celebration for Kuan Kong
	The 15th day, birthday of Siong Guan Tai Teh (scholar) and Chap Goh Meh; end of New Year's celebrations
16th day	birthday of Ts'oi T'in Tai Seng Yeh (Sun-heu-tze; The Great Sage of All Heavens, in English irreverantly called the Monkey God) [Feb. 12-13, 1979]
18th day	celebration for the Star God
Second month	
2nd day	birthday of Toa Peh Kong
15th day	celebration for Kuan Ti Kong

251

Appendix 5

19th day	birthday of Kuan Yin
23rd day	2nd birthday of Ts'oi T'in Tai Seng Yeh (see also 16th day of first month)
Third month	
3rd day	birthday of Siong Teh, celebrated for three days
1st week	Ching Ming (cleaning one's relatives graves)
23rd day	birthday of T'ien-hou (Queen of Heaven, also called Ma Chu P'oh or Ma Tsu, a Sea Goddess) (see Case 7)
Fourth month	
8th-9th day	birthday of Nor Cha Sam T'ai Tze (The Third Prince) [May 3-4, 1979]
Fifth month	
5th day	Dragon Boat Festival** [May 30, 1979]
11th day	birthday of Seng Ong Kong
13th day	birthday of Kuan Kong***
Sixth month	
6th day	consecration of Kam T'ien Siong Teh's temple (see Case 1)
19th day	2nd birthday of Kuan Yin (actually the day when she entered the nunnery) [July 22-23, 1978]
23rd day	celebration for the God of Fire, Hwo-shen Sheng-tan
Seventh month	(month of the "hungry ghosts")
1st day	opening of the Gates of Hell
6th day	celebration for the Weaver God
15th day	celebration for the Lord of Earth, also Feast of the Souls
21st day	celebration for Yama, God of Hell
24th day	consecration of Seng Ong Kong
Eighth month	
3rd day	birthday of the Kitchen God, Tsao-shen
15th day	moon festival# [Oct. 6, 1978]
15th-16th day	3rd birthday of Ts'oi T'in Tai Seng Yeh (see also 16th day of first month and 23rd day of second month) [Oct. 6-7, 1978]

Ninth month
1st-9th day   Festival of the Nine Imperial Gods [Oct. 21-29, 1978]## (see Case 7)
1st-15th day   pilgrimages to Kusu Island (Toa Peh Kong Temple and a Muslim keramat)
19th day   3rd birthday of Kuan Yin (day of her enlightenment)

Tenth month
15th day   birthday of Har Kuan Tai Teh (scholar)
18th day   celebration for the 18 Lohans (Buddhist saints)

Eleventh month
7th day   celebration for Kuan Peng Yak
15th day   celebration for Tung Chet
17th day   birthday of O-mi-t'o-fo (Amitābha Buddha)

Twelfth month
8th day   birthday of Mi-lo-fo (Buddha-to-come, Maitreya)
12th day   birthday of Kam T'ien Siong Teh
24th day   celebration for the Kitchen God, Tsao Chen; sending the gods off to heaven

---

*   According to the lunar calendar. Brackets indicate the dates according to the solar calendar, as celebrated in Singapore in 1978/1979.

**   The statesman and poet K'üh-yuen 屈原 (332-295 B.C.), native of the state of Ch'u 楚 (a large principality in the provinces of Hupeh and Honan), drowned himself in protest against injustice and corruption. Rice dumplings are eaten and also thrown into the water to symbolically lure fish away from the body of the martyr wherever Chinese live inside or outside of the borders of Mainland China. Dragon boat races are also held to reenact the search for his corpse in the waters of the Mih-lo 抇羅. See among others, Doré, First Part, Vol. V, 1918, pp. vii, 466, note 2, and pp. 649-50.

*** Actually the birthday of his son, Kuan-ping, but as a son's birthday should not be celebrated before his father's, Kuan Kong's birthday which is the 24th day of the sixth month was rescheduled.

\#   Moon cakes are eaten. In times of revolt against the Mongol dynasty, secret messages had been smuggled back and forth inside such cakes.

\#\#   The Nine Imperial Gods are Star Lords of the Northern Dipper and two invisible stars nearby. They cure ailments, bring luck and bestow wealth and longevity.

Appendix 6
Malay-Muslim Fextivals*

December
1st day of 1st month**   *Awal Muharram*
during the month   *Pesta Pulau Pinang* (carnival on the Island of Penang)

March
12th day of 3rd month   *Mawlid Al-Nabi* (Muḥammad's birthday)***
                         [March 3, 1979]

April
during the month   cultural festival at the seaport of Tanjung Kling

May
during the month   *Main Pantani* (rice harvest festival around Kuala Trenganu)
12th-13th day   harvest festival of the Kadazan in Sabah

June
1st-2nd day   Dayak harvest festival in Sarawak
6th day   birthday of H.M. the Yang Di Pertuang Agung, Head of State

---

*   As celebrated in Singapore, Malaysia, and Thailand in 1979. The dates vary from year to year according to the lunar calendar.

**   According to the Muslim calendar.

*** At Muḥammad's birthplace, a dome and minaret was first built by Khayzurān, mother of the Abbasid Caliph Harūn al-Rashid. It remained a place of sanctity till the Wahhabis took Mekka in 1344 (1425 A.D.). Dome and minaret were taken down and all ornaments removed in the firm belief that such representations are expressions of idolatry. Everything should be associated only with the worship of God. Legists and theologians opposed the celebration of Muhammad's birthday which is a later development, and was gradually adopted by many countries to satisfy public sentiment. Wahhabis oppose the day on principle. The day is usually celebrated with special prayers, recitation of the entire Qur'ān and literary compositions, called *mawlids*. There will be processions and almsgiving See S.G.F. Brandon, ed. *Dictionary of Comparative Religion*. New York: Charles Scribner's Sons, 1970.

Appendix 6

July
during the month [1979]   *Ramaḍān* (fasting from sunrise to sundown)

August
9th day   National Day in Singapore#
10th day *Dhul H'jza*   *Id Al-Adha* or *ab-id al Kabir*##
24th day   *Hari Raya Puasa* (end of fasting)
                Id Al-Fitr; in Thailand, *al-id al-saghir*###
31st day   *Hari Kebângsaan* (Malaysia National Day)

November
11th day   *Hari Raya Haji* (completing the last phase of one's pilgrimage)

\# Although Singapore became independent in 1965 and only 15 per cent of the population are Malay, this day is important for Singaporean Malay-Muslims.

\#\# This festival is an essential part of the pilgrimage rites, but is not confined to pilgrims alone. The rejoicing extends at some places in the Muslim world up to four days. People put on at least one new piece of clothes. Being the only occasion when Muslims sacrifice, Muslims are reminded of Abraham's readiness to obey God's command to sacrifice his son, Ishmael, at Mānā (place of pilgrimage). At that time, the Archangel Gabriel substituted a broadtailed sheep for Ishmael. When a Muslim family observes this sacrifice the animal is divided into three portions — one for relatives, one for the poor, and one for the family (see Brandon 1970).

\#\#\# On this day the breaking of the fast is celebrated. It is observed on the 1st *Shanwāl,* the end of *Ramadān.* Alms are given and gifts of food are exchanged with friends. People congregate for worship. There is an air of general rejoicing and mutual congratulations. The festival may extend to four days celebration. People will try again to wear at least one piece of new clothes (see Brandon 1970).

Appendix 7
Hindu, Mainly Tamil, Festivals

Month	Time	Festival	Location*	Temple
Chithirai** (April-May)	full moon	*Chithirai Paruvam* (prayers to the dead, also propitiating Citragupta, recordkeeper of Yama)	Teluk Anson	Subramanya
	9 days of bright half when sun enters Medam (Aries)	*Srī Rāma Navami* Hindu New Year (*Ugathi*, Telegu New Year; *Varasha Prappu*, Tamil New Year; *Vishu*, Malayalee New Year)	Parit Buntar	Jevi
Vaikasi (May-June)	full moon	*Vaikasi Visakam* (prayers to Viṣṇu; Yama, and Dharmagupta)	Ipoh	Subramanya
Aani (June-July)	***	*Śiva*; also *Varalakṣmī Viratham* (prayers to Lakṣmī)		All Śiva temples
Aadi (July-Aug.)	8th day of dark half	*Srī Krisna Jayanti* (Krisna's birthday)	Taiping	Chettiar
	***	*Adi Puram*		Subramanya
		Adi Vel		Vinayaga
Aavani (August-September)	14th day of bright half asterism Thiruvanam in ascendance#	*Vinayaga Chathurthi* (creation of Ganesa) harvest	Seremban	
	full moon	*Onam* (Malayalee harvest festival; also commemorating Mahabali)		
Puratassi (September-October)	***	*Navarātri* (nine nights; three nights each to Pārvatī, Lakṣmī, Sarasvātī, manifestations of the same goddess)	Singapore	Tiru Mariamman Thandayuth
	***	*Timiti*# (fire walking)	Singapore	Tiru Mariamman
Aippasi (October-November)	14th day of dark half	*Dipavali* (festival of lights)		
	6th day of bright half	*Kantha Shashti* (in honor of Subramanya/Murugan)	Kuala Pilah	Kandasamy
Karthikai (November-December)	full moon	*Kartikai Dipam* (fire walking)	Singapore	Subramanya
		Tirukarthukai		
Markali (December-January)	***	*Thiruvembavai*		

257

Appendix 7

Month	Time	Festival	Location*	Temple
Thai (January–February)	first four days	*Makara Sankranti*, *Thai Pongal* (agricultural festival) *Thamilar Vila* (Tamil festival)		
	when asterism Pūṣam is on ascendance##	*Thaipusam* (keeping vows made to Murugan/Subramanyam)	Kuala Lumpur Penang Singapore	Batu Malai Thannirmali Thandayuthapani
Masi (February–)	14th day of dark half	*Mahā Śivarātri* (prayers to Śiva)		
	when asterism Māgha is on ascendance##	*Māsi Magham* (prayers to Murugan/Subramanyam)	Malacca Muar Johore	Sannyasi Malai Subramanya Mariamman
Panguni (March–April)	full moon	*Panguni Uttaram*, *Kalyana Viratrham* (celebrating the marriage of Subramanya and Theivanai)	Singapore Sentul (Selangor) Kuantan	Balasubramma Subramanya Marathandavan

Source: Arasaratnam (1966) and the priests of the various temples, also Cooper and Kumar (1979)

* These festivals may be celebrated at any other location too, but the celebrations at these locations draw a larger crowd from different regions. This list contains only places in Malaysia and Singapore.

** These are the Tamil names for the twelve months. Other Hindus use the following Sanskrit names: Caitra (March-April), Vaiśākha (April-May), Jyaiṣṭa (May-June), Āṣāḍha (June-July), Śrāvana (July-August), Bhādrapada (August-September), Aśvina (September-October), Kārttika (October-November), Mārgaśira (November-December), Pauṣa (December-January), Māgha (January-February), Phālguna (February-March). According to the occasion, names appear either in Tamil or in Sanskrit.

*** These festival days are set down in an almanac *(Panchangam)* which is published at the beginning of each year.

\# Timiti is celebrated after six weeks of preparations (on the first Monday the flag of Hanuman is hoisted in front of the shrine of Draupadi, there will be processions, and readings of the Mahābhārata at night, every following Monday. On the second Monday, e.g., the engagement of Draupadi to Arjuna; on the third Monday, Draupadi's marriage to Arjuna; on the fourth Monday, the undressing of Draupadi; on the fifth Monday, Aravan Pujai, etc will be the themes.

\#\# The lunar zodiac is divided into twenty-seven *nakṣatras* (asterisms).

258

Appendix 8
Thai Festivals*

April
6th day   Chakri Day (the present dynasty was founded on this day)
13th-15th day   *Songkran* or *Pi Mai* (lunar New Year)

May
5th day   anniversary of the coronation of Rama IX (the present king)
full moon   *Visakha Pūja* (commemorating Buddha's birth, enlightenment, and death)
one week later   Buddha's cremation is commemorated

June
**   *Raek Na* (First Ploughing)
**   first fruit are offered to monks
24th day   National Day

July
**   Wai Khru (paying respect to one's teachers)
full moon   *Khao Phansa* (beginning of Buddhist Lent; 21-year-old men may be ordained for one rainy season)
**   rice planting

August
**   rice planting may continue until the middle of this month
12th day   Queen's Birthday

September
**   presentation of milk and honey to monks; *Og Phansa* (end of rainy season; young men leave monkhood)

October
23rd day   Chulalongkorn Day
**   *Kathin* (presentation of robes to monks)

November
full moon   *Loy Krathong* (festival of lights), *Chalong Trai Pi* (royal presentation of robes to monks)

Appendix 8

December
5th day — King's Birthday
10th day — Constitution Day
January
1st day — *Pi Mai* (solar New Year)
February
full moon — *Magha Pūja****
March
** — Blessing the Rice Seed
January through March, pilgrimages are made to distant *wats* (monasteries)

Sources: Rama V *Account of the Royal Ceremonies of the Twelve Months* [Ruang Phra Rajabidhi Sip Song Dyang], 1888, and a mimeographed publication of the Christian Student Movement, Chiang Mai, 1969-70.

* Most of the Thai festivals are calculated according to the lunar calendar.
** These ceremonies are conducted on auspicious days determined by the Court brahmin.

Notes

Part 1
Theoretical Considerations

Chapter 1
Who Is a Shaman?

[1] I decided not to use the regular plural "media" to avoid confusion between "mass media" that are technological means to disseminate information and "mediums" who, as human agents, relay messages from the spiritual world.

[2] During the Tamil month of Thai (*Thaipusam*, January–February), Hindu devotees carry *kavadis*. A *kavadi* may be anything from a relatively small wooden yoke to a sixty-pound steel frame, attached with 108 hooks to the body of the devotee. The shape of the frame is supposed to symbolize Lord Murgam's steed, the peacock.

In Singapore, devotees walk, for example, from the Perumai Temple on Serangoon Road to the Thandayuthapani Temple on Tank Road (see also Babb 1976). In Malaysia, they walk from the Maha Mariamman Temple at High Street in Kuala Lumpur to the Batu Caves, eight miles outside of the city, and, in Penang, to the temple on Waterfall Road.

[3] In October, Hindu devotees practice *Timiti* (*Pookulittal*, "walk on a bed of flowers," i.e., walk on fire). In Singapore, 1979, for example, at Sri Mariamman Temple, South Bridge Road, over eight hundred Hindu walked on fire (personal observation; see also Figs 1 and 2, and Babb 1974a).

[4] Especially during the Lenten season, Jesus Christ "comes" to some Chinese mediums in Singapore. They are also "visited" by Nepalese Buddhas, even Amitābha Buddha. When Christ "arrives," the mediums assume the posture of Christ on the Cross. They are then given water to drink to ease their pain. The manifestation of Christ's suffering is the only function of such events (personal observation at several occasions with different mediums at a temple on Upper Serangoon Road in 1978/1979, see also Part 2, Case 5).

[5] As has been said before, it cannot be proven scientifically whether a spirit enters, i.e., "possesses," the body of a medium or whether the spirits are projections of the

medium's unconscious. Psychiatrists will talk about "split personality" or "dissociation," without recognizing that such alternate states of consciousness are accessed and exited at will and may indicate a transition, necessary for the mental and spiritual growth of that individual. (See also Chapter 3.4.3–4, and the Glossary).

[6] See, among others, Bourguignon (1966) who distinguishes between trances with and without the element of possession.

[7] On September 12, 1978, I witnessed a tiger possession in Pattani, southern Thailand (see Part 2, Case 14e and Fig.37).

Horse possession are reported among Malay, e.g., in Johore Bahru and Singapore. See also Zainul-Abidin Bin Ahman (1922), *The Citizen* (September 16, 1978), and Part 2, Case 10; also Figs 30–32).

Chapter 2
The Social Setting

[1] These data have been extracted from available Thailand Yearbooks, issued by the Thai government.

[2] Three per cent (approximately 21 million) of the over 700 million Muslims today live in China, mainly in the Provinces of Shensi and Kansi. Muslims entered China on the trade routes across Central Asia from the 9th century A.D. on. Kublai Khan (1260–1294) also recruited Muslims to suppress Tibetan rebels. See, among others, Forces (1976).

[3] Ninety-nine per cent of the Thai Muslims are Sunn'ites and only 1 per cent Shi'ites ("Partisans of Ali"). Shi'ites recognize only the descendants of Ali, Muhammad's son-in-law, the fourth caliph, as legitimate successors of the prophet. They believe in continued revelations and have messianic expectations. Sunn'ites, in contrast, are dedicated to the *Sunna* (Law). They adhere to the orthodox Muslim traditions and believe in historical succession.

[4] When not indicated otherwise, facts and figures were taken from *Information Malaysia*, the Incorporating Malaysia Year Book 1976/77.

[5] These facts and figures can be found in the Singapore Census 1976 and in Chen (1978).

Chapter 3
Elements of Shamanism

[1] For different kinds of alternate states of consciousness, see Sections IV:3–4 of

this chapter and the Glossary.

² *Brahmins* inherit their caste and office. Not all Hindu shamans and mediums in Malaysia and Singapore, however, belong to the *brahmin* caste. Even when they do not master the proper *brahmin* rituals, they will attempt to simulate brahmanical customs and repeat what they saw *brahmins* perform in Hindu temples. The same is valid for Thailand.

³ *T'ang* means actually a household altar.

⁴ The money for the Kiew Lee Tong Temple on Upper Thompson Road, Singapore, inaugurated on March 12, 1979, was, for example, donated by a member of parliament, Mr. Yeo Toon Chie. The old temple on Queen Street had to be torn down in the course of city planning and the place of worship was relocated several miles away from the old site.

⁵ These HDB flats are subsidized by the government. Where workers and employees with low salaries cannot afford a HDB apartment, the government will pay the difference.

⁶ Malays believe "that every letter, word and verse in the Holy Qur'an has two meanings — the one generally taught by religious instructors and an esoteric one, hidden from most eyes, but revealed to certain adepts . . . . This esoteric knowledge, if coupled with complete faith in the unlimited power inherent in the Holy Word, enables the possessor to achieve results that are generally classified as miracles." Such concepts are known to other ethnic groups and other religions as well, e.g., "through the knowledge of a secret Great Name of God . . . . Moses was able to divide the Red Sea" (Shaw 1975:3).

⁷ On divining blocks, see also Elliott (1955:39) and Dore (Part ONE, III, 1916:353).

⁸ For use of charm papers, see also Comber (1957:47) and Dore (Part ONE, III, 1916:ii–iii).

⁹ When an individual was not able to solve a predicament himself, the Buddha suggested to recite a *sutta* (Pāli; Sanskrit, *sūtra*). A *sutta* is one of the 84,000 sermons of the historical Buddha, memorized during his life time. The Buddhist canon was then codified at different Buddhist Councils after his death. Together with the *Vinaya* (rules of discipline) and the *Abhidhamma* (metaphysical teachings), the *suttas* were transmitted orally for over four hundred years to be finally written down on Sri Lanka in the first century B.C. The *suttas* are the second "basket" of the *Tipitaka* (The Three Baskets of the *Theravāda* Canon).

On *pareitta suttas* (magical passages from the Buddhist Canon), see, among others, Spiro (1967), Tambiah (1968, 1970, 1973) and Heinze (1982a).

Notes

[10] See, among others, Benjamin (1974:2), Danaraj (196) and Winstedt (1961).

[11] The Koran 53:19–22 condemns the worship of three pre-Islamic deities, however, *Sura 71*, revealed to the Prophet at Mecca approximately in 620 A.D., some two years before his *hijra* (flight to Medina), is entitled, *The Jinn*. The word *jinn* comes from the Arabic *jann* ("covering, covertness, veiling and darkness," but also "something that lies hidden in the womb like an embryo"). "The extent of a jinn's power and knowledge is great . . . although . . . hidden from humans. While a few jinns (who are 'believers') are benevolent, many of them are destructive and highly amoral beings . . . . Jinn . . . having a logic of their own . . . also belong to the covered part of the human nature . . . the id" (Kakar 1982:25).

Twenty-two verses of the Koran mention *jinns*, sixty-eight verses speak of *al-Shaitan* (Satan, singular) and seventeen of *al-Shaiatin* (devils, plural).

Shah Wali-Allah Dihlawi (1703–1762), a great orthodox Muslim reformer, advised which verses from the *jinn* chapter of the Koran should be recited to expel *jinns* from a house (see S.A.A. Rizvi, "Aspects of Islamic Folk Traditions in the Indian Subcontinent," paper presented at the Xth International Congress for Anthropological and Ethnological Sciences, Delhi, December 1978). - About the magical quality of verses from the Koran, see also footnote 10 in Chapter 3.

The *hadith* literature on *jinns* is enormous. (The *hadith* are sayings of the Prophet and traditional stories that aid in governing Islamic life. They interpret the Koran.)

It is believed that *jinns* have airy or fiery bodies. They can assume whatever shape they wish.

[12] Although the caste system has been declared unconstitutional in 1948, caste still plays a role in Indian life, e.g., in selecting a spouse and in religious rituals.

[13] Pāli, "those who adhere to the Word of the Elders." The *Theravadin* are the only extant school of the early eighteen Buddhist schools of thought. See also, Glossary, under *Buddhism*.

[14] The Three Worlds are *kama loka* (World of Desire), *rupa loka* (World of Form), and *arupa loka* (World Without Form). Deities can be reborn in one of the six heavens of *kama loka* or one of the sixteen heavens of *rupa loka*.

[15] For more detailed explanations of technical terms, see the Glossary.

[16] Liu-pei is said to have been a native of Choh-chow in the north of Chihli (see Dore, Part One, V, 1918:497–499).

[17] Chapters One to Forty of this novel have been translated into German by Wilhelm Grube under the title *Metamorphosen der Goetter* (see, Comber 1958:28–29; Manson 1965; and personal communication, Professor Wolfram Eberhard, Berkeley, March 1980).

Chapter 4
Socio-Psychological Considerations

[1] See, "How bomohs work," *The Asia Magazine*, Part 2, 2 April 1975, and the report on the Symposium on Neurological Sciences in Kuala Lumpur, 11 April 1975.

[2] See, Part 2, Case 3, also Ackerman and Lee (1978:24–35), Kok (1975:35–38), and Lewis (1971:32) who spoke of peripheral cults which "commonly embrace downtrodden categories of men who are subject to strong discrimination in rigidly stratified societies." He found "peripheral cults" are "far from being a secure female monopoly." Important is that he felt such cults "cannot be explained plausibly in terms of any innate tendency in hysteria on the part of women." Kok (1975) also mentioned that in some cases he studied the women did not show any previous symptoms of hysteria. Furthermore, mass hysteria is a phenomenon not a cult.

[3] See, Hinderling (1973) who got similar answers when he studied communication between doctors and patients in Thailand. Kleinman reported that "Chinese medicines have fewer side effects than Western medicines. Western medicine works much quicker, but it only removes symptoms. It does not, like Chinese medicine, remove the underlying cause of illness. . . . Chinese medicine may not help you sometimes, but it won't hurt you. Western medicine may remove your symptoms or illness, but sometimes the treatment is worse than the illness" (1980:87).

[4] A social worker at Woodbridge Hospital told me in Spring 1979 that she works monthly on 400 cases. She has to talk to families to take former mental patients back. She assists patients to be trained in skills according to their faculties, and she attempts to find employers willing to give them a chance.

[5] See, Heinze (1974:125–34 and 1982a-94–109); also Spiro (1965) on "Religious Systems as Cultural Constituted Defense Mechanisms."

Part 2
Shamanic Practices:
A Case History Approach

[1] Whether the language of the spirit was actually medieval Hokkien was not confirmed by outside observers.

[2] The Siong Lim Temple is located in Jalan Tao Payo. It is one of the largest Chinese temples in Singapore. Built in 1902 by two Hokkien merchants who came

from Amoy, it has been restored at a cost of 1 million Singapore dollars. The temple is dedicated to the 18 Lohans (allegedly former bandits who became converted to Buddhism; see also Dore, Second Part, VII, 1922:332–287).

[3] He speaks of the temple described in Case 3. The name *Namoputaya* can be translated with "Hail Buddha." His first visit to this temple took place in 1976, three years before he wrote this account.

[4] Outside the liminal state of *communitas* shared with shamans, mediums, and healer, client hesitate to talk about their problems. Kleinman (1980) confirmed the difficulties in following up healing and other success stories.

[5] This calculation is based on the lunar calendar. In the solar calendar, it is approximately beginning of October.

[6] The word "dipper" refers not only to the stellar constellation and the residences of the Nine Imperial Gods but means also a bowl with a handle, used in temples for offerings. Schafer (1977) mentions, furthermore, that Chinese saw the constellation of Ursa Major as being the chariot of celestial beings.

[7] See Dore who mentioned that when Marīcī is represented with three heads in China and Japan, the one on the right will be a sow's head. The sow head in India is always on the left. "Besides being the Goddess of Dawn, she is also deemed to protect nations from the fury of war" (Second Part, VII, 1922:303–311).

[8] Chun-ti appears as a Taoist in Chapter 65 of the novel *Feng-shen yen-i* (Metamorphoses of the Gods). He allegedly lived at the end of the Shang and the beginning of the Chou Dynasty (according to the new chronology around 1050 B.C.). In Chapter 71 of the above-mentioned novel he rides a peacock and in Chapter 78 he presents the "Doctrine of the West." A modern "Study of the Landman Organizations" (*Tung-hsang tsu-chih-chi yen-chiu*), p.45, mentions him as a deity in the clubhouse of the businessmen of Kiangsu, Chekiang. I would like to express my gratitude to Professor Wolfram Eberhard who brought these references to my attention.

[9] Schipper reported that, at a Taoist ceremony in Taiwan, five or more votive oil lamps played an important part. They were called "*tou-teng*, bushel lamps . . . . These lamps symbolize *fate*: bushel = measure = the Dipper = the controller of Destiny." There is a connection between representatives of the community and the bushel lamps, "because each lamp represents the destiny of a given representative; together they stand for the fate of the community." In general, there will be five main dignitaries, "The title of the last of the five, Head of the Lamp of Heaven, refers to another votive lamp, which unlike the tou-teng is placed outside, in front of the temple, where it hangs on a long bamboo pole" (Schipper 1974:318).

¹⁰ For a discussion of the custom of tying the wrists (a) to keep out evil, (b) to keep one's vital essence inside, and (c) to seal a contract with a god or gods, see Heinze (1982a: 76–84).

¹¹ A printed version of this speech was distributed during the ceremonial dinner to which I had been invited by the temple committee. I am grateful to Professor Wolfram Eberhard and Stephen Bokenkamp who assisted in preparing this translation.

¹² The ten Buddhist precepts can be compared with the Ten Commandments in Judaism and Christianity, the first Buddhist precept being "to abstain from taking life" (do not kill). Buddhist laymen usually keep the first five precepts. Only on special days, they vow to observe all ten. Buddhist monks and nuns, of course, observe many more precepts, *Theravāda* monks, for example, observe 227 rules of discipline.

¹³ The sun, the moon and the five planets, plus Rahu and Ketu.

¹⁴ In the *Dictionary of Chinese Buddhist Terms* (Soothill 1975) we find the explanation that (1) all those who observe the first five percepts will be reborn in the world of man; (2) all those who practice the ten forms of good action will be reborn in one of the heavens, i.e., will become gods; (3) all those who practice the Four Noble Truth will become Buddhist disciples; (4) all those who practice the twelve *nidānas* will become Pratyeka Buddhas, and (5) all those who practice the five *paramitas* (perfections) will become Buddhas or *bodhisattva*. The speaker in Singapore put men and gods into the same category but *bodhisattvas* and Buddhas into two different groups.

¹⁵ It is believed that many Buddhas have manifested on this earth before the historical Buddha appeared. According to *Theravāda* tradition, he lived from 623–543 B.C. in Magadha, the present Indian state of Bihar (other scholars say he lived from 563–483 B.C.). It is believed that more Buddhas will materialize in the future and Maitreya will be the next Buddha-to-come.

¹⁶ Sanskrit, "Earth Treasure," one of the eight *dyani* (transcendent, produced by meditation) *bodhisattvas*. Probably first a female deity, Kṣitigarbha became the guardian of the earth. He is associated with Yama who rules over the dead in the ten hells. From the 5th century A.D. on, Kṣitigarbha started to play the role of a savior who delivers sufferers from the hells which, in Chinese belief, are located in Central China.

¹⁷ In Sanskrit, *anuttara samyak sambodhi.*

¹⁸ As has been mentioned in Part 1 of this book that Hindu deities became the protectors of Buddhism. They live in one of the 22 heavens and are in need of

salvation themselves. After they have enjoyed the fruit of their good *karma,* they are reborn on earth to cultivate themselves until all defilements have been removed and they enter *nirvāṇa.*

[19] During the festival, vendors of fish and birds are available to give devotees an opportunity "to release life."

[20] Harada mentionsed especially Liu Kuo Win, a scholar residing in Penang, as well as Chu Chin T'ao. Citing Taoist scriptures, he talks about Yun Chi Ch'i Ch'ien, Chiu Huang Tou Mu Shuo, Chieh Sha Yen Sheng Chen Chin, and Chiu Huang Hsian Ching Chu Chieh.

[21] The society observes Spring Day as the Day of Celebration for three significant events, namely, (1) the founding of the World Red Swastika Society, (2) the taking of the Holy Picture, and (3) the revelation of the Sacred Scriptures. Readers will note that Spring Day celebrations do not correlate with the date (November 21, 1921) when the Holy Picture was taken.

[22] The ouija board got its name from the word "yes" which in French is "oui" and in German "ja." It was invented after the planchette had already been used for similar purposes. The letters of the alphabet are arranged in a half circle on the board, while a movable piece, touched lightly by two individuals, will start sliding into the direction of certain characters and spell out the answer.

[23] Among them was Charles E. Cory, chairman of the Department of Philosophy, Washington University, who investigated Mrs. Curran for three years and published his report in the September issue of *Psychological Review* (Litvag 1972:278–288).

[24] IPL is the abbreviation used for the inferior temporal lobule of each of the two hemispheres of the human brain.

[25] See also Isaiah 28.11, Joel, the four Gospels, the Psalms (e.g., 51:10, 11:63:3, 5, 139:1, 5, 1, 150), the Acts and Paulus (Corinthians I, 14:21, etc.).

[26] The other groups in Singapore are located at Balestier Road, Aljunied Road, Jurong Road, Onraet Road, Sime Road, Pasir Panjang, and Henderson Road.

[27] The present Thai king, Rama IX, was ordained for two weeks in 1946, shortly before his coronation.

[28] God of the Hindu trinity; Brahmā being the creator, Śiva the destroyer (of the corrupted world so that a new world can be created), and Viṣṇu the preserver.

[29] A famous monk who became Sangharaja during the reign of King Monkut in the middle of last century (see also Case 17).

[30] Ceylonese chronicles report that, in approximately 250 B.C., the Indian Emperor Asoka sent his son, Prince Mahinda, and his daughter, Princess Sanghamitta,

to Sri Lanka to spread Buddhism on this island. When the two Indian envoys arrived, many nature spirits converted to Buddhism.

[31] A mythical serpent. *Nāgas* are believed to preserve esoteric knowledge and to act as protectors of the *Dhamma*.

[32] Whoever can afford it in Thailand, has not only concubines but also a second wife. A law has already been passed which grants children of second wives part of their father's inheritance.

Glossary

Aboulis - Loss of will power.
Acculturation - in contrast to enculturation:
  1. acquisition of cultural items from other ethnic groups;
  2. process of becoming adapted to a new or different culture;
  3. process of wittingly or unwittingly assuming behavioral patterns and modes of thinking from other in-groups.

Agnosis (first used by Freud) - Absence of recognition.
Allotheism - Worship of foreign or unsanctioned gods.
Alter - Concept of other self or person as distinct from the individual self.
Altered states of consciousness (ASC) - "Any mental state(s), induced by various physiological, psychological, or pharmacological maneuvers or agents, which can be recognized subjectively by the individual himself (or by an objective observer of the individual) as representing a sufficient deviation in subjective experience or psychological functioning from certain general norms for that individual during alert, waking consciousness. This sufficient deviation may be represented by a greater preoccupation than usual with internal sensations or mental processes, changes in the formal characteristics of thought, and impairment of reality testing to various degrees" (Ludwig in Tart, 1969:9–10).

Each ASC has state-specific properties (Tart, 1969, 1986).

Amnesia - Partial or total loss of memory (sometimes including personal identity), due to brain injury, shock, fatigue, repression, illness, or induced by anesthesia.
Analgesis - Loss of the sense of pain.
Anesthesia -
  1. Partial or total loss of the sensation of pain, esp. to touch, resulting from a lesion in the nervous system or from some other abnormality;
  2. partial or total loss of sensation and consciousness without loss of vital functions, artificially produced by the administration of one or more agents to block the passage of pain impulses along the nerve pathways to the brain, causing temporary dullness of perception or sensitivity.

Animism -
  1. a. Attribution of conscious life to nature and natural objects;

b. doctrine that all life is produced by a spiritual force separate from matter;
   c. belief in the existence of spirits separable from bodies;
2. a. worship of the souls of men and animals (necrolatry);
   b. worship of spiritual beings who are not permanently associated with certain bodies or objects (spiritism);
   c. worship of spiritual beings who cause permanent or periodically recurring phenomena of nature (naturism; Hastings 1921).
3. Belief in spirits presumably standing "behind" and determining the behavior of natural objects, artifacts, animals, and men. This is the first level of abstraction from the pre-animist magical belief in extraordinary, i.e., charismatic, forces (Weber 1951:298).

Aphasia -
1. Incapacity of coherent utterances, not caused by structural impairment of the vocal organs, but by lesion of the cerebral centers for speech. Distinguishable from
2. congenital or acquired *aphonia*, due to paralysis or imperfect approximation of the vocal cords, and
3. hysterical mutism, when the patient is obstinately and involuntarily silent, although the vocal organs are uninjured and the cerebral centers of speech are only functionally affected.

Aphonia - Loss of voice due to an organic or functional disorder.

Apotheosis -
1. Raising a human being to the rank of a god, deification;
2. glorification of a person, thing or idea.

Apotropaic - Designed to ward off evil.

Apport - Object moved by non-physical means from one place to another; sometimes, allegedly, passing through walls.

Archetype -
1. Original pattern or model from which all other things of the same kind are fashioned;
2. in scholastic philosophy: idea of the divine intellect determining the form of an object;
3. in psychoanalysis: "The unconscious [is] the totality of all psychic phenomena that lack the quality of consciousness. These psychic contents might fittingly be called 'subliminal' on the assumption that every psychic content must possess a certain energy value in order to become conscious" (first used by Jung 1960:133).

Jung called factors and motifs "that arrange the psychic elements into certain images" archetypal. They can be "recognized only from the effects they produce . . . . They may be compared to the invisible presence of the crystal lattice in a saturated solution. As *a priori* conditioning factors they represent a special, psychological instance of the biological 'patterns of behavior,' which give all living organisms their specific qualities" (1958:149).
4. Archetypes can be called energy potentials which are culturally conditioned during the process of rising to the conscious level of individuals and groups (Heinze 1996).
5. Archetypes have been compared with the Platonic *eidos,* taught by Dionysius the Areopagite. They are mentioned also in the Corpus Hermeticum (Jung 1960:136, footnote 8).
6. When Harding (1965:136) recognized the patterns of continuous action in the modes of nesting and migration of birds, she tried to establish the connection to the mythologem of man.

Asceticism -
1. Rigorous abstention from self-indulgence;
2. voluntary renouncement of sensual pleasures;
3. disciplinary course of action toward an intellectual, moral, and/or religious goal (for a monk otherwordly, for a puritan innerworldly; Weber 1951:291).

Astral body - In theosophy: subtle contour of the physical body, usually not separating from it in life but surviving after death.

Astral plane - In theosophy: plane from where various intelligences (e.g., souls of dead people, demons, and fire-born spirits) control the movements of stars and planets.

Aura -
1. Particular atmosphere or quality that seems to arise from and surround a person or thing;
2. commonly: colors around a person which reflect his/her personal characteristics and mood;
3. in medicine: warning sensation which precedes a seizure or other neurological disorders. It may be a feeling of light air, or tingling, ascending from within the body or the limbs to the head; or it may be flashes of light, noises in the ear, etc.;
3. in occultism: form of astral body (or astral spirit) allegedly visible to those who declare it to be so. Wallnofer (1965:178) agrees that this is open to

argument, but mentions an indefinable aura which makes it sometimes possible to diagnose a person's condition.

Autism -
1. Brain disorder which causes inability to use language or filter and process information;
2. extreme withdrawal from others, excluding reality while indulging in wishful thinking, and bizarre behavior like spinning and head-banging.

Automatism -
1. Physiologically: action of an organ or living body which is not immediately due to any change in the circumstances in which the organ or the body is placed but is the result of changes arising in the organ or the body itself, determined by causes other than the influences of the circumstances of the moment, e.g., the working of the will;
2. psychologically: action determined in an organism apart from the central will or control of that organism, e.g., visual or auditory hallucinations; messages written without intention; glossolalia; automatic writing; reflex cerebral action or unconscious cerebration.

Automatic Writing - see **Automatism**.

Automnesia - Spontaneous revival of memories of an earlier condition of life.

Autonomic Nervous System - Located in the cranial region near the pituitary gland, it regulates bodily functions autonomously, i.e., it cannot be controlled by the will. Closely related to the hormone-forming glands, it consists of the sympathetic system (acting mainly as the "stimulator") and the parasympathetic system ("preserver of the finer, constructive functions") of the body. Both regulate the nervous control and balance of the viscera—such as heart, lungs, guts—by traveling to the organs together and interacting there, often antagonistically. Sometimes the parasympathetic nerves become stimulators, and vice versa; for instance, the intestinal movement of contracting waves is effected by the stimulating action of the parasympathetic nerves on the smooth muscles of the gut, and the inhibiting action of the sympathetic nerves (Wallnofer 1965:175).

Recent research, however, has revealed that the autonomic nervous system is only relatively independent and can be influenced by imagery (Achterberg 1985).

Autopoiesis - Concept of self-organization.

Belief - Emotional acceptance of a proposition or doctrine, implicitly considered to be adequate, with varying degree of subjective certitude.

Glossary

Bibliolatry -
1. Excessive veneration or absolute dependence on sacred writings, considered to be infallible;
2. maintaining the view that no revelation is possible outside the Bible.

Bioplasma - Fifth state of matter (the other four being—solid, liquid, gaseous, plasma): part of each organisms' biofield, consisting of ions, free electrons, and free protons, highly conductive and providing opportunities for the accumulation and transfer of energy within the organism as well as among different organisms; concentrated in the brain and the spinal cord.

Black hole - Collapsed star which creates a gravity well so powerful that light cannot escape and the star becomes invisible.

Buddhism - Teaching of the historical Buddha who lived from 623 to 543 B.C. in Magadha (presently the State of Bihar in northern India). He taught that suffering is inherent in life and can only be eliminated through mental and moral self-purification (The Four Noble Truths, the fourth being the Eightfold Noble Path).

Theravåda ("The Word of the Elders") is derogatively called *H¥nayåna* ("The Lesser Vehicle") by Mahåyåna Buddhists. Codified after the death of the Buddha in a series of councils, the canonical language is Påli. After an oral tradition of nearly 500 years, the Påli Canon was put into writing on Ceylon during the reign of King Vattagamani (89–77 B.C.). The first 300 years after the Buddha's death, the practice of Buddhism was limited to the regions in which the Buddha had taught in Northern India. Approximately 250 B.C., after having conquered and unified all provinces of India, Emperor Asoka began to sponsor missionary activities. According to Ceylonese chronicles, one of his sons, Mahinda, went to Ceylon and two monks, Phra Sona and Phra Uttara, were sent to *Suvarnabhumi* (the "Golden Territories," presumably southern Burma, Sumatra or Takuapa on the east coast of the Malayan Peninsula). - At present, only 0.2 per cent of all Indians are Buddhists. Buddhism was absorbed into Hinduism and had declined in India already before Muslims (Ghorid Turks) began to invade the subcontinent in 1175. Revival movements during the 1800s were mainly sparked by Ceylonese monks. The fact that Dr. Ambedkar, together with a large number of untouchables, converted to Buddhism in 1956, marks another phase of Buddhist developments in India. *Theravåda* traditions have been kept alive mainly on Sri Lanka (Ceylon), in Burma, Thailand, Laos, and Cambodia, though Laotian and Cambodian Buddhists

Glossary

have suffered during the reign of socialist governments in the second half of the 20th century.

Mahāyāna ("The Greater Vehicle") consolidated approximately 200 years after the Buddha's death. First written down in the 1st century A.D. in Sanskrit, *vaipulya* ("expanded") *sūtras* ("thread; discourse") expounded on the metaphysics of the Buddha's teachings and basic concepts were reinterpreted. *Mahāyāna* Buddhists, e.g., speak of a *bodhisattva* ("Buddha-to-be") who forgoes his own salvation to save all sentient beings while *Theravadin* remind of the last words of the Buddha, "work out your own salvation with diligence" (*Digha Nikaya, Mahaparinibbana Sutta*). - *Mahāyāna* was introduced to Central Asia along the trade routes to China when the Kushans ruled India in the 1st century A.D. From Central Asia, it spread to China and later to Siberia, Korea, and Japan. In the 7th century A.D., *Mahāyāna* entered Tibet from India. From the 8th to the 13th century A.D., it was also practiced in Cambodia, Vietnam, Java, Sumatra, and on the Malayan Peninsula. Because the Khmer ruled at that time over part of the Central Plain and the northeast of Thailand, and the supremacy of Sailendra (predominantly Malay) rulers was recognized in southern Thailand, traces of *Mahāyāna* remained in these regions. *Mahāyāna* continued to be practiced in Vietnam, side by side with Confucian, Taoist, and later Christian beliefs.

Tantrayana, also called *Vajrayana*. developed in the 6th century A.D. in northern India. It promised health, wealth, and power as well as full enlightenment in this life (some schools included the actual consummation of wine, meat, and sexual intercourse). When Padmasambhava brought Buddhism to Tibet in the 8th century, it absorbed features of the earlier Bon religion and developed a rich culture of visualizations, guiding, e.g., the souls of the dead through the Bardo (period between reincarnations).

Catalepsy - Intermittent neurosis, characterized by the inability to change the position of a limb, sometimes induced as a stage of hypnosis.

Catharsis -
1. Purification of emotions (pity, fear, etc.) that leads to honestly facing the cause of difficulties, facilitating spiritual renewal;
2. satisfying release of tension which brings repressed feelings and ideas to the surface (into consciousness).

Channeling - (in new-age belief) Conveying messages from the spiritual world.

Charisma -
1. Greek: "gift of love";

2. supernatural power attributed to a person or office regarded as having a special relationship to what is considered to be of ultimate value;
3. faculty of a leader capable of eliciting enthusiastic, popular support, symbolically unifying and directing human affairs;
4. in theology: spiritual gift or talent, divinely granted to an individual as token of grace, e.g., in Christianity: the power of healing, speaking in tongues, and prophesying.

Chrematistic - Pertaining to the acquisition of wealth.

Chronomantics - Magical belief and practice believing in "auspicious" and "inauspicious" hours and times.

Clairvoyance - Perception of objects and objective events without any known sensory process.

Clinical -
1. In medicine: pertaining to direct, analytical and dispassionate observation and treatment of a patient as distinguished from experimental or laboratory studies;
2. in psychology: pertaining to laboratory tests in contrast to observation.

Communitas -
1. Unstructured or rudimentarily structured and relatively undifferentiated community of individuals who enjoy equal status during a ritual (Turner 1969:96) and who have been led to a level of experience where the unexpected (change) can happen (Heinze, 1991).
2. anti-structure in the sense of being undifferentiated, egalitarian, direct, extant, nonrational, existential, not shaped by norms, not institutionalized, not abstract, tending to ignore, reverse, cut across or occur outside of structural social relationships (Turner 1974:64–65).

Confucianism - System of teaching attributed to the Chinese philosopher Confucius (551–479 B.C.); characterized by the emphasis on the cardinal virtues of filial piety, kindness, righteousness, propriety, intelligence, and faithfulness. In Chinese, called *fu chiao*. Historically, Confucianism formed the basis of much of Chinese ethics, education, statecraft and religion.

Confucianism has neither a statement of faith nor an authoritative doctrine. It never developed a specialized priesthood, priestly functions were either performed by the head of state or clan or designated to scholarly officials. Confucianism frowns upon monasticism and asceticism. Its scriptures—the Analects—though revered, were never thought of as "revelation" in the same sense as the Bible, the Koran or the Vedas. With no rites of initiation into a religious community, Confucianism is also without a distinctive doctrine of the afterlife and lacks an eschatology. Yet, if religion is broadly defined as man's recognition of, belief in, and attitudes toward a higher spiritual power or powers, if religion is concerned with the ultimate meaning of human life and destiny, Confucianism could be classified as a religion and not simply an ethico-political philosophy (Smith 1971:33). - Orthodox Confucian Chinese perform rites for the sake of their fate in this world: for long life, children, wealth, and to a small degree for the good of the ancestors, but not at all for the sake of their fate in the "hereafter" (Weber 1951:144).

Conjurer -
1. User of magic spells to evoke spirits;
2. magician, sorcerer, person skilled in legerdemain, possibly an early shaman (see also, *Shaman*);
3. originally: person who solemnly entreats or appeals to someone.

Consciousness -
1. Awareness or perception of a physical, psychological, intellectual, social, or spiritual fact;
2. concerned awareness;
3. in psychology: totality of sensations, perceptions, ideas, attitudes, and feelings of which an individual or a group is aware at a given time;
4. waking life;
5. part of mental life or psychic content, immediately available to the ego.

Contemplation -
1. Thoughtful inspection of a particular object;
2. mystical meditation and awareness of God and his presence.

Cosmogony -
1. creation, origination or manner of coming into being of the universe;
2. theory or account of the origin of the universe;

Cosmology -
1. Branch of systematic philosophy that deals with the character of the universe as a cosmos by combining speculative metaphysics and scientific knowledge, e.g., treating the universe as a physical system;
2. particular theory or body of doctrine relating to the natural order.

Cryptesthesia - Power of perceiving without use of any sensory mechanism.

Cryptomnesia - Submerged or subliminal memory of events forgotten by the supraliminal self. Memory is not experienced as such but considered to be an original production.

Cult - Group of individuals who organize to worship a particular deity or deities. Practicing mutually agreed upon rituals, a cult is not always sanctioned by organized (world) religion.

Delirium -
1. Mental disturbance characterized by confusion, disordered speech and hallucinations;
2. frenzied excitement.

Delusion - Belief which, by socio-cultural standards, is demonstrably false, but held with complete conviction.

Dementia - Condition of deteriorated mentality.

Demiurge -
1. An autonomous creative force or decisive power;
2. Plato: subordinate deity who fashions the sensible world in the light of eternal ideas;
3. Gnosticism: subordinate deity who is the creator of the material world.

Demon -
1. Any of the secondary deities on the level between gods and men;
2. evil spirit;
3. superhuman being believed to be capable of manifesting in men, generally regarded to be evil;
4. any person who has great energy or skill.

Depression -
1. State of feeling sad;
2. psychoneurotic or psychotic disorder, marked by sadness, inactivity, difficulty in thinking and concentration, significant decrease or increase of appetite, time spent sleeping, feelings of dejection and hopelessness, sometimes suicidal tendencies;
3. lowering of vitality and functional activity.

Dissociation - Mental mechanism whereby a split-off part of the personality temporarily possesses the entire field of consciousness and behavior.

Dissociative Identity Disorder (DID) - see **Multiple Personality Disorder**.

Divination - Practice of foretelling the future or the unknown by using implements, e.g., divining rods, sortilege, dice, shells, yarrow sticks, cards, cloud formations, intestine of sacrificed animals, etc.

Diviner - Somebody who practices divination. See also, *Shaman*.

Dogma -
1. Rigidly held, collective, and authoritative opinion, tenet or belief;

Glossary

    2. doctrine or body of doctrines of a theology or religion, formally stated and authoritatively proclaimed by a church, to be accepted on faith.

Dowsing - Art of using a hand-held instrument, such as a Y-shaped rod or a pair of L-shaped rods, or a pendulum, to look for water and other objects or to answer yes/no questions.

Drug - Chemical substance that affects the performance of the body and/or the mind, originally intended for use as medicine.

Dynamogency - Increase of nervous energy by appropriate stimuli; often opposed to inhibition.

Dyesthesia -
1. Any impairment of the senses, esp. of the sense of touch;
2. diminished, excessive or inappropriate sensitivity to pain.

Eclectic - Gathered from different sources, systems and/or doctrines.

Eclesiolatry - Maintaining the view that no salvation is possible outside the church.

Ecmnesia - Memory gap, remembering only occurrences prior to a given date, but not remembering what happened for a certain time period after that date.

Ecstasy -
1. State of overwhelming joy and rapture;
2. state of intense emotional excitement, pain or other sensations, beyond reason and self-control;
3. state of intense absorption in divine and cosmic matters, with loss of sensory perception and voluntary control (vital functions are depressed);
4. violent dissociation and madness.

Ecumenical -
1. General or universal, esp., concerning the Christian church as a whole;
2. promoting worldwide Christian unity.

    Having originated in Protestantism, the ecumenical movement of the 20th century is working toward an interconfessional Christian unity, focussing on a World Council of Churches. Supported by many Protestant, Eastern, Orthodox, and other church bodies, the movement promotes functional organizations which cooperate on such common tasks as missionary work among students and conferences that foster mutual understanding on fundamental issues in belief, worship and polity (i.e., world problems).

Ego -
1. The "I," as distinguished from others;

2. "center" of the conscious self to which all psychological activities and qualities refer.

Enchantment -
1. Use of charms to influence and gain power over others;
2. something that charms or delights.

Enculturation - in contrast to acculturation
Adaptation to prevailing patterns of one's own culture through primary learning and basic induction by parents, teachers, and peers.

Energy -
1. Intrinsic, vital force;
2. physical quantity which measures the capacity for doing work.
   Greek, *energeia*; Chinese, *ch'i*; Japanese, *ki*: Thai, *khwan*; Sanskrit, *prana, kundalini*; Reichenbach, *od*.

Entelechy - Seeding, coding, dynamic propulsion.

Entheogen - Psychedelic substance traditionally used in a religious context.

Epigenetic development - Biological growth directed by features of the developing organism beyond the influence of the genes.

Eschatology -
1. Science of dealing with the ultimate destiny or purpose of man;
2. branch of theology or doctrine dealing with death, resurrection, immortality, judgment day.

Esoteric -
1. Designed for and understood only by a select circle of initiates;
2. beyond the understanding and knowledge of most people.

Eucharist -
1. Consecrated meal of a religious community, communion;
2. act of giving thanks.

Euphoria -
1. State of emotional exaltation;
2. feeling of vigor, well-being or high spirits;
3. in psychology: exaggerated feeling without obvious cause.

Exorcism - Practice of expelling evil spirits by adjuration, often by using a holy name or magic rite. A vestige of this lives on in the *exsufflatio*, e.g., the baptismal rites of the Catholic Church (Wallnofer 1965:177, see also, the *Rituale Romanum* 1976).

Exorcist - Somebody who practices exorcism. See also *Shaman*.

Glossary

Expressive behavior - In psychology: behavior which seeks immediate satisfaction by expressing emotions and feelings in interpersonal relationships.

Extrasensory perception (ESP), coined by J.B. Rhine -
1. Communications by other means than the five senses, e.g., clairvoyance, clairaudience, clairsentience;
2. response to an event not perceived by any known sense.

Faith -
1. Firm and unquestioned belief;
2. something believed and adhered to with conviction, i.e., cherished values, ideas, beliefs, etc.,
3. something not requiring proof or evidence because individuals and groups completely trust and rely on it.

Fugue -
1. Pathological disturbance of consciousness during which patients perform acts of which they apparently are conscious but of which, after recovery, they have no recollection;
2. temporary flight from reality.

Geomancer - Somebody who practices geomancy. See also *Shaman*.

Geomancy -
1. Chinese: *feng shui*;
2. divination by using contours of rocks and mountains, shapes of trees, flow of water, etc.;
3. science of bringing into harmony natural forces, e.g., determining the site of a house or a grave to prevent future problems.

Ghost -
1. Disembodied soul;
2. dead person, believed to inhabit an unseen world, but appearing to the living in bodily likeness.

Glossolalia -
1. State of falling into trance, mainly during church services and "speaking in tongues," unknown to the individual during waking consciousness;
2. ecstatic utterances of unintelligible speech-like sounds, considered to be manifestations of a deep religious experience.

Gnosticism -
1. Reliance on mystic and esoteric religious insights with emphasis on knowledge rather than faith;
2. belief that matter is inherently evil;

3. practice of any of various cults of late Pre-Christian and early Christian centuries, declared heretical by the Church.

Hallucination - Any sensory perception which has no objective counterpart within the field of vision, hearing, etc., but is connected with a compulsive sense of reality.

Hallucinogenic - Means causing hallucinations, alterations or distortions of perception.

Hermeneutic - Pertaining to interpretation, esp., of biblical texts.

Herolatic - Pertaining to hero worship.

Heteraesthesia - Sensibility decidedly different from any of the known senses, e.g., perception of a magnetic field, running water, crystals, metals, etc.

Heterodoxy - Belief deviating from established doctrines and official standards.

Hierocracy - Priestly rule or influence by ministering or withholding grace.

Hierogamy - Divine marriage.

Hinduism - Complex body of social, cultural, and religious beliefs and practices of Hindus, developed and practiced mainly on the Indian subcontinent but having large communities all over the world. Though its caste system has been abolished in 1948 by constitution, caste is still observed in religious context, choice of spouses, inheritance, etc.

From appr. 1,500–600 B.C., *brahmins* (priestly caste), were divinely inspired and collected the four Vedas—*Ṛg, Sama, Yajur*, and *Atharva* (mainly hymns to nature gods and instructions how to worship them). From the 6th century B.C. on, philosophical systems were taught by *brahmins* in ashrams outside of cities. Over time, all forms and theories were viewed as aspects of one eternal being (Brahmā, Atman), including the belief in *ahimsa* (non-violence), *karma* (the quality of each thought, word, and action determines the quality of one's future life), *dharma* (universal law) and *mokṣa* (release). The Way of Action (*karma yoga*), the Way of Knowledge (*jnana yoga*) or the Way of Devotion (*bhakti yoga*) lead toward the release from the round of rebirths (*samsara*). The various *upanisads* (philosophical treatises) and *puranas* (legends of gods, also containing cosmological and cosmogenic observations) were transmitted orally and later written down in Sanskrit, adding to the basic Vedic scriptures. Patanjali, for example, collected the 196 *yoga sūtras* (Prabhavananda 1953).

The trinity of Hinduism are Brahmā (creator), Viṣṇu (Preserver, and his 10 *avatāras*, e.g., Rāma, Krishna, Buddha), and Śiva (destroyer, with his sons, the elephant-headed Ganesha and Kārtikeya or Murgam and his *vel*, "spear"). In one form, Śiva is an ascetic and his wife Pārvatī the daughter of the Himalayas, in another form Śiva dances the cosmic dance of creation in a ring of fire, destroying demons. His wife Mahākālī is the Great Mother who ultimately is the only one who can defeat the strongest demons.

Hubris - Insolence or arrogance resulting from excessive pride or passion.

Hyperboulia - Increased power over the organism resembling the power which we call "will" when it is exercised over the voluntary muscles and seen in the bodily changes effected by self-suggestion.

Hypermnesia - Overactivity of one's memory, a condition in which past acts, feelings or ideas are brought vividly to the mind, which, in its natural condition, has wholly lost the remembrance of them. It has been suggested that the subliminal memory retains these remembrances throughout, and their supraliminal evocation implies an increased grasp of natural faculties.

Hyperphrenia - Condition in which energy has been withdrawn from ego functions and from complexes that govern everyday activities, e.g., the emotions, concentrating instead on the deeper levels of the psyche which are composed of emotionally laden, symbolic affect images.

Hyperpromethia - Supernormal power of foresight, hypothetically attributed to the subliminal self to explain premonitions without assuming either that the future scene is shown to the percipient by any mind external to his/her own, or that circumstances which we regard as future are in any sense already existent.

Hypnagogig -
1. Pertaining to the state preceding sleep;
2. reduced awareness of environment, but increased awareness of subconscious thoughts, feelings, and sensations.

Hypnopompic -
1. Pertaining to the semi-conscious state preceding waking;
2. awareness of subconscious thoughts, feelings, and sensations which can be brought into waking consciousness.

Hypnosis -
1. State of reduced awareness of environment but focussed on specific objects, verbally induced by another person (hypnotist), though self-hypnosis is also possible;
2. trance state in which the subject remains in rapport and responsive to suggestions. It may induce anesthesia or paralysis and may also have curative value.

Hypochondria - State of marked concern and anguish due to a pathological change in self-experience during which an individual's attention is continuously or principally directed toward his/her own physical and mental states, exaggerating every trifling symptom.

Hysteria -
1. Psychoneurosis marked by emotional excitability involving disturbances of psychic, sensory, vasomotoric, and visceral functions;
2. conduct or outbreak of wild and uncontrollable behavior of individuals or groups exhibiting unmanageable fear, fits of laughter or crying.

The symptoms of hysteria "consist of an autoplastic attempt to discharge the tension created by intrapsychic conflict, expressing drive and defense simultaneously, short-circuiting conscious perception of conflict related to the oedipus complex" (Abse 1959).

"The secondary gain, the importance of which Abse believes is often underestimated, involves the individual's use of his symptoms to attract attention, gain sympathy, and manipulate other people" (Freed 1959).

Hysteria was defined by Fish (1964) as the presence of mental or physical symptoms to gain an advantage, usually motivated unconsciously. Slater (1965) considered hysteria not to be a disease because whether it was studied either from the perspective of genetical or personality clusters, its syndromes fragmented during investigations.

Epidemic hysteria usually refers to a variety of irrational fear or bizarre behavior affecting a few up to hundreds of people in close proximity to each other. The clinical picture does not conform to the description of a typical hysteria and is usually transient; clients recover spontaneously or respond to any form of suggestive treatment (Kok 1975:35; see also "mass hysteria, Case 3, Part 2).

Id -
1. Unconscious or deepest part of the psyche;
2. part of the psyche from which impersonal instincts and impulses arise that demand immediate gratification of primitive needs;
3. instincts and impulses which are not in contact with the world but only with the body, dominated by the pleasure principle. They are not an entity but merely a description of a system of potentials.

Illusion -
1. False idea or conception; belief or opinion not in accord with facts;

2. unreal, deceptive or misleading appearance of image;
3. misinterpretation of some object actually seen or heard, e.g., taking a rope for a snake or a snake for a rope.

Impulse -
1. Sudden inclination or incitement of mind or spirit arising either directly from feelings or from some outer influence and prompting some unpremeditated action;
2. tendency to act in a particular way;
3. readiness or impulsion to act;
4. awareness of one's reactions.

Inhibition - Mental or psychological process that restrains or suppresses an action, emotion or thought.

Instinct -
1. Naturally inherent aptitude, tendency, impulse, capacity;
2. complex and special responses on the part of an organism to environmental stimuli, largely hereditary and unaltered through the pattern of behavior; can be modified by learning;
3. in Yoga: involved reason, when experience becomes subconscious;
4. in psychoanalysis: primal biological urge (e.g., hunger), impelling a response (eating) which brings relief of tension.

 Human instincts are seen as being self-preservative, sexual, and, sometimes, aggressive.

Introspection -
1. Examination of one's own thoughts and feelings;
2. self-analysis.

Instrumental behavior - In psychology: behavior which seeks to change things in the object world by manipulating them, usually to benefit oneself.

Intuition -
1. Act or process of coming to direct knowledge or certainty without reasoning or inferring;
2. immediate cognizance or conviction without rational thought;
3. revelation through insight or innate knowledge.

Islam - "Submission" to God. Muhammad, the prophet of God, was born about 570 A.D. in Mekka. He engaged in caravan trade, married a well-to-do widow, Khadija, and had three daughters with her. In his 40th year, he developed contemplative habits and received the call to break with the prevailing polytheism and to proclaim the worship of the One God, Allah. The sacred book of all

Muslims is the Koran. Written down in Arabic, it contains the word of God, revealed to Mohammed by the Archangel Gabriel. After ten years of preaching, Muhammad was invited to come to Yathrib (later called al-Madina). He followed the invitation in 622. The Muslim calendar begins with the year of Muhammad's *hegira* (emigration). In 630, Mecca was won back and its sanctuary rededicated to Allah. After the prophet's death in 632, disputes arose about his succession and schools developed. The Sunn'ites (followers of the tradition) believe that Muhammad's successor should be elected (85 per cent of all Muslims today are Sunn'ites). The Shi'ites (partisans of Ali) recognize Ali (Muhammad's cousin and son-in-law) and his descendants as the only legitimate successors. Shi'ites also believe in continuing revelations.

At present, Islam is the second largest religion in the world with over 700 million believers not only in Arab countries but also in Pakistan, Indonesia, Malaysia, Thailand, Singapore, the Philippines, Africa, Russia, and China.

Kairos - Liminal condition in which a person becomes ready for profound changes in values and attitudes.

Karma -
1. Sanskrit; *kamma*, Pāli: what has been done;
2. Hindu (and Buddhist) belief that the quality of an individual's thoughts, words, and deeds determines his/her present and future.

Kirlian photography - Semyon and Valentina Kirlian generated a high-frequency field between two electrodes and placed an object directly on a film resting within the field and producing a photograph of the object without using a camera or a lens. The surrounding corona represents the ionized air (i.e., electrons torn from the object when the high-frequency field is created).

Legend -
1. Story from the past, though not verifiable, usually regarded as historical;
2. Person or thing that inspires legends.

Levitation - Raising of objects or persons by supernormal means.

Liminality -
1. Transitional period, when participants have temporarily entered a sacred space where the unexpected can happen. After leaving the sacred space, they have to be reincorporated into their social environment and may be given a new status (Van Gennep 1960; Heinze 1991).
2. State, outside of time and space, used by shamans to shift attention out of an illness pattern into a state where change becomes possible, e.g., the the self-healing powers of patients are triggered.

Logotherapy (used by Frankl 1978) - Healing through meaning.
Lycantrophy -
1. Form of insanity during which an individual imagines him- or herself to become a wolf or a dog;
2. Human being assuming the form of a wolf or a dog, e.g., through magic.

Macrobiotics - Art of striving for long life through a special diet or by magical means.

Magic -
1. Use of charms, spells, and rituals to control events or to monitor natural or supernatural forces;
2. any mysterious, seemingly inexplicable or extraordinary power or influence.

Magical Flight -
1. Mind-expanding state,
2. in folklore, shamanic excursion to different levels of consciousness
   a. to retrieve otherwise not accessible information and
   b. to find lost souls.

Magician -
1. Expert in magic, see also *Shaman, Sorcerer, Wizard;*
2. performer of baffling tricks, producing concealed objects or making objects disappear, mainly by skillfully using his/her hands (sleight of hand, legerdemain).

Manichaeism - Religious philosophy, taught from the 3rd to the 7th century A.D. by the Persian Mani or Manichaeus and his followers, combining Zoroastric, Gnostic, Christian, and pagan elements. Manichaeism is based on the doctrine of the two contending principles of good (light, God, the soul) and evil (darkness, Satan, the body).

Mantic -
1. Pertaining to divination;
2. having prophetic powers.

Meditation - Methods of
1. cultivating the mind by focussing on a specific object of thought (one-pointedness);
2. clearing the mind of preoccupation with self-interest;
3. completely letting go of all thoughts and emotions by simply watching or witnessing whatever arises in consciousness;
4. non-attachment to contents of the mind with an increasing ability to exercise choice in how to use the mind, i.e., developing a greater sense of self-mastery, well-being, equanimity, and reduced stress;

5. cultivation of heightened awareness to penetrate mundane *(lokiya)* levels of consciousness to reach supermundane otherworldly, transcendental *(lokuttara)* levels in pursuit of the "ultimate truth."

Medium see **Spirit medium**, also **Shaman**.

Melancholy -
1. Sadness and desperation of spirit;
2. in the middle ages: the black hole; one of the four humors of the body, coming from the spleen or the kidneys and causing gloominess, irritability and/or depression.

Mental health -
1. Relatively enduring state during which
   a. an individual's body, mind, and soul are well balanced, and
   b. the individual has zest for life, and works toward self-realization,
2. ability to receive and give love and to take responsibility, i.e., to be loving and productive (Kildahl 1972:48).

Metamorphosis - Aside from botanical, zoological, and pathological interpretations, the complete change of form and structure or substance of humans, animals, even unanimate objects as if transformed by magic or witchcraft.

Metastasis - Change of location of a bodily function from one place (e.g., the brain center) to another location in the body.

Metempsychosis -
1. At death: passing of the soul into another body, either human or animal;
2. transmigration.

Monk -
1. Somebody who has been ordained and accepted into the order of an official religion;
2. somebody who has taken a vow to lead an ascetic life (e.g., vow of celibacy) and is devoted to prayer, healing, missionary or other altruistic activities;
3. somebody who has retired from the world and exercises self-denial for religious reasons.

Multiple Personality Disorder (MPD) - Disorder of adaptation in which natural defense mechanisms called up under past extreme conditions of abuse and vulnerability persist into the present; now commonly known as *Dissociative Identity Disorder (DID)* because the personalities are understood to be separated from one another as though by impermeable walls. They may not know of each other's existence, but there may be evidence accumulating of black-outs, lovers they don't remember, phone calls about incidents they don't recall, food they don't like in the refrigerator, unremembered suicide attempts that land them in the hospital, and other incomprehensible phenomena. DID personalities, known as "alters," may even have different biochemistries.

Muslim - Follower of Islam, submitting to the will of God (Allah).

Mysticism -
1. Experience of union or direct communion with ultimate reality;
2. belief that direct knowledge of God, of spiritual truth, of ultimate reality, etc., is attainable through intuitive insight different from sensory perception or rationalization.

Myth - Traditional story that explains natural phenomena or prehistoric events and serves as basis for worldview, ideals and the institutions of a culture.

Mythology -
1. A body of myths that deals with the gods, demigods and legendary heroes of a culture;
2. an interpretation of myths.

Narcotic -
1. Originally: substance that dulls the senses and induces sleep;
2. legally: drug which causes chemical dependence or addiction.

Necromancy - Practice of foretelling the future through alleged communication with the dead.

Neurosis - Functional disorder of the central nervous system, having one of the following reactions—anxiety, hysteria, phobia, obsession, and compulsion.

Occultism -
1. Attempt to control natural processes by secret and magical procedures or belief in possessing such control;
2. secret, mysterious, esoteric knowledge.

Od - (first used by K. von Reichenbach, 1788–1809) Hypothesized force or natural power, thought to manifest itself in certain individuals or things, also connected with hypnotism and magnetism.

Oneirocritic - Somebody who interprets dreams.

Oneiromancy - Practice of interpreting dreams (e.g., to foretell the future).

Ontology - Metaphysical study of the ultimate nature of being.

Orgiasticism - Pursuit of an altered state of consciousness—revelry, ecstasy, frenzy—through excessive indulgence in intoxicants, sex, dance, music, etc.

Glossary

Orgone - (first used by Wilhelm Reich, 1897–1957) Life energy, pervading nature and allegedly restorable by having, e.g., an individual sitting in a specially designed box. See also *Energy*.

Orthodoxy - State of conformity to an official formulation of truth, esp., religious belief, custom or doctrine.

Osmosis -
1. In chemistry: tendency of a solvent to pass through a semi-permeable membrane (like the wall of a living cell) into a solution of higher concentration, equalizing concentrations on both sides of the membrane.
2. in religion: the permeability of belief systems, see also *Syncretism*.

Pareidolia - Misconception of an external stimulus, like seeing pictures in the fire or in cloud formations.

Paraphasia - Erroneous and involuntary use of one word for another or of one syllable for another, sometimes also called Freudian slip.

Paraphysics - Investigation of nature, modes of action, and forms of energy, not described in traditional Western physics.

Parapsychology -
1. Study of phenomena involving the transfer of information by non-sensory means (extra-sensory perception) or matter being affected by non-physical means (psychokinesis);
2. investigation of electromagnetic and geomagnetic influences, based on the theory of vibrations, mainly used for healing.

Pathology -
1. Branch of medicine that deals with the nature of diseases, esp. structural and functional changes caused by disease;
2. all conditions, processes or results of a particular disease; and
3. any abnormal variation from a healthy or proper condition.

Pentecost - Christian festival on the 7th Sunday after Easter, celebrating the descent of the Holy Spirit upon the Apostles.

Phobia - Exaggerated and often disabling fear of a particular thing or situation, inexplicable to the subject, having occasional a logic of its own; using illogical symbolic objects which serve to protect, e.g., against anxiety originating from unexpressed aggressive impulses.

Placebo -
1. Substance which has no pharmacological effect but is administered to cause an individual to believe s/he is receiving treatment;

Glossary

2. Latin, "I shall please."

Pneuma - Wind, air, soul, spirit.
The ancient Greek believed *pneuma* to be the vital soul or principle that regulates man's pulse and breathing (similar to the Chinese *ch'i*). In sense and significance, *pneuma* is often used interchangeably with *aura* (literally: breeze, air). Both are probably best translated with "life-giving breath" or "life-giving force" (Sanskrit: *prana*; see also *energy*).

Pneumatic - In theology: pertaining to spirit and/or soul, esp. used by gnostics for the highest of the three classes into which mankind is divided.

Poltergeist -
1. Noisy or mischievous ghost;
2. spirit producing mysterious noises, e.g., rapping, also moving objects; manifests usually where there are teenagers in the house. See also, phenomena connected with *Psychokinesis*.

Possession -
1. Condition of being possessed or dominated by something or someone, e.g., a strong personality, demon, passion, idea, or purpose;
2. in psychology: dissociative state where an individual's personality is replaced by another, e.g., multiple personality disorder which requires treatment and possibly integration of the different personalities;
3. in Asian belief: intrusion of a spirit/deity to do "salvation work." Integration is not attempted, because it is believed that
   a. spirits (who do not or cannot reincarnate) manifest for a certain time on demand while the "soul" of the possessed individual allegedly visits heavens and returns naturally after the departure of the spirit;
   b. the spirit of a past state oracle selects a monk who falls into trance easily (i.e., has a permeable ego axis) to become his successor (i.e., that the strength of shamans originates on a level where there is no ego.) The monk is then trained and, when in trance, will advice the Dalai Lama in affairs of state (see, Nechung oracle, Heinze 1991:102–106 and Avadon 1984).

Prayer -
1. Any action designed to bring an individual into contact with the Divine;
2. solemn, humble approach to divinity in word and thought, e.g., petition, confession, thanksgiving, adoration, praise, and communion;
3. devotional service.

Precepts - Commands or moral principles intended to be general rules of action for a certain group of people, e.g., the 227 precepts for *Theravāda* monks.

Glossary

Precognition - Perception of future events without rational inference.

Premonition - Supernormal perception of an event which is still part of the future.

Prestidigitation - Performance of tricks by quick and skillful use of the hands (sleight of hand, legerdemain).

Priest -
1. Somebody who performs sacrificial, ritual, mediating, interpretative, and ministerial functions;
2. ordained religious functionary of an official religion, claiming authority through the powers invested in him/her by God.

Priesthood - Specific group of leaders who officiate at regular times at fixed places according to codified beliefs and norms on behalf of a religious community.

Promnesia - Paradoxical sensation of recollecting a scene which is only now occurring for the first time.

Prophecy -
1. Function or vocation of a prophet;
2. inspired declaration of divine will and purpose;
3. a prediction of something to come.

Psi -
1. Twenty-third letter of the Greek alphabet;
2. blanket name for the psychic in general;
3. whole family of phenomena and experiences, real or alleged, for which no physical cause has as yet been discovered.

Psychedelic -
1. Greek: *psyche* ("soul") and *delos* ("to reveal");
2. quality of mind-expanding substances (natural: Peyote, Ayahuasca; or chemical: LDS), causing temporary changes in consciousness: hallucinations, delusions, intensification of awareness, and sensory perception, etc.

Psychoactive - Substance affecting the mind, inducing changes of mood, thinking, and behavior.

Psychoanalysis -
1. Method of inquiry (free association, dream analysis, etc.) into psychic content and mechanisms to render them readily accessible to voluntary explanation by the conscious mind;
2. therapy developed by Sigmund Freud (1856–1939) who suggested that the instinctual life-impulse (*id*) of a human being is inhibited by education, conventions, etc., and that thereby internal, emotional experiences are

repressed into the subconscious. Freud restricted his speculations to two instincts: the sex-instinct *(libido)* and the death-instinct *(thanatos)*. Even his closest disciples felt that these restrictions prevented further discussion of other issues.

In principle, a cure is attempted by the patient talking freely and without restraint to the psychoanalyst. The patient is expected to transmit his spontaneous thoughts, association of ideas—coherent or not—and his dreams. The chance of unburdening one's mind and soul is in itself a release of tension which is helpful in coping more successfully with anxieties.

Since Freud, psychoanalytic techniques have been further developed, e.g., by Alfred Adler (1870–1937), working with the principle of power; Carl Gustav Jung (1875–1961), see *Archetype*; Victor M. Frankl (1905–), see *Logotherapy*; and others.

Psychokinesis - Influence exerted on a physical system without the use of any known form of physical energy.

Psycholytic -
1. Greek: *psyche* ("soul") and *lysis* ("to loosen");
2. "mind-freeing" or "mind-loosening," releasing emotional and cognitive inhibitions.

Psychometry - Extrasensory perception of facts concerning an object or its owner through direct contact with the object.

Psychopath - Somebody who pretends to suffer from a mental or emotional disorder and attempts to exploit the sympathy of others.

Psychopomp -
1. Soul guide;
2. somebody who conducts the souls of the dead safely into other worlds or who calls back the wandering souls of the living.

Psychosis -
1. Profound disorder of the mind and behavior that results from inability to tolerate the demands of one's environment whether the imposed stress is felt to be too great or there exists a primary inadequacy or acquired debility of the organism, esp., in regard to the nervous system, manifesting in disorder of perception, thinking, etc.; pressured withdrawal from external reality with an incomplete return;
2. major mental disorder in which the personality of an individual is seriously disorganized and contact with reality is impaired.

There are two kinds of psychoses: (a) functional (characterized by lack of apparent organic cause, and mainly of the schizophrenic or manic-depressive type); and (b) organic (characterized by a pathological organic condition, such as brain damage or disease, metabolic disorders, etc.).

Psychoses, similar to drug-induced or mystical states, are retreats to the mythic or collective, deeper layers of the psyche where they lose their individual uniqueness and become increasingly collective. Unless they are universalized, they may assume autonomous functional systems (see, among others, Jung 1961, *Psychological Reflections*, cited by Fischer in Pelletier 1976:87).

Psychosomatic -
1. Physical disorder of the body originating in or aggravated by psychic or emotional processes;
2. interactions between mind or emotions and body, resulting from emotional stress or neurotic symptoms.

Psychotomimetic - Mimicking or inducing psychosis.

Psychotropic - Mind-altering (into a different state of consciousness).

Radiesthesia - Detection of subtle influences which affect a person's health.

Radionics - Instrumental form of radiesthesia, using electrical or other devices with adjustable dials.

Rapid eye movements (REM) - indicate
1. a dream state in humans and animals,
2. not a deep unconscious state but a state of inward concentration in which the sleeper is insensitive to external or peripheral stimulation (Furst 1972:263).

Ratiocination - Process of exact thinking and reasoning, using formal logic.

Regression -
1. Trend or shift toward a lower or less perfect state;
2. progressive decline, manifesting a disease;
3. gradual loss of differentiation and function of a body part, esp. physiological change as in aging;
4. gradual loss of memories and acquired skills;
5. reversion to an earlier mental or behavioral level.

Religion -
1. Latin: *relego* ("tie together again");
2. reunion of temporarily estranged elements to one functional unit, to reunite (with the Divine);

3. system of attitudes, practices, rites, ceremonies and beliefs by which individuals or communities put themselves into relation to God or to a supernatural world. This includes sets of values by which events in the world should be judged;
4. doctrines or customs adopted on faith.

The sociologist Bellah saw religion "as a set of symbols that may be institutionalized, considered as normative in a society or internalized in a personality . . . . They state or suggest what reality ultimately is, what the source of order (and often disorder) in the universe is, what sort of authority in the most general terms is acceptable to men, and what sorts of action by individuals make sense in such a world" (1965:71).

The anthropologist Lessa found, e.g., that religion is also concerned with "threats to these central values, or to social or individual existence." Religion then "has important *defense* functions in providing ways of managing tensions and anxieties." Therefore, "religion both maintains the ultimate values of a society and manages tensions in the personalities of individual members of a society" (1965:1).

Repression -
1. Active avoidance of input from the internal world;
2. process or mechanism of ego defense whereby wishes or impulses an individual is incapable of fulfilling are made inaccessible to consciousness, except in disguised form, e.g., conversion neurosis, sublimation or symbolization.

Retrocognition - Extrasensory perception of past events.

Ritual -
1. Conventionalized act during which individuals express their respect and regard for some object of ultimate value;
2. devotional service, established by tradition or sacerdotal precepts, to be performed at intervals and regarded as having a special, e.g., religious, significance;
3. creation of a sacred space where the unexpected (e.g., meeting with the Divine) can happen. During the ritual participants are in a *liminal state*, have equal status and experience *communitas*, so that a shift of attention out of an old, unproductive pattern into a new, more productive frame of mind becomes possible (See Heinze 1991, also Van Gennep, *Rites of Passage*, 1960, and Victor Turner, *The Ritual Process*, 1966).

Glossary

Sacerdotal - Relating to priests and priesthood, characterized by the belief in the divine authority of the priesthood.

Schizophrenia - Mental disorder of unknown cause, characterized, e.g., by the splitting of an individual personality, with fundamental disturbances in the perception of reality.

Scotoma -
1. Dark area in the visual field;
2. blind spot.

Semiotic - General theory of signs and symbols, esp. the analysis of the nature and relationships of signs in language.

Sentient -
1. Capable of sensation or at least rudimentary consciousness;
2. conscious capacity of distinguishing and perceiving.

Shaman - Practitioner who can access different states of consciousness at will and acts as priest, diviner and/or healer, but most of all, as mediator to the spiritual world in response to pragmatic (physical, emotional, mental as well as social, and spiritual) needs of individuals and groups. Shamanism did not become an organized and codified religion, on the contrary, shamans are able to operate in the framework of world religions and complement other social systems. See also *Conjurer, Diviner, Exorcist, Geomancer, Magician, Oneirocritic, Sorcerer, Spirit Medium, Warlock, Witch,* and *Wizard*.

Shamanic practices - See *Automatic Writing, Clairvoyance, Conjuring, Divination, Enchantment, Exorcism, Geomancy, Legerdemain, Magic* (black/malevolent or white/benevolent), *Magical Flight, Necromancy, Oneiromancy, Possession, Prestidigitation, Prophesy, Sleight of Hand, Sorcery, Trance,* and *Witchcraft*.

Shrine -
1. Consecrated or hallowed place;
2. tomb of a holy man (e.g., a Muslim *keremat)*.

Sign -
1. Token or indiction;
2. conventional or arbitrary mark, figure or symbol, used as an abbreviation for a word or words it represents;
3. a motion or gesture, used to express or convey an idea, command, decision.

Somatic -
1. Pertaining to the body, as distinguished from the soul, mind or psyche; 2. corporal; physical.

Sorcerer -
1. Somebody who uses black magic to harm people and who can also counteract the black magic of others;
2. new-age practitioner who maintains s/he has knowledge and power to influence the course of events.

Sortilege - Divination or prophesy by casting lots.

Soteriology - Religious teaching of salvation and a redeemer.

Soul -
1. Immaterial essence or substance;
2. vital life principle, actual cause of life;
3. immortal part of man.

   Like the word "spirit," "soul" can stand for "breath, life, self, ghost, the Absolute." Probing into Indo-European languages, there is the word "atmosphere" (Greek: *atmos* ["vapor"] and *sparis* ["sphere"]) which indicates a pervading or surrounding influence or spirit and brings us closer to the Sanskrit *atman* which has been interpreted differently by Vedic, Upanisadic, Sankhyan, Jain, Buddhist, and Vedanta philosophers. From the empirical self in dreams, it became the object or subject of change, until it stood for the unchangeable absolute. There is, furthermore, the Sanskrit word *prana* (mostly used in connection with "breath").

Spirit -
1. breath of life;
2. immaterial, intelligent or sentient part of man;
3. immortal part of man;
4. supernatural being;
5. active essence of a deity serving as invisible, life-giving, inspiring power. See also *Soul* and *Pneuma*.

Spirit medium -
1. Individual who claims to be temporarily "possessed" by a disembodied spirit;
2. individual who mediates between alternate states of consciousness for those who seek immediate personal experience of locally accessible spiritual powers to find solutions for individual physiological, psychological, mental, social, and spiritual needs which cannot be satisfied otherwise. See also, *Shaman*.

Spiritism -
1. Theory that mediumistic phenomena are caused by spirits of the dead;
2. belief that natural objects possess indwelling spirits.

Glossary

Sublimation - Elevating basic drives and desires to another level of consciousness where they can be used creatively.

Subliminal - Quality of thoughts, feelings, etc., lying beneath the ordinary threshold (*limen*) of consciousness, as opposed to *supraliminal*, lying above the threshold.

Superstition -
  1. Irrational or unfounded belief or practice;
  2. unreasoning awe or fear of something unknown, mysterious or imaginary;
  3. tenet, scruple, habit, etc., founded on fear or ignorance.

Suppression -
  1. Retardation or stoppage of growth;
  2. conscious intention of excluding certain thoughts and feelings from consciousness.

Symbol -
  1. Something that stands for or suggests something else by reason of relationship, association, convention or accident;
  2. word, phrase, or image having a complex of associated meanings, perceived as having inherent values, separable from those which it symbolizes and performing its normal function of standing for or representing that which it symbolizes; usually conceived as deriving its meaning chiefly from the structure in which it appears.

  Tillich mentioned that symbols may have some characteristics in common with signs,
  a. they point beyond themselves to something else;
  b. they participate in that to which they point;
  c. they open up levels of reality which otherwise are closed for us;
  d. they unlock dimensions and elements of our soul;
  e. they cannot be produced intentionally and cannot function without being accepted by the unconscious dimension of our being;
  f. they cannot be invented and, like living beings, they grow and die. (They die because they can no longer produce responses in the group in which they originally found expression; 1965:40–43).

Synchronicity - Meaningful co-occurrence of a subjective experience and an objective physical event in a manner that transcends the laws of causality and identity, as in precognition and clairvoyance.

Syncretism -
  1. The origin of this word can be traced back to the inhabitants of the Greek island of Crete who rallied around a common cause and "syncretized" to

Glossary

withstand external foes;
2. presently used when elements of different belief systems reconcile to form an integrated pattern.

Synergy - Series of actions correlated or combined into a group.

Taoism -
1. Chinese philosophy: Founded by Lao-tzu in the 6th century B.C. He taught conformity to the *Tao* (Way) by unassertive action and retirement from the world. The key to Lao-tzu's teachings is, indeed, the *Wei-Wu-Wei*, "doing by not doing," which does not mean to do nothing. According to Lao-tzu, man should be still and passive before the doings of nature, i.e., the *Tao*. Man should perform his small daily tasks and not tackle problems when they have become overwhelmingly huge. People should also not interfere in the politics of kings. In the *Tao Te Ching*, 81 brief poems, Lao-tzu probes into the essence of the *Tao*. Other Taoist writers, e.g., Lieh-tzu (5th or 4th century B.C.) and Chuang-tzu (4th century B.C.) present their ideas in the form of allegories, usually satirical. Some scholars think Lieh-tzu is an imaginary figure who was created by Chuang-tzu (Wallnofer 1965:176) and that the *Tao Te Ching*, although it may contain earlier material, was put together in the 3rd century A.D.
2. Folk-religious beliefs and practices: Socio-religious movements, political dissidence and utopian ideas led, in the 2d century A.D., to revelations of "Lord Lao the Most High," received by Chuang Tao-ling. Celestial masters introduced the concepts of sin and disease and taught therapeutic rites. The visionary tradition continued with Yang Hsi who met the "Perfected Ones" on Mt.Mao Shan near Nanking, Central China, from 364 to 370 A.D. Taoism soon became a highly syncretic religion, concerned with obtaining longevity and immortality through magical means. Temples were built and a pantheon of deities developed which was propitiated an organized group of priests who practiced alchemy, divination and sorcery, drawing many ideas from the Yin-Yang.

   Compiled and printed in the middle of the 15th century, the Taoist Canon comprises presently 1,120 volumes. Taoism has been called "Chinese folk religion." The revelations continued and Taoist schools developed lineages and ritual text traditions (personal communication, Professor Wolfram Eberhard, 1980).

Telekinesis - Movement of objects allegedly not due to any known force; synonym for *psychokinesis*.

Glossary

Teleology -
1. Study of acts considered as being related to purpose or being;
2. purposive study of behavior with reference to a future situation.

Telepathy - Transmission of information from mind to mind, without using sensory channels.

Temple - Building dedicated to sacred services (e.g., worship of a deity, ordination of monks), usually taken care of by an organized priesthood.

Thaumaturge - Individual who supposedly works miracles.

Totemism -
1. Natural object or animated being (e.g., animal, bird), used as the emblem of a clan, family or group;
2. object or natural phenomenon to which individuals, families or siblings consider themselves closely related;
3. representation of such an object, serving as a distinctive mark of a clan or group.

Trance -
1. State of partially suspended animation or inability to function;
2. state characterized by limited sensory and motor contact with the surroundings and subsequent lack of recall; resembles (or is), in extreme form, coma;
3. ego mechanism designed to allow for the discharge of basic drives in a goal-oriented (adaptive or defensive) manner;
4. esp. in Asia: professionally used in shamanic and artistic performances (in the West we know of highway trances and different states of consciousness used by actors, artists, and hypnotists).

   Trance experiences comprise a variety of different states: dissociation, hypnagogig or hypnopompic states, dreams, ecstasies, fugue states, hallucinations, hypnosis, hysteria, illusions, visions, physical collapse with obsessive ideas and/or compulsive actions, etc.

   "During a trance, the hypothalamus, the nervous centre for primitive physical and emotional behavior, becomes inactive, though the people still respond to speech and social communication" (Wavell 1955:16).

Transactional - Realized in actuality.

Transference - In psychoanalysis: emotional attachment a patient may develop toward the therapist. It is assumed that the perceptions and feelings of the patient toward the therapist replicate previous patterns of interaction, such as those experienced in early childhood.

Glossary

Vision -
1. Something imaginary, supernatural, or prophetic, experienced other than by ordinary sight;
2. ultimately, temporary experience of reunion with the Divine; interconnectness.

Warlock - Somebody with supernatural power and knowledge by an alleged pact with evil spirits. See also *Conjurer, Magician, Sorcerer, Witch*, and *Wizard*.

Witch - Somebody who uses magic for benevolent or malevolent purposes. In folk belief, witches cannot die until they have transmitted their faculties to a successor. See also *Conjurer, Magician, Sorcerer,* and *Wizard*.

Wizard -
1. Originally, wise man;
2. magician, sorcerer, or conjurer.

Yoga -
1. Sanskrit: *yuj* ("to bind together, to hold fast");
2. English: *yoke*;
3. Aside from numerous forms of popular, nonsystematic, nonbrahmin as well as Buddhist and Jain practices, the classical *yoga* is an Indian system of philosophy (see Patanjali's collection of 196 *yoga sūtras*, Prabhavananda 1953), emphasizing effort and self-discipline to obtain concentration, before asking for divine aid. The purpose of *yoga* is to unify body and spirit, so that dispersion and automatisms that characterize profane consciousness are eliminated. For the devotional (mystical) schools of *yoga*, this "unification" precedes the true union of the human soul with God (Eliade 1969).

Zoroastrianism - A prophetic religion maintaining that Zarathustra (628–551 B.C.) spoke with God face to face. After his first revelation at the age of 30, Zarathustra fled to Chorasmia where he established his religion. Only a fraction of his sacred book, the *Avesta,* survived. We know about the liturgy (*Yasna*), sacrificial hymns (*Yashts*), the *Videvnat Law* against demons and about the One God, Ahura Mazdah, the "Wise Lord." Basic are the dichotomies of truth-falsehood, righteousness-wickedness, order-disorder. After the founder's death, the belief system included again ancient gods.

Zoroastrianism was the national religion of the Persian Empire from the 3rd to the 7th century A.D. It lost its impact before the coming of Islam. Presently, there are no more than 120,000 believers in Zoroastrianism known to follow the tradition.

Bibliography

Abbott, J. *The Keys of Power*. London: Methuen & Co., Ltd., 1932.
Abele, David F. "'Arctic Hysteria' and Latah in Mongolia," *Transactions of the New York Academy of Science*, Series 2, *14:7* (1952):291–297.
Abse, D.W. "Hysteria," *American Handbook of Psychiatry*, ed. S. Arieti. New York, 1959.
Achterberg, Jean "Mind and medicine: The role of imagery in healing," *Journal of American Society for Psychical Research*, 83:2 (1989):93–100.
———, B. Dossey and L. Kolkmeier. *Rituals of Healing: Using Imagery for Health and Wellness*. New York: Bantam Books, 1994.
Ackerknecht, Edwin H. "Medical Practices," *Handbook of South American Indians*. vol.5, ed. Julian Steward. Washington: U.S. Government Printing Office, Bureau of American Ethnology Bulletin 143, 1949, pp. 621–543.
Ackerman, S.E. and Raymond L.M. Lee. "Mass Hysteria and Spirit Possession in Urban Malaysia: A Case Study," *Journal of Sociology and Psychology*, vol.1 151 (1978):24–35.
Al-Attas, Prof Syed Naguib. *Some Aspects of Sufism as Understood and Practised among the Malays*. Singapore: Malaysian Sociological Research Institute, Ltd., 1963.
Alexseev, Vasilli M. *The Chinese Gods of Wealth*. Hertford, England: S. Austin, 1928.
Ames, Michael M. "Magical-animism and Buddhism: A structural analysis of the Singhalese religious system," *Religion in Southeast Asia*, ed. E.B. Harper. Seattle, WA: University of Washington Press, 1964.
———. "Tovil Exorcism by White Magic," *National History*, *86:1* (January 1978):42–49.
Andrew, E. *The People Called Shakers*. New York: Oxford University Press, 1953.
Annandale, Nelson. "A magical ceremony for the cure of a sick person among the Malays of Upper Perak," *Man*, *3* (1903a):100–103.
———. "Notes on the popular religion of the Patani Malays," *Man*, *3* (1903b):27–28.

Bibliography

Anon. "Belief in spirits and demons," *Journal of the Straits Branch of the Royal Asiatic Society, 17,* Notes & Queries, 4 (1886):126–130.

_____. "'Spirits' and their somewhat serious consequences," *Malayan Police Magazine, 4* (1931):202–203.

Arasaratnam, S. *Indian Festivals in Malaya.* Kuala Lumpur: University of Malaya, Department of Indian Studies, 1966.

Avadon, John F. *In Exile from the Land of Snows.* New York: Alfred A. Knopf, 1984.

Babb, Lawrence A. *Walking on Flowers in Singapore, A Hindu Festival Cycle..* Singapore: University of Singapore, Department of Sociology, Working paper No.27, 1974a.

_____. "Hindu Mediumship in Singapore," *Southeast Asian Journal of Social Science, 2:1–2* (1974b):29–43.

_____. *Thaipusam in Singapore: Religious Individualism in a Hierarchical Culture.* Singapore: University of Singapore, Department of Sociology, Working Paper No.49, 1975.

Baity, Philip Ch. *Religion in a Chinese Town.* Taipei: Asian Folklore and Social Life Monograph 64, 1975.

Balys, J.B. "Der Schamanismus in Malakka und Indonesien," Vienna, Austria: University of Vienna, Institute of Ethnology, unpublished doctoral dissertation, 1933.

Banks, David J. *Trance and Dance in Malaya: The Hindu-Buddhist Complex in Northwest Malay Folk Religion.* Buffalo, N.Y.: SUNY, Special Studies Series, Council on International Studies, January 1976.

Bartlett, Harvey Harris. "The Labors of the Datoe: Part 1: An Annotated List of Religious, Magical and Medical Practices of the Batak of Asahan," repr., *Papers of the Michigan Academy of Sciences, Arts and Letters, XXII,* 1929, publ. 1930, and Part 2, "Directions for the Ceremonies, XIV, 1930, publ. 1931.

Basham, A.L. *The Wonder That Was India, A Survey of the Culture of the Sub-Continent Before the Arrival of the Muslims.* New York: Grove Press, 1959.

Bastide, R. *Sociologie et Psychoaanlyse.* Paris: Presses universitaires de France, 1950.

Becker, A.L. and Aram A. Yengoyan, eds. *The Imagination of Reality, Essays in Southeast Asian Coherence Systems.* New York: Ablex Publishing Corporation, 1979.

Bellah, Robert N. "Religious Evolution," *American Sociological Review, XXIX* (1964):358–374.

Belo, Jane. *Trance in Bali*, preface by Margaret Mead. New York: Columbia University Press, 1960.
Benjamin, Geoffrey. *Indigenous Religious Systems of the Malay Peninsula*. Singapore: University of Singapore, Department of Sociology, Working Paper No.29 (1974) and in Becker (above) 1979:9–27.
Berkowitz, Morris I., Frederick P. Brandauer, and John H. Reed. *Folk religion in an Urban Setting*. Hong Kong: Christian Study Centre on Chinese Religions and Culture, 1969.
Berreman, G.D. "Brahmins and Shamans," *Religion in South Asia*, ed. E.B. Harper. Seattle, WA: University of Washington Press, 1964.
Bharati, Agehananda. *The Tantric Tradition*. London: Allen & Unwin, Ltd., 1968.
Blacker, Carmen. *The Catalpa Bow, A Study of Shamanistic Practices in Japan*. London: George Allen and Unwin, Ltd., 1975.
Blagden, C.O. "Notes on the folklore and popular religion of the Malays," *Journal of the Straits Branch of the Royal Asiatic Society, 29* (1896):1–2.
Blumer, Herbert. *Symbolic Interactionism; Perspective and Method*. Englewood Cliffs, NJ: Prentice-Hall, Inc., 1969.
Bogoras, Waldemar. *The Chukchee Religion*. New York: Memoirs of the American Museum of Natural History, N.ii, Part 2, 1907.
_____. "K psikhologii shamanstva u naradov severovostochnoi," *Ethonografischeskoe obsoreniye, 94–95* (1910):1–36.
Bosch, F.D.K. *The Golden Germ: An Introduction to Indian Symbolism*. S-Gravenhage, Netherlands: Mouton and Co., 1960.
Bourguignon, Erika. "The Self, the Behavioral Environment, and the Theory of Spirit Possession," *Context and Meaning in Cultural Anthropology*, ed. Melford E. Spiro. New York: The Free Press, 1965, pp.39–60.
_____. "World Distribution and Patterns of Possession States," *Trance and Possession States*, ed. Raymond Prince. Montreal, Canada: Proceedings, Second Annual Conference, R.M. Bucke Memorial Society, 4–6 March 1966, pp.3–34.
_____. "Spirit Possession and Altered States of Consciousness, The Evolution of an Inquiry," *The Making of Psychological Anthropology*, ed. George D. Spindler. Berkeley, CA: University of California Press, 1978, pp.447–515.
Browne, Charles. "Mediums with a Message," *Bangkok Post*, Sect.II (April 15, 1979):15 and 24; (April 22, 1979):22.
Burr, Angela. "Religious Institutional Diversity — Social Structural and Conceptual Unity: Islam and Buddhism in a Southern Thai Coastal Fishing Village," *The Journal of the Siam Society, 60* (1972):183–215.

Bibliography

———. "Buddhism, Islam and Spirit Beliefs and Practices and Their Social Correlates in Two Southern Thai Coastal Fishing Villages," Ph.D. dissertation. London School of Oriental and African Studies, 1973.
Burridge, K. "Kuda Kepang in Batu Pahat," *Man, 61* (1961):33–36.
Cavendish, R., ed. *Man, Myth and Magic.* London: R. Parnell, 1970–72.
Cardena, Etzel. "The Phenomenology of Possession: An Ambiguous Flight," *Proceedings of the Fifth International Conference on the Study of Shamanism and Alternate Modes of Healing, 1988,* ed. Ruth-Inge Heinze. Berkeley, CA: Independent Scholars of Asia, Inc., 1989.
Chakravarty, Nilmani. "Spirit belief in the Jakata Stories," *Journal of the Royal Asiatic Society, Bengal Branch*, new series, *10:7* (1931)257–263.
Chard, Robert L. Master of the Family: History and Development of the Chinese Cult to the Stove. Berkeley, CA: University of California, Ph.D. dissertation, 1990.
Chen, Peter S.J. "Strategies for the Development of a Singapore Identity," *Journal of Sociology and Psychology, 1* (1978):1–8.
——— and Hans-Dieter Evers. *Studies in ASEAN Societies, Urban Society and Social Change.* Singapore: Chopmen Enterprises, 1977.
Ciba Foundation. *Transcultural Psychiatry.* London: J. and A. Churchill, Ltd., 1965.
Cicourel, Aaran V. *Cognitive Sociology, Language and Meaning in Social Interaction.* Harmondworth, Middlesex: Penguin Books, 1973.
Clark, Kathleen. "Yap Ah Loy's Temple," *Straits Times Annual* (1961):66–69.
Claus, Peter. "The Siri Myth and Ritual: A Mass Possession Cult of South India," *Ethnology, XIV:1* (January 1975):47–58.
Clements, Forrest E. "Primitive Concepts of Disease," *University of California Publications in American Archaeology and Ethnology, 32* (1932):185–252.
Clifford, Hugh. *In Court and Kampong.* London: Grant Richards, 1897.
———. *Studies in Brown Humanity.* London: Grant Richards, 1898.
Closs, Alois. "Das Religioese im Schamanismus," *Kairos, 2* (1960).
Comber, Leo. *Chinese Magic and Superstition in Malaya.* Singapore: Donald More, 1957.
———. *Chinese Temples in Singapore.* Singapore: Eastern Universities Press, 1958.
———. *Chinese Ancestor Worship in Malaya.* Singapore: Eastern Universities Press, Malayan Heritage Series No.1, 1963.
Connor, Linda H. "Ships of Fools and Vessels of the Divine: Mental Hospitals and Madness, A Case Study," *Social Science and Medicine, 16* (1982):783–794.

Cooper, Robert G. and Rengaraju Raj Kumar. "Anti-Structure and Ethnic Identity Change: An Evaluation of Changing Emphases in Indian-Hindu Calendrical Ceremonies in Singapore," *Journal of Sociology and Psychology*, 2 (1979):11–27.

Cuisinier, Jeanne. *Danses magiques de Kelantan*. Paris: Travaux et memoires de l'Institut d'ethnologie, Universite de Paris, 1936.

_____. *Sumangat, l'Ame et Son Culte en Indochine et en Indonesie*, preface de Louis Massignon. Gallimard: L'Espece Humain Librairie 7, 1951.

Czaplicka, Marie Antoinette. *Aboriginal Siberia: A Study in Social Anthropology*. Oxford, England: Clarendon Press, 1914.

Dacher, Elliott S. "Old Landscapes, New Eyes: From Treatment to Healing," *Bridges* (Magazine of the International Society for the Study of Subtle Energies and Energy Medicine), *6:4* (Winter 1995):1,9–11.

Danaraj, Alain. *Hindu Polytheism*. New York: Bollingen Foundation, 1964.

Dato' Sedia Raja, Abdullah. "The Origin of Pawang and the Berpat Ceremony," *Journal of the Royal Asiatic Society, Malay Branch*, 2 (1927):310–313.

Davidson, W.D. "Psychiatric Significance of Trance Cults," Paper read at the 121st Annual Meeting of the American Psychiatric Association, 3–7 May 1965, New York.

Davis, Richard. "Tolerance and Intolerance of Ambiguity in Northern Thai Myth and Ritual," *Ethnology, XIII* (1974):7–24.

Dean, Stanley R., ed. *Psychiatry and Mysticism*. Chicago, IL: Nelson Hall, 1975.

De Groot, J.J.M. *The Religious System of China*. Leiden, Netherlands: Brill, 1892–1910, 6 vols.

_____. "Les Fetes Annuellement Celebres a Emoui (Amoy), Etude Concernant La Religion Chinois," *Annales Musee Guimet, XI–XII*. Paris: Ernest Leroux, 1886.

De Heusch, Luc. "Culte de possession et religions initiatiques de salut en Afrique," *Religions de salut*. Brussels: Annales du Centre d'Etudes des Religions, 1962.

Delaney, William P. "Northern Thai Spirit Mediums, Relationships Among Health, Possession Trance, and Polity," paper read at the 26th Annual Meeting of the Midwest Conference on Asian Affairs at Northern Illinois University, De Kalb, IL, October 15, 1977.

Demetrio, Francisco, S.J. "The Shaman as Psychologist," *Asian Folklore Studies* (1977):55–73.

Denzin, Norman K. "Symbolic Interactionism and Ethnomethodology: A Proposed Synthesis," *American Sociological Review, 34:6* (1969):992–934.

Bibliography

Deren, M. *Divine Horsemen.* Chicago, IL: Aldine, 1970.
Devereux, George. *Normal and Abnormal in Some Uses of Anthropology, Theoretical and Applied.* Washington, DC: The Anthropological Society of Washington, 1956, pp.23–48.
_____. *From Anxiety to Method in the Behavioral Sciences.* The Hague/Paris: Mouton & Co., 1967.
De Zoete, Bernd and Walter Spies. *Dance and Drama in Bali.* London: Faber and Faber, 1938.
Dicker, R. "The Defensive Function of an Altered State of Consciousness," *Journal of the American Psychoanalytical Association*, 11 (1965):356–401.
Dole, Gertrude E. "Shamanism and Political Control among the Kuikuru," *Voelkerkundliche Abhandlungen*, 1 (1964):53–62.
Dore, Henri, S.J. *Researches into Chinese Superstitions*, transl. M. Kennelly. Reprinted, Taipei, Taiwan: Ch'eng Wen Publishing Company, 1966–1967. First edition: Shanghai: T'usewei Printing Press, 1914–1929, 15 vols.
Dorsainvil, J.C. *Vodou et Nervrose.* Port-au-Prince, Haiti: Imprimerie La Pressed, 1911.
Douglas, Mary. *Natural Symbols, Explorations in Cosmology.* London: Barrie and Rockliff, The Cresset Press, 1970.
Dubois, Abbe, J.A. *Hindu Manners, Customs and Ceremonies*, transl. Henry K. Beauchamp. Oxford, England: Clarendon Press, 1905, 3rd ed.
Durand, Maurice. "Technique et Pantheon des Mediums Vietnamiens (Dong)," *Publication de l'Ecole francaise d'Extreme Orient*, 45 (1959):1–333.
Duerkheim, Emile. *The Elementary Forms of the Religious Life*, transl. Joseph Ward Swain. New York: The Free Press, 1965; London: Allen & Unwin, 1958; First ed, 1915.
Duerrenberger, E.P. "A Lisu Shamanistic Seance," *The Journal of the Siam Society*, 64:2 (July 1976):151–160.
Eberhard, Wolfram. *Chinese Festivals.* New York: Henry Shuman, 1952.
_____. *Guilt and Sin in Traditional China.* Berkeley and Los Angeles, CA: University of California Press, 1967.
_____. *The Local Cultures of South and East China*, transl. Alide Eberhard. Leiden, Netherlands, E.J. Brill, 1968.
Eder, Matthias. "Schamanismus in Japan," *Paideuma, VI:7* (May 1958):367–380.
Edsman, Carl-Martin, ed. *Studies in Shamanism,* based on papers read at the Symposium on Shamanism held at Abo from the 6th to 8th of September,

1962. Stockholm, Sweden: Almquist & Wiksell, Scripts Instituti Donneriani Aboensia, I, 1967.

Eister, Allen W., ed. *Changing Perspectives in the Scientific Study of Religion.* New York: A Wiley-Interscience Publication, John Wiley and Sons, 1974.

Eliade, Mircea. *Shamanism, Archaic Techniques of Ecstasy*, transl. Willard R. Trask. Princeton, NJ: Princeton University Press, Bollingen Series LXXVI, 2nd printing, 1974; First edition: *Le Chamanism et les techniques archaique de l'extase.* Paris: Payot, 1946.

―――. *Yoga, Immortality and Freedom.* Princeton, NJ: Princeton University Press, Bollingen Series LVI, 1969.

Eliot, Sir Charles. *Hinduism and Buddhism, A Historical Sketch.* London: Edward Arnold & Co., 1921, 3 vols; 2nd vol. repr. New York: Barnes & Noble, Inc., 1968.

Elliott, Alan J.A. *Chinese Spirit Medium Cults in Singapore.* London: London School of Economics and Political Science, 1955.

Endicott, Kirk Michael. *An Analysis of Malay Magic.* Oxford, England: Clarendon Press, 1970.

English, H.B. and A.G. *An Comprehensive Dictionary of Psychological and Psychoanalytical Terms.* New York: Longmans, Green, 1958.

Evans-Pritchard, E.E. *Witchcraft, Oracles and Magic Among the Azanda.* London, England: Oxford University Press, 1937.

Evans-Wentz, W.Y., comp. and ed. *The Tibetan Book of the Dead.* London: Oxford University Press, paperback, 1960.

Fabrega, Horacio, Jr. "Concepts of disease: logical features and social implications," *Perspectives in Biology and Medicine.* Chicago, IL: The University of Chicago Press, vol.15, no.4, Summer 1972.

Fairchild, E.P. "Shamanism in Japan," *Folklore Studies, 21* (1962).

Favas, Ref.P. "Pawangs," *Journal of the Indian Archipelago, 3* (1849):115–116.

Festinger, Leon and H.H. Kelley. *Changing Attitudes Through Social Contact.* Ann Arbor, MI: Research Center for Group Dynamics, 1951.

Festinger, Leon, H.S. Riecken, and Stanley Schachter. *When Prophecy Fails.* Minneapolis, MN: University of Minnesota Press, 1956.

Field, M.M. *Search for Security: An Ethnopsychiatric Study of Rural Ghana.* Evanston, IL: Northwestern University Press, 1960.

Findeisen Hans. *Schamanentum, dargetellt am Beispiel der Bessenheitspriester nordeurasiatischer Voelker.* Zurich/Wien: Europa Verlag, 1957.

Firth, Raymond. "Ritual and Drama in Malay Spirit Mediumship," *Comparative Studies in Society and History*, 9 (1967):190–207.
_____. *Symbols: Public and Private*. London: Allen and Unwin, 1973.
_____. "Faith and Scepticism in Kelantan Village Magic," *Kelantan: Religion, Society and Politics in a Malay State*, ed. William Roff. Kuala Lumpur, Malaysia: Oxford University Press, 1974.
Fischer, R.W. "A Cartography of the Ecstatic and Meditative States," *Science* (1974):897–904; also, *Understanding Mysticism, its methodology, interpretation in world religions, psychological evaluations, philosophical and theological appraisals*, ed. Richard Woods. Garden City, NY: Image Books, 1980, pp.286–305.
Forbes, Andrew D.W. "The Muslim national minorities of China," *Religion, Journal of Religion and Religions*, VI (Spring 1976):57–87.
Frank, J.D. *Persuasion and Healing: A Comparative Study of Psychotherapy*. Baltimore, MD: The Johns Hopkins Press, 1961.
Frankl, Victor E. *Psychotherapy and Existentialism, Selected Papers on Logotherapy*. New York: Washington Square Press, Inc., 1967.
_____. *The Unheard Cry for Meaning. Psychotherapy and Humanism*. New York: Simon and Schuster, 1978.
Frazer, Sir James George. *The Golden Bough, A Study in Magic and Religion*. London: McMillan, 3rd ed., 1955; New York: The McMillan Co., 1951.
Freed. Stanley A. and Ruth S. "Spirit Possession as Illness in a North Indian Village," unpublished paper, 1959.
Freedland, Nat. *The Occult Explosion*. New York: Putnam, 1972.
Freeman, D. "Fire-walking at Ampang, Selangor," *Journal of the Malay Branch of the Royal Asiatic Society*, 2 (1924):74–76.
Freud, Sigmund. *The Basic Writings of Sigmund Freud*, transl. and ed. Dr.A.A. Brill. New York: The Modern Library, 1938.
_____. "Obsessive Acts and Religious Practice," *Collected Papers*, 2. London: Hogarth Press, 1948, p.50.
_____. "A Case of Demonical Possession," *Collected Papers*, 4. London: Hogarth Press, 1958, 9th impr., pp.436–476.
Frigerio, Alejandro. "Levels of Possession and Awareness in Afro-Brazilian Religions," paper presented at the 5th Annual Conference of the Association for the Anthropological Study of Consciousness, Pacific Palisades, CA, March 1–5, 1989.

Freed, Stanley A. and Ruth S. "Spirit Possession as Illness in a North Indian Village," unpublished paper, 1959.
Freedland, Nat. *The Occult Explosion*. New York: Putnam, 1972.
Freeman, D. "Fire-walking at Ampang, Selangor," *Journal of the Malay Branch of the Royal Asiatic Society*, 2 (1924):74–76.
Freud, Sigmund. *The Basic Writings of Sigmund Freud*, transl. and ed. Dr.A.A. Brill. New York: The Modern Library, 1938.
_____. "Obsessive Acts and Religious Practice," *Collected Papers*, 2. London: Hogarth Press, 1948, p.50.
_____. "A Case of Demonical Possession," *Collected Papers*, 4. London: Hogarth Press, 1958, 9th impr., pp.436–476.
Frigerio, Alejandro. "Levels of Possession and Awareness in Afro-Brazilian Religions," paper presented at the 5th Annual Conference of the Association for the Anthropological Study of Consciousness, Pacific Palisades, CA, March 1–5, 1989.
Fromm, Erich. *The Sane Society*. New York: Rinehart & Co., 1956.
_____. *Psychoanalysis and Religion*. New Haven, CN: Yale University Press, 1958.
Geertz, Clifford. "Religion as a Cultural System," *Anthropological Approaches to the Study of Religion*, ed. Michael Banton. London: Tavistock Publications, 1966, pp.1–46.
Gerini, Col. G.E. *Chulakantamangala or The Tonsure Ceremony as performed in Siam*. Bangkok, Thailand: Bangkok Times Office, 1895; Bangkok: The Siam Society, 2d ed., 1976.
Gill, M.M. and M. Brenman. *Hypnosis and Related States*. New York: International Universities Press, Inc., 1961.
Gimlette, Dr. John D. *Malay Poisons and Charm Cures*. London/Kuala Lumpur/New York/Melbourne: Oxford University Press, 1975; First ed., 1915.
Goldammer, Kurt. *Die Formenwelt des Religioesen, Grundriss der systematischen Religionswissenschaft*. Stuttgart, Germany: Alfred Kroner Verlag, 1960.
Goudenough, Erwin. *Psychology of Religious Experience*. New York: Basic Books, 1965.
Goodman, Felicitas. *Speaking in Tongues*. Chicago, IL: The University of Chicago Press, 1972.
_____. Jeannette H. Henney and Esther J. Pressell. *Trance, Healing, and Hallucination: Three Field Studies in Religious Experience*. New York: A Wiley Interscience Series, John Wiley and Sons, 1974.

Bibliography

Gould, Julius and William Kolb, eds. *A Dictionary of the Social Sciences*. New York: Free Press, 1964.
Graham, David Crockett. *Folk Religion in Southwest China*. Washington, D.C.: Smithsonian Press, 1961.
Hale, A. "How Mir Hasan Became a Pawang," *Straits and States Annual* (Singapore, 1920):108–114.
Halifax, Joan. *Shaman, the Wounded Healer*. New York: Crossroad, 1982.
Hallett, Holt S. *A Thousand Miles on an Elephant in the Shan States*. London: William Blackwood and Sons, 1890.
Hallowell, A. Irving. "The Social Function of Anxiety in a Primitive Society," *American Sociological Review*, 6 (1941):869–881.
Hamer, J. and Irene Hamer. "Spirit Possession in Its Sociopsychological Implications Among the Sidamo of Southwest Ethiopia, *Ethnology*, 5 (1966):392–408.
Hand, Wayland D. "The Folk Healer: Calling and Endowment," *Journal of the History of Medicine*, 26 (1971):263–275.
Hansen, Valerie. *Changing Gods in Medieval China, 1127–1276*. Princeton, NJ: Princeton University Press, 1990.
Harada, Masami. "The Faith of Kew Ong Yeah in Malaysia," *The Toho Shukyo* [The Journal of Eastern Religions], *53* (May 1979):1–21.
Harding, M. Esther. *The "I" and the "Not-I," A Study in the Development of Consciousness*. New York: Pantheon Books, 1965.
Harner, Michael J., ed. *Hallucinogens and Shamanism*. New York: Oxford University Press, 1973.
_____. *The Way of the Shaman*. New York: Bantam Books, 1980.
Harrison, T. "Gawal Antu: Great Spirit Festival," *Straits Times Annual* (1966):74–77.
Hartog, J. "The Intervention System for Mental and Social Deviants in Malaysia," *Social Science and Medicine*, 6 (1972a):211–220.
_____ and G. Resner. "Malay Folk Treatment — Concepts and Practices with Special References to Mental Disorders," *Ethnomedicine*, *1:3–4* (1972b):353–372.
Hassan, Riaz. *Singapore, Society in Transition*. Kuala Lumpur, Malaysia: Oxford University Press, 1976.
Hastings, James, ed. *Encyclopedia of Religion and Ethnics*. New York: Charles Scribner's Sons, 1921.

Heinze, Ruth-Inge, "Stages of Spiritual Development," *Visakha Puja* (1974):125–134.

―――. "The Nature and Function of Some Therapeutic Techniques in Thailand," *Asian Folklore Studies*, 2 (1977a):85–104.

―――. transl. and ed. *The Biography of Ahjan Man*. Taipei, Taiwan: Orient Cultural Series, Asian Folklore and Social Life Monograph Series, 89, 1977b.

―――. *The Role of the Sangha in Modern Thailand*. Taipei, Taiwan: Orient Cultural Series, Asian Folklore and Social Life Monograph Series, 93, 1977c.

―――. "Mediumship in Singapore Today," *Journal of Sociology and Psychology*, 2 (1979a):54–70.

―――. "The Social Implications of the Relationships Between Mediums, Entourage and Clients in Singapore Today," *Southeast Asian Journal of Social Sciences*, VII:2 (1979b):60–80.

―――. "The Nine Imperial Gods in Singapore," *Asian Folklore Studies*, XL:2 (1981):151–171.

―――. *Tham Khwan, How to Contain the Essence of Life, A Socio-Psychological Comparison of a Thai Custom*. Singapore: Singapore University Press, 1982a.

―――. "Glossolalia in Singapore," *Folklore*, VII (January 1982b):33–38.

―――. "Shamans or Mediums, Toward a Definition of Different States of Consciousness," *Phoenix, Journal of Transpersonal Anthropology*, VI:1–2 (1982c):25–44.

―――. "The Ritual Process: Translating the Ineffable Into Ritual Language," *Proceedings of the 7th International Conference on the Study of Shamanism and Alternate Modes of Healing*, ed. Ruth-Inge Heinze. Berkeley, CA: Independent Scholars of Asia, 1990, pp.1–17.

―――. *Shamans of the 20th Century*. New York: Irvington Publishers, Inc., 1991.

―――. "Role et Fonctions actuels des chamanes en Asie du Sud-Est: les etats alterne de la conscience," *Diogene*, 158 (Paris, Gallimard, Avril–Juin, 1992):119–129. [English translation, Providence: Berg Publishers, 1992, pp.133–144.]

―――. "The Relationship Between Folk and Elite Religions: The Case of Thailand," *The Realm of the Sacred, Verbal Symbolism and Ritual Structure*. ed. Sitakant Mahapatra. Delhi: Oxford University Press, 1992, pp.13–30.

―――. "The Dynamics of Chinese Religion: A Recent Case of Spirit Possession in Singapore," *Chinese Beliefs and Practices in Southeast Asia*, ed. Cheu Hock-Tong. Petaling Jaya, Malaysia: Pelanduk Publications, 1993, pp.187–197.

———. "Alternate States of Consciousness," *Silver Threads*, ed. Jean Milay, Dean Brown and Beverly Kane. New York: Praeger, 1993, pp.201–209.

———. "The Lotus and the Serpent: Signs and Symbols, Archetypes and Myths, *Society for the Anthropology of Consciousness*, (March 1995); expanded manuscript to be published in 1997.

Henderson, James. "Exorcism and Possession in Psychotherapy Practice," *Canadian Journal of Psychiatry*, *27* (1982):129–134.

Hilgard, E.R. "Automatic writing and divided attention," *Divided Consciousness: Multiple Controls in Human Thoughts and Action*, by E.R. Hilgard. New York: John Wiley and Sons, 1977, pp.131–154.

Hinderling, Paul. *Communication Between Doctors and Patients in Thailand*, Part 3, Interviews with Traditional Doctors. Saarbruecken, Germany: University of the Saar, Report from the South Asia Programme, 1973.

Hitchcock, John T. and Rex L. Jones, eds. *Spirit Possession in the Nepal Himalayas*. New Delhi: Vikas Publishing House, 1976.

Hoffmann, Helmut. *Symbolik der Tibetischen Religionen und des Schamanismus*. Stuttgart, Germany: Anton Hiersemann, 1967.

Homans, George C. "The Function of Religion in Modern Society," *Reader in Comparative Religion*. eds W.A. Lessa and E.Z. Vogt. Evanston, IL, and White Plains, NY: Row, Peterson and Co., 1958.

Honegger, B. "A Neuropsychological Theory of Automatic Verbal Behavior," *Parapsychology Review* (May/June 1980).

Houtsma, M.Th., ed. *The Encyclopedia of Islam*. London: Luzac & Co., 1913–1938.

Howells, William. *The Heathens*. New York: Doubleday, 1956.

Hsu, Francis L.K. *Religion, Science and Human Crises*. London: Routledge & Kegan Paul, 1952.

———. *Psychological Anthropology, Approaches to Culture and Personality*. Homewood, IL: Dorsey Press, 3rd ed., 1961.

Huey, Ju Shi. "Chinese Spirit Mediums in Singapore, An Ethnographic Study," University of Singapore, Department of Sociology, unpublished M.A. Thesis, December 1977.

Hullett, Arthur. "Bringing the Gods Down to Earth," *The Asia Magazine* (September 15, 1979):3, 14, 17, 18, 21.

Hyman, Stanley Edgar. "The Ritual View of Myth and the Mystic," *Journal of American Folklore*, *68* (1955):462–472.

I Ging, Das Buch der Wandlungen, transl. and ed. Richard Wilhelm. Duesseldorf/Koeln: Eugen Diederichs Verlag, Taschenausgabe, 6, 1960.

Irwin, J.A. "Some Siamese Ghost-Lore and Demonology," *The Journal of the Siam Society*, IV (1907):19–33.
Isherwood, C. *Ramakrishna and His Disciples*. New York: Simon and Schuster, 1965.
Jacobi, H. "Cosmogeny and Cosmology, Indian," *The Encyclopedia of Religion and Ethics*, IV (1911):1452–161.
Jahoda, Gustav. *The Psychology of Superstition*. Hammondsworth, Middlesex: Penguin Books, Ltd., 1970.
James, William. *The Varieties of Religious Experience*. New York: Modern Library, Inc. 1950.
Janet, P. *L'Automatism Psychologique*. Paris: Felix Alcan, 1889.
Jilek, Wolfgang. "From Crazy Witch Doctor to Auxiliary Psychotherapist — The Changing Image of the Medicine Man," *Psychiatria Clinica*, 4 (1971):200:220.
———. *Indian Healing*. Surrey: Handbook House Publishers, 1982a.
———. "Altered States of Consciousness in North American Indian Ceremonials," *Ethos*, 10:4 (Winter 1982b):326–243.
Jordan, David K. *Gods, Ghosts and Ancestors*. Berkeley, CA: University of California Press, 1972.
———. "How to become a Chinese Spirit Medium," paper read at the Association for Asian Studies at the Pacific Coast Meeting, Eugene, Oregon, June 1977.
Jung, Carl G. *The Archetypes and the Collective Unconscious*, transl. R.F.C. Hull. New York: Pantheon Books, Bollingen Series, IX, 1959.
———. *The Structure and Dynamics of the Psyche*, transl. R.F.C. Hull. New York: Pantheon Books, Bollingen Series, VIII, 1960.
———. *Civilization in Transition*, transl. R.F.C. Hull. New York: Pantheon Books, Bollingen Series, X, 1964.
———. *Psychology and Religion*, transl. R.F.C. Hull. Princeton, NJ: Princeton University Press, Bollingen Series, XI, 2d ed., 1969.
———. "The Psychological Foundations of Beliefs in Spirits," *Psychology and Extrasensory Perception*, ed. Raymond Van Over. New York: Mentor Books, 1972.
Kakar, Sudhir. *Shamans, Mystics and Doctors, A Psychological Inquiry into India and its Healing Traditions*. Boston, MA: Beacon Press, 1982.
Kaplan, Bert and Dave L. Johnson. "The Social Meaning of Navaho Psychopathology and Psychotherapy, "*Magic, Faith, and Healing*, ed. Ari Kiev. New York: The Free Press, 1964, pp.203–229.
Kardiner, Abram. *The Psychological Frontiers of Society*. New York: Columbia University Press, 1945.

Kendall, Laurel. "Caught Between Ancestors and Spirits: Field Report of a Korean Mansin's Healing Kut," *Korea Journal, 17:8* (August 1977):8–23.

Kennedy, J. "Nubian Zar Ceremonies as Psychotherapy," *Human Organization, 4* (1967):185–194.

Keupers, Joh. "A Description of the *Fa-ch'ang* Ritual as Practiced by the *Lu Shan* Taoists of Northern Taiwan," *Buddhist and Taoist Studies, I*, ed. Michael Saso and David W. Chappell. Oahu, HI: The University of Hawaii Press, Asian Studies at Hawaii, No.18, 1977, pp.79–94.

Keyes, Charles F. "The Power of Merit," *Visakha Puja, 2516* (May 16, 1973):95–101.

Kiev, Ari, ed. *Magic, Faith, and Healing, Studies in Primitive Psychiatry Today*. New York: The Free Press, 1st paperback, 1974.

Kildahl, John. *The Psychology of Speaking in Tongues*. New York: Harper and Row, 1972.

Kirsch, A. Thomas. "Phu Thai Religious Syncretism, A Case Study of Thai Religion." Cambridge, MA: Harvard University, unpublished Ph.D. dissertation, 1967.

Kleeman, Terry F. Wenchang and the Viper: The Creation of a Chinese National God. Berkeley, CA: University of California, Ph.D. dissertation, 1980.

Kleinman, Arthur. *Patients and Healers in the Context of Culture. An Exploration of the Borderland between Anthropology, Medicine, and Psychiatry*. Berkeley, CA: University of California Press, 1980.

Kok, Lee Peng. "Epidemic Hysteria, A Psychiatric Investigation," *Singapore Medical Journal, 16:1* (March 1975):35–38.

Krippner, Stanley. "Altered States of Consciousness," *The Highest State of Consciousness*, ed. J. White. New York: Doubleday, 1972.

_____. *Song of the Siren, A Parapsychological Odyssey*. New York/San Francisco: Harper Colophon Books, 1977.

_____. and Alberto Villoldo. *The Realms of Healing*. Milbrae, CA: Celestial Arts, 1952.

Kris, Ernst. *Psychoanalytic Explorations in Art*. New York: International Universities Press, 1952.

Kroeber, Alfred L. "Totem and Taboo: An Ethnological Psychoanalysis," *American Anthropologist, XXII* (1920):48–55.

_____. "Psychosis or Social Sanctions," *The Nature of Culture*. Chicago, IL: The University of Chicago Press, 1952.

Kuhn, Manfred H. "Major Trends in Symbolic Interaction Theory in the Past Twenty-Four Years," *Sociological Quarterly, 5* (Winter 1964):61–84.

La Barre, Weston. *The Ghost Dance, Origins of Religion*. New York: Dell Publications, 1978, 3rd printing.

Laderman, Carol C. "Taming the Wind of Desire, The concept of angin appears as useful in Malaysia as ego and superego in the West," *Asia* (January/February 1980):34–39.

_____. *Taming the Wind of Desire, Psychology, Medicine, and Aesthetics in Malay Shamanistic Performance*. Berkeley, CA: University of California Press, 1991.

Lambert, G.W. "Studies in the automatic writing of Mrs. Verall: X. Concluding reflections," *Journal of the Society for Psychical Research* (1971):217–222.

Landolt, H. "Mystical Experience in Islam," *Personality Change and Religious Experience*. Montreal, Canada: Proceedings of the 1st Annual Conference, R.M. Bucke Memorial Society, 1965.

Laotze's Tao-te Ching, with introduction, transliteration and notes by Dr. Paul Carus. Chicago, IL: Open Court Publications, 1898.

Laski, M. *Ecstasy*. London: Cresset Press, 1961.

Laufer, Berthold. "The Development of Ancestral Images in China," *Journal of Religious Psychology*, 4 (1913):111–123.

_____. "Origin of the Word Shaman," *American Anthropologist*, 19 (1917):361–371.

Laurentin, Rene. *Catholic Pentecostalism*, transl. Matthew J. O'Connell. New York: Doubleday/Image, 1978.

La Vallee-Poussin, Louis. "Cosmogony and Cosmology, Buddhist," *The Encyclopedia of Religion and Ethics*, IV (1911):129–138.

_____. "Magic, Buddhist," *The Encyclopedia of Religion and Ethics*, VIII (1911):255–257.

_____. "Nature, Buddhist," *The Encyclopedia of Religion and Ethic*, IX (1911):209–214.

Law, Bimala Charan. *The Buddhist Conception of Spirits*. Calcutta and Simla, India: Thacker, Spink & Co., 1923.

Leary, T. *The Politics of Ecstasy*. London: McGibbon & Kee, 1970.

Le Bar, Frank, Gerald Hickey and John K. Musgrave, eds. *Ethnic Groups of Mainland Southeast Asia*. New Haven, CN: Human Relations Area Files Press, 1964.

Lederer, Wolfgang. "Primitive Psychotherapy," *Psychiatry*, 22 (1959):225–265.

Leslie, Charles, ed. *Anthropology of Folk Religion*. New York: Vintage Books, 1960.

Bibliography

Lessa, William A. and Evon Z. Vogt. *Reader in Comparative Religion, An Anthropological Approach.* New York: Harper and Row, 3rd ed., 1972.
Leuba, J.H. *A Psychological Study of Religion.* New York: Macmillan, 1912.
Levi-Strauss, Claude. "The Effectiveness of Symbols," and "The Sorcerer and His Magic," *Structural Anthropology*, transl. Claire Jacobson and Brooke Grundfest. New York: Basic Books, 1963, pp.167–185 and 186–205.
Levy-Bruhl, Lucien. *The "Soul" of the Primitive*, transl. Lilian A. Clare. London: George Allen & Unwin, Ltd., 1965.
Lewis, I.M. *Ecstatic Religion, An Anthropological Study of Spirit Possession and Shamanism.* Harmondworth, Middlesex: Penguin Books, Ltd., 1971; repr. 1975.
_____. "Spirit Possession or Deprivation Cults, *Man, I:2* (1966).
Lieban, R.W. "Shamanism and Social Control in a Philippine City," *Journal of the Folklore Institute, II:1* (1965).
Litvag, I. *Singer in the Shadows: The Strange Story of Patience Worth.* New York: Macmillan, 1972.
Locke, A. *The Tigers of Trengganu.* London: Museum Press, Ltd., 1954.
Loeb, E.M. "Shaman and Seer," *American Anthropologist, 31* (1929):60–84.
Lommel, Andreas. *Shamanism: The Beginning of Art*, transl. Michael Bullock. New York: McGraw-Hill Book Co., 1967.
Ludwig, Arnold M. "Altered States of Consciousness," *Archives of General Psychiatry, 16* (1966):225–234; also, *Altered States of Consciousness*, ed. Charles T. Tart. New York: John Wiley & Sons, Inc., 1969, pp.9–22.
Machado, A.D. "On the supposed evil influences exercised by ghosts in the Malay Peninsula," *Journal of the Straits Branch of the Royal Asiatic Society, 35* (1903):208–209.
MacKenzie, D.A. *The Migration of Symbols.* London: Kegan Paul, Trench, Trubner & Co., Ltd., 1926.
Malinowski, Bronislaw. *Magic, Science and Religion.* New York: Doubleday Anchor Books, 1948.
Mandelbaum, David G. "Transcendental and Pragmatic Aspects of Religion," *American Anthropologist, 68:5* (October 1966):1174–1191.
Manis, J.G. and B.N. Meltzer, eds. *Symbolic Interaction: A Reader in Social Psychology.* Boston, MA: Allyn & Bacon, 1967.
Manson, Joy. *Festivals of Malaysia.* Singapore: Eastern Universities Press, 1965.
Marasinghe, M.M.J. *Gods in Early Buddhism, A Study in Their Social and Mythological Milieu as Depicted in the Nikayas of the Pali Canon.* Kelaniya, Sri Lanka: University of Sri Lanka, Vidyalankara Campus Publication Board, 1974.

Maringer, J. *The Gods of Prehistoric Man*. London: Weidenfeld, 1960.
Marriott, McKim. "Little communities in an indigenous civilization," *Village India*, ed. M. Marriott. Chicago, IL: University of Chicago Press, 1955, pp.171–222.
Matthews, R.H. *Chinese-English Dictionary*. Cambridge, MA: Harvard University Press, 1945.
Maulana, Mohammad Ali. *The Holy Qu'ran*, Arabic text, Engl.transl. and comm. Chicago, IL: Specialty Promotions Co., Inc., 6th ed., 1973.
Maxwell, William E. "Shamanism in Perak," *Journal of the Straits Branch of the Royal Asiatic Society*, *XII* (1883):222–232.
McDonnell, Kilian, ed. *The Holy Spirit and Power and the Catholic Charismatic Renewal*. Garden City, NY: Doubleday, 1975.
McHugh, J.M. *Hantu Hantu: An Account of Ghost Belief in Modern Malaya*. Singapore: Donald More, 1955.
Morton, Robert K. *Social Theory and Social Structure*. New York: Free Press, 1957.
Messing, S. "Group Therapy and Social Status in the Zar Cult of Ethiopia," *Culture and Mental Health*, ed. M.K. Opler. New York: Macmillan Publishing Co., Inc., 1958.
Metraux, A. *Religion and Shamanism, Handbook of South American Indians*, 5, ed. J.H. Stewart. Washington, DC: Smithsonian Institution, Bureau of American Ethnology, Bulletin 43, 1949, pp.559–599.
_____. *Voodoo in Haiti*. New York: Oxford University Press, 1959.
Michael, H.N. *Studies in Siberian Shamanism*. Toronto, Canada: The Arctic Institute of North America, University of Toronto, Anthropology of the North, transl. from Russian sources, 4, 1963.
Miller, Casper J., S.J. *Faith-Healers in the Himalayas*. Kathmandu, Nepal: Tribhuvan University Press, 1979.
Mischel, Walter and Frances M. Psychological Aspects of Spirit Possession," *American Anthropologist*, 60 (1958):249–260.
Miyakawa, H. and A. Kollautz. "Zur Ur- und Vorgeschichte des Schamanismus," *Zeitschrift fuer Ethnologie*, *91*:2 (1966):161–193.
Mohammed, Aris, Normah. "The Syncretic Basis and 'Functions' of Spirit Beliefs and Institutions in a Malay Village Community," University of Singapore, Department of Sociology, unpublished B.A. Honors Academic Exercise, 1973.
Monier-Williams, Monier. *Brahmanism and Hinduism*. London: John Murray Publication, Ltd., 1891.

_____. *Indian Wisdom or Examples of the Religious, Philosophical and Ethical Doctrines of the Hindu.* Varanasi, India: Chowkhamba, 1975.

Morechand, George. "Notes sur les chamanes et mediums de quelques groupes Thai," *Bulletin de l"Ecole Francaise d'Extreme Orient, 64* (1968).

Muehl, Anita. *Automatic Writing.* Dresden and Leipzig, Germany: Theodor Steinkopf, 1930; New York: Helix Press, 2nd ed., 1963.

Mustapha, Siti Hanifah. "Malay Magic and Folk Medicinal Practice Among the Malays in Singapore," University of Singapore, Department of Malay Studies, unpublished M.A. thesis, 1977.

Myers, F.W.H. "Automatic Writing III," *Proceedings of the Society for Psychical Research, 4* (1887):209–261.

_____. *Human Personality and Its Survival of Bodily Death.* London: Longmans, Green, 1003, 2 vols.

Myers, John.T. "A Hong Kong spirit-medium temple," *Journal of the Hong Kong Branch of the Royal Asiatic Society, 15* (1975):15–27.

_____ and Davy Leung. *A Chinese Spirit-medium Temple in Kwun Tong: A Preliminary Report.* Hong Kong: Social Research Centre, Chinese University of Hong Kong, 1974.

Nagata, Judith A. "What is a Malay?" *American Ethnologist, 1:2* (1974):331–350.

Needham, Joseph. *Science and Civilization in China.* Cambridge, MA: Harvard University Press, 1956.

Needleman, J. *The New Religions.* Garden City, NY: Doubleday, 1970.

Neher, Andrew A. "Auditory Driving Observed with Scalp Electrodes in Normal Subjects," *EEG and Clinical Neurophysiology, 13* (1961):449–451.

_____. "A Physiological Explanation of Unusual Behavior in Ceremonies Involving Drums," *Human Biology, 34* (1962):151–160.

Neumann, Erich. *The Origins and History of Consciousness,* 2 vols, with a foreword by C.G. Jung, transl. R.F.C. Hull. New York: Harper & Brothers, 1962; Princeton, NJ: Princeton University Press, 1954.

Newell, W.H. *Treacherous River: A Study of Rural Chinese in North Malaya.* Kuala Lumpur, Malaysia: University of Malaya Press, 1962.

Ng, Cecilia. "The Sam Poh Neo Keramat, A Study of a Baba Chinese Temple," University of Singapore, Department of Sociology, unpublished Bachelor of Social Science Honors thesis, 1976.

Nioradze, George. *Der Schamanismus bei den sibirischen Voelkern.* Stuttgart, Germany: Strecker und Schroeder, 1925.

Nowak, Margaret and Stephen Durrant. *The Tale of the Nisan Shamaness. A Manchu Folk Epic*. Seattle/London: University of Washington Press, 1977.

Nyce, Ray. "Chinese Folk Religion in Malaysia and Singapore," *The South East Asia Journal of Theology*, 12 (Spring 1971):81–91.

_____. *Chinese New Villages in Malay, A Community Study*. Singapore: Malaysian Sociological Research Institution, Ltd., 1973.

Obeyesekere, Gananath. "The great tradition and the little in the perspective of Sinhalese Buddhism" *The Journal of Asian Studies*, 22 (1963):139–153.

_____. "The Idiom of Demonic Possession: A Case Study," *Social Science & Medicine, 4* (1970):97–111.

_____. "Psycho-Cultural Exegesis of a Case of a Spirit Possession from Sri Lanka," *Contributions to Asian Studies, 8, The Psychological Study of Theravada Societies*, ed. Steven Piker. Leiden, Netherlands: E.J. Brill, 1975, pp.41–89.

O'Brien, E. *Varieties of Mystic Experiences*. New York: Holt, 1964.

O'Dea, Thomas F. *The Sociology of Religion*. Englewood Cliffs, NJ: Prentice-Hall, 1966.

Oesterreich, Traugott Konstantin. *Die Besessenheit*. Langensalza, Germany: Wendt & Klauwell, 1921; *Possession and Exorcism*. New York: Causeway Books, 1974.

Olson, Jon L. and Marc Cramer. "Spirits and Structure: The Possession of Jose C." Unpublished paper, California State University, Los Angeles, 1982.

Ornstein, R. *The Psychology of Consciousness*. New York: Penguin Books, 1972.

Osman, Mohammed Taib. "The Bomoh and the Practice of Malay Medicine, Indigenous, Hindu, and Islamic Elements in Malay Folk Beliefs," Bloomington, IN: Indiana University, Folklore Institute, unpublished Ph.D. dissertation, 1967.

_____. "How bomohs work," *The Asia Magazine, II* (April 2, 1975).

Overmyer, Daniel L. *Folk Buddhist Religion, Dissenting Sects in Late Traditional China*. Cambridge, MA and London: Harvard University Press, 1976.

_____. "Spirit-writing (fu-chi) texts, Values in Sectarian Literature, Mid Ming to the Twentieth Century, Part 2," Paper delivered at the annual Meeting of the Association for Asian Studies, Toronto, March 13, 1981.

Pang, Duane. "The P'u-Tu Ritual," *Buddhist and Taoist Studies, I*, ed. Michael Saso and David W. Chapell. Oahu, HI: The University of Hawaii Press, Asian Studies at Hawaii, No. 18, 1977, pp.79–94.

Parsons, Talcott. *Societies: Evolutionary and Comparative Perspectives*. Englewood Cliffs, NJ: Prentice -Hall, 1966.

Pavlov, L.P. *Lectures on Conditioned Reflexes*. London: Lawrence & Wishart, vol.2, 1941.

Pelletier, Kenneth R. and Charles Garfield. *Consciousness: East and West*. New York/San Francisco/London: Harper Colophon Books, 1976.

Peters, Larry. *Ecstasy and Healing in Nepal: An Ethnopsychiatric Study of Tamang Shamanism*. Malibu, CA: Undena Publications, 1981.

—— and D. Price-Williams. "Towards an experiential analysis of shamanism," *American Ethnologist* (1980):397–413.

Piyasilo, Phra. "A Flashing of the Shield, Youth in Search for Religious Experience," *World Fellowship of Buddhists Review* (Bangkok, November–December 1977):26–28.

Popov, A.A. *Materialy dlja bibliografii russkoi literatury po izuceniyu samanstva severno-aziarisikh narsdov*. Leningrad, Russia: Academic Nauk, 1932 (650 studies).

Poree-Maspero, Eveline. "Notes sur les particularities du culte chez les Cambodgiens," *Bulletin de l'Ecole Francaise d'Extreme Orient, 44:2* (1954):619–641.

——. "La ceremonie de l'appel des esprits vitaux chez les Cambodgiens," *Bulletin de l'Ecole Francaise d'Extreme Orient, 45:1* (1955):145–183.

——. *Etudes sur les rites agraires des Cambodgiens*. Paris: 1969, 3 vols.

Potter, Jack M. "Cantonese Shamanism," *Religion and Ritual in Chinese Society*, ed Arthur Wolf. Stanford, CA: Stanford University Press, 1974.

Pottier, Richard. "Notes sur les chamanes et mediums de quelques groupes Thai," *Asie de Sud-est et le Monde Insulindien, 4:1* (1973):99–109.

Prabhavananda, Swami and Christopher Isherwood. *How to Know God, the Yoga Aphorisms of Patanjali*. New York: The New American Library, 1953.

Prince, M. *The Dissociation of Personality*. New York and London: Longmans, Green, 1906.

——. "Awareness, Consciousness, Co-Consciousness, and Animal Intelligence from the Point of View of the Data of Abnormal Psychology," *Pedagogical Seminar, XXXII* (1925):106–188.

Prince, Raymond, ed. *Trance and Possession States*. Montreal, Canada: Proceedings of the Second Annual Conference, R.M. Bucke Memorial Society, 4–6 March 1966, publ. 1968.

Quah, Stella. "Accessibility of Modern and Traditional Health Services in Singapore," *Social Science and Medicine*, vol.11 (1977a):33–340.

_____. *The Unplanned Dimensions of Health Care in Singapore: Traditional Healers and Self-Medication*. Singapore: University of Singapore, Department of Sociology, Working Paper No.62, 1977b.

Quebedeaux, Richard. *The New Charismatics*. Garden City, NY: Doubleday, 1976.

Rahmann, R. "Gottheiten und Schamanismus bei den Mundavoelkern und ihren dravidischen Nachbarn." Vienna, Austria: University of Vienna, Institute of Ethnology, unpublished doctoral dissertation, 1935.

Rajadhon, Phya Anuman. "The Phi," *The Journal of the Siam Society*, XL:2 (January 1954):153–178.

_____. *Life and Ritual in Old Siam. Three Studies of Thai Life and Customs*, transl. and ed. William J. Gedney. New Haven, CN: Human Relations Area Files Press, 1961.

_____. "Thai Charms and Amulets," *The Journal of the Siam Society*, LII:2 (July 1964):171–198.

Rank, Gustav. "Shamanism as a Research Subject," *Studies in Shamanism*, ed. Carl Martin Edsman. Stockholm, Sweden: Almquist and Wiksell, 1962.

Rao, T.A. Gopinatha. *Elements of Hindu Iconography*. Madras, India: The Law Printing Housek 1914–1916, 4 vols.

Raybeck, Douglas. "Main Peteri: The Healing Ceremony as Means of Reducing Social Stress," paper read at the conference of the American Anthropological Association, 1970.

Reik, Theodor. *Ritual: Psycho-Analytic Studies*. London: Hogarth Press and Institute of Psycho-Analysis, 1931.

Rituale Romanum (The Rites of the Catholic Church), as Revised by the Second Vatican Ecumenical Council). New York: Pueblo, 1976 (first published 1614).

Robert, Katherine. "The Role of Malay Magicians and Medicine Men, A Study of the Practice, Their Clients and Their Relations to Their Clients in Singapore," University of Singapore, Diploma of Social Studies Exercises, 1959.

Robinet, Isabelle. "Radonees extatique des Taoistes dans les astres," *Monumenta Serica*, 32 (1976:159–273.

_____. "Metamorphosis and Deliverance from the Corpse in Taoism," *History of Religions* (1979):37–70.

Roheim, Geza. "Psychoanalysis of Primitive People," *International Journal of Psychoanalysis*, 13 (1932):1–221.

Bibliography

Rose, L. *Faith Healing.* London: Penguin Books, 1971.
Rouget, G. *Music and Trance: A Theory of the Relations between Music and Possession.* Chicago, IL: University of Chicago Press, 1985.
Sachner, R.C. *Mysticism, Sacred and Profane.* Oxford, England: Oxford University Press, 1961.
Salmon, G. *A Sermon on the Work of the Holy Spirit.* Dublin, Ireland: Hodges, Smith, 1859.
Sargant, W. *Battle for the Mind.* London: Pan Books, 1964.
Saso, Michael R. *Taiwan Feasts and Customs.* Hsinchu, Taiwan: Chabanel Language Institute, 1965.
_____. *The Teachings of Taoist Master Chuang.* Hew Haven and London: Yale University Press, 1978.
Schafer, Edward H. *Pacing the Void. T'ang Approaches to the Stars.* Berkeley, CA: University of California Press,, 1977.
_____. "The Jade Woman of Greatest Mystery," *History of Religions, 17* (1978):387–398.
Schipper, Kristofer M. "The Written Memorial in Taoist Ceremonies," *Religion and Ritual in Chinese Society,* ed. A.P. Wolf. Stanford, CA: Stanford University Press, 1974, pp.309–324.
Schroeder, Dominik. "Zur Struktur des Schamanismus," *Anthropos, 50* (1955):848–881.
Scupin, Raymond. "Transformation in Islam Ideology: The Thai Muslim Case," paper presented at the American Anthropological Association meeting in Washington, DC, December 7, 1980.
Sears, Robert. *Survey of Objective Studies of Psychoanalytic Concepts.* New York: Social Science Research Council, 1943.
Shaw, William. "Aspects of spirit-mediumship, trance and ecstasy in Peninsular Malaysia," *Federation Museums Journal* (New Series), *18* (1963):71–176.
_____. *Aspects of Malaysian Magic.* Kuala Lumpur, Malaysia: Muzium Negara, 1975.
Shirokogoroff, S.M. *Psychomental Complex of the Tungus.* London: 1935.
Shuttleworth, Charles. *Hutan Rimba. Safaris in the Malayan Jungle.* Singapore: Malayan Publication, 1963.
Sills, David L., ed. *International Encyclopedia of the Social Sciences.* New York: Macmillan Co., and The Free Press, 1968.
Silverman, Julian. "Shamans and Acute Schizophrenia," *American Anthropologist, 69* (1967):21–31.

Skeat, Walter William. *Malay Magic: An Introduction to the Folklore and Popular Religion of the Malay Peninsula.* London: Macmillan & Co., Ltd.,1900; London: Frank Cass & Co., Ltd., 2d ed., 1965.
Smith, Adam. *Powers of Mind.* New York: Random House, 1975.
Smith, D. Howard. *Chinese Religions. From 1000 B.C. to the Present Day*, gen.ed. E.O. James. New York: Holt, Rinehart and Winston, History of Religion Series, 1968.
Soothill, William Edward and Lewis Hodous, comp. *A Dictionary of Chinese Buddhist Terms.* London: Kegan Paul, Trench, Trubner, and Co., Ltd., repr. by Ch'eng Wen Publishing Co., Taipei, 1975.
Sources of Chinese Tradition, ed. Wm. Theodore de Bary. New York: Columbia University Press, 1966.
Spencer, S. *Mysticism in World Religion.* London: Penguin Books, 1963.
Spiro, Melford E. "Religious Systems as Cultural Constituted Defense Mechanisms," *Context and Meaning in Cultural Anthropology*, ed. Melford E. Spiro. New York: The Free Press of Glencoe, Inc., 1965.
_____. "Religion: Problems of Definition and Explanation," ed. Michael Banton. London: Tavistock Publications, 1966, pp.85–126.
_____. *Burmese Supernaturalism, A Study in the Explanation and Reduction of Suffering.* Englewood Cliffs, NJ: Prentice-Hall, 1967.
_____ and Roy G. D'Andrade. "A Cross-Cultural Study of Some Supernatural Beliefs," *American Anthropologist*, 60 (1958):456–466.
Starbuck, E.D. *The Psychology of Religion.* London: Scott, 1901.
Stevenson, I. "Some comments on automatic writing," *Journal of the American Society for Psychical Research*, 72 (1978):35–332.
Stirling, W.G. "Chinese Divining Blocks and the "Pat Kwa' or Eightsided Diagram," *Journal of the Malayan Branch of the Royal Asiatic Society*, 2 (1924a):72–73.
_____. "Chinese Exorcists," *Journal of the Malayan Branch of the Royal Asiatic Society*, 2 (1924b):41–47.
Strickman, Michel. "Taoism, History of," *Encyclopedia Britannica*, 17 (1981):1044–1050.
Sweeney, Amin. "The Shadow Play of Kelantan. Report on a period of field research," *Journal of the Malayan Branch of the Royal Asiatic Society*, 43:2 (1970):53–80.
Tambiah, Stanley J. "The Magical Power of Words," *Journal of the Royal Asiatic Institute*, III:2 (1968).

_____. *Buddhism and the Spirit Cults in Northeast Thailand.* Cambridge, England: University Press, Comparative Studies in Social Anthropology, 1970.

_____. "Form and Meaning of Magical Acts: A Point of View," *Modes of Thought,* eds Robin Horton and Ruth Finnegan. London: Faber & Faber, 1973.

_____. *The Buddhist Saints of the Forest and the Cult of Amulets: A Study in Charisma, Hagiography, Sectarianism and Millennial Buddhism.* Cambridge, NY: Cambridge University Press, 1984.

Taylor, Sarah E.L., ed. *Fox-Taylor Automatic Writing 1869–1892,* unabridged record. Minneapolis, MN: Tribune-Great West Printing Co., 1932.

Tart, Charles T. *Waking Up, Overcoming the Obstacles to Human Potential.* Boston, MA: New Sciences Library, Shambhala, 1986.

_____, ed. *Altered States of Consciousness.* New York: John Wiley Sons, 1969.

Textor, Robert B. *Patterns of Worship: A Formal Analysis of the Supernatural in a Thai Village.* New Haven, CN: Human Relations Area Files, 1973a.

_____. *Roster of the Gods: An Ethnography of the Supernatural in a Thai Village.* New Haven, CN: Human Relations Area Files, 1973b.

The Citizen, "Galloping 'horses'!" *7:18* (September 16, 1978):14–15.

The Malay Mail (February 18, 1970).

The Straits Times (October 1, 1975).

Thomas, E.S. "The Fire Walk," *Proc.Social Psychiatry Research, 42* (193)):292–309.

Thomas, M. Ladd. "Thai Muslim Separatism in South Thailand," paper presented at the Association for Asian Studies at the Pacific Coast Meeting, Santa Cruz, June 26, 1982.

Tillich, Paul. *Dynamics of Faith.* New York: Harper Torchbook, 14th printing, 1965; 1st printing, 1957.

_____. "The Meaning of Health," *Religion and Medicine, Essays on Meaning, Values and Health,* ed. David Belgum. Ames, IO: The Iowa State University Press, 1967, pp.3–12.

Titiev, Mischa. "A Fresh Approach to the Problem of Magic and Religion," *Southeastern Journal of Anthropology, 16* (1960):292–298.

Topley, M. "Chinese Rites for the Repose of the Soul; with special reference to Cantonese custom," *Journal of the Malayan Branch of the Royal Asiatic Society, 25:1* (1952):149–160.

_____. "Chinese Women's Vegetarian Houses in Singapore," *Journal of the Malayan Branch of the Royal Asiatic Society, 27:1* (1954).

Torrey, E.F. *Witchdoctors and Psychiatrists: The Common Roots of Psychotherapy and Its Future.* New York: Harper and Row, 1986.

Trueblood Brodzky, Anne, Rose Danesewich, and Nick Johnson, eds. *Stone bones, and skin, ritual and shamanic art.* Toronto, Canada: The Society for Art Publications, 1977.

Turner, Victor. *The Ritual Process, Structure and Anti-Structure.* Chicago, IL: Aldine Publishing Co., 1966.

_____. "Myth and Symbol," *International Encyclopedia of Social Science, 10.* New York: The Macmillan Co., and The Free Press, 1968, pp.576–582.

_____. "Metaphors of Anti-Structure in Religious Culture," *Changing Perspectives in the Scientific Study of Religion,* ed. A.W. Eister. New York: Wiley, 1974, pp.63–84.

Turton, Andrew, "Matrilineal Descent Groups and Spirit Cults of the Thai-Yuan in Northern Thailand," *The Journal of the Siam Society,* 60 (1972):217–256.

Underhill, Evelyn. *Mysticism: A Study in the Nature and Development of Man's Spiritual Consciousness.* New York: Noonday Press, 1955; London: Methuen & Co., Ltd., 16th ed., 1949; 1st ed. 1911.

Van Gennep, Arnold. *The Rites of Passage,* transl. Monika B. Vizedom and Gabrielle L. Cafees, introd. Solon T. Kimball. Chicago, IL: University of Chicago Press, 1960; Paris: *Les Rites de Passage,* 1st ed.

Wach, Joachim. *Types of Religious Experience.* Chicago, IL: University of Chicago Press, 1951.

Waddell, L.A. "Demons and spirits, Buddhist," *The Encyclopedia of Religion and Ethics, IV* (1911):571–572.

_____. *The Buddhism of Tibet or Lamaism.* Cambridge, England: W. Heffer & Sons, Ltd., repr. 1939.

Wagner, Nathaniel N. and Tan Eng Seon, eds. *Psychological Programs and Treatment in Malaysia.* Kuala Lumpur, Malaysia: University of Malaysia Press, 1971.

Wallace, Anthony F.C. "Cultural Determinants of Response to Hallucinatory Experience," *Archives of General Psychiatry, 1* (1959):59–69.

_____. *Religion: An Anthropological View.* New York: Random House, 1966.

Wan Ho, Poh. "Chinese Spirit Medium Divination in Penang, A Study of Performance Structure," Universiti Sains Malaysia, School of Humanities, Term Paper, March 1979.

Watts, Alan W. *The Wisdom of Insecurity, A Message for an Age of Anxiety.* New York: Pantheon Books, 1951.

Bibliography

Wavell, Stewart, Audrey Butt, and Nina Epton. *Trances.* London: Allen & Unwin, 1966.
Wayman, Alex. "Trance and Possession States, with Indo-Tibetan Emphasis," *Proceedings Second Annual Conference, R.M. Bucke Memorial Society*, ed. Raymond Prince. Montreal, Canada, March 4–6, 1966, publ. 1968.
Wetherhead, L. *Psychology, Religion and Healing.* New York: Abingdon, 1951.
Weber, Max. *The Religion of China: Confucianism and Taoism*, transl. and ed. Hans H. Gerth. Glencoe, IL: The Free Press, 1951.
_____. *The Religion of India, Sociology of Hinduism and Buddhism*, transl. and ed. Hans H. Gerth and Don Martindale. Glencoe, IL: The Free Press, 1960.
_____. *The Sociology of Religion*, transl. Ephraim Fischoff. London: Methuen, 1965, 1st ed., 1922.
Webster's Third New Dictionary of the English Language. Springfield, MA; G. & C. Merriam Co., 1971.
Wee, Vivienne. "'Buddhism' in Singapore," *Singapore: Society in Transition*, ed. Riaz Hassan. Kuala Lumpur, Malaysia: Oxford University Press, 1976, pp.155–188.
_____. "Religion and Ritual among the Chinese of Singapore. An Ethnographic Study," University of Singapore, Department of Sociology, unpublished M.A. thesis, 1977.
_____. *Chinese Religion in Singapore and Peninsular Malaysia.* Kuala Lumpur, Malaysia: Oxford University Press, 1980.
Werner, E.T.C. *A Dictionary of Chinese Mythology.* New York: Julian Press, 1961.
Wilkins, W.J. *Hindu Mythology; Vedic and Puranic.* Calcutta, India: Thacker, Spink & Co., 3rd ed., 1900.
Wilkinson, R.J. *Malay Beliefs.* London: Luzac & Co., 1906.
_____. *A Malay-English Dictionary* (romanized). London: MacMillan & Co., Ltd., 1957.
William, C.A.S. *Encyclopedia of Chinese Symbolism and Art Motives.* New York: Julian Press, 1960.
Wilson, P.J. "Status Ambiguity and Spirit Possession," *Man*, 2 (1967):155–378.
Winstedt, R.O. "Propitiating the Spirits of a District (menjamu negeri)," *Journal of the Federated Malay States Museum*, 9 (1920):93–95.
_____. "Karamat: sacred places and persons in Malaya," *Journal of the Malay Branch of the Royal Asiatic Society*, 2 (1924):264–279.
_____. *Shaman, saiva and sufi: a study of the evolution of Malay magic.* London: Constable & Co., 1925; *The Malay magician: being shaman, saiva and sufi.*

London: Routledge & Kegan Paul, Ltd. 1961.
Winthrop, Robert H. "Norm and Tradition in American Benedictine Monasticism," unpublished Ph.D. dissertation, University of Minnesota, Minneapolis, Department of Anthropology, 1981.
Wirz, Paul. *Exorcism and the Art of Healing in Ceylon.* Leiden: E.J. Brill, 1954.
Wolf, Arthur P., ed. *Religion and Ritual in Chinese Society.* Stanford, CA: Stanford University Press, 1974, esp. his essay on "Gods, Ghosts, and Ancestors."
Wong, C.S. *A Cycle of Chinese Festivals.* Singapore: Malaysia Publishing House, 1967.
Wright, Th. *The Open Door: A Case History of Automatic Writing.* New York: John Day Company, 1970.
Yaacob, Mohamed Fauz. *Main Puteri.* Singapore: Malaysia Publishing House, 1967.
Yang, C.K. *Religion in Chinese Society.* Berkeley, CA: University of California Press, 1961.
Yap, P.M. "The Possession Syndrome: A Comparison of Hong Kong and French Findings," *Journal of Mental Science, 106* (1960):114–137.
Zaehner, R.D. *Mysticism, Sacred and Profane, An Inquiry Into Some Varieties of Preaternatural Experience.* London: Oxford University Press, 1967.
Zainul-Abidin Bin Ahmad. "The tiger-breed families," *Journal of the Straits Branch of the Royal Asiatic Society, 75* (1922):36–39.
_____. "The Akuan or Spirit Friends," *Journal of the Straits Branch of the Royal Asiatic Society, 86* (1925a):378–384.
_____. "Dato Parao, Were-Tiger," *Journal of the Malayan Branch of the Royal Asiatic Society, 3:1* (1925b):74–78.
_____. "The Work of the Bomohs in Kelantan," B.A. Honors thesis, University of Malaysia, Singapore, 1957.
Zaretsky, Irving I. *Bibliography on Spirit Possession and Spirit Mediumship.* Evanston, IL: Northwestern University Press, 1966.
Zinberg, Norman E., ed. *Alternate States of Consciousness, Multiple Perspectives of the Study of Consciousness.* New York: The Free Press, 1977.
Zuehlsdorf, Volkmar. "The Witch Doctors of Chiangmai," *Zeitschrift fuer Kultur und Geschichte Ost- und Suedostasiens, 112* (1972): 79–87.

Index

Abhidhamma, 263
Abse, 285
Achterberg, J., 228, 229, 274
Ackerknecht, E.H., 4
Ackerman, S.E. and R.L.M. Lee, 265
acupuncture, 105
Adler, A., 294
Ahjan Man, 37
alienation, 112
Allah, 73, 107, 241, 286, 289
alternate states of consciousness, xxiii, 7, 58, 59, 61-64, 67, 68, 182, 227, 262, 271, 298
altruistic, 42, 45, 111
Amitābha (O-mi-t'o fo), 76, 80, 89, 125, 134, 136, 150, 151, 156-158, 162, 253, 261
amnesia, 176, 271
amulets, charm (joss) papers, 40, 72, 155
ang pow (red envelope), 45, 126, 135, 144, 154, 231, 251
angin (wind), 190, 191, 237
animism, xix, 271
animistic, 33, 34, 198
apron, see siu-to
arahant (enlightened one), xxiii, 37
arati (waiving of lights), 130
archetype, 12, 272, 273, 294
Atharva Veda, 103, 283

auditory driving, 60
automatic writing, 63, 68, 86, 87, 163-166, 172, 226, 297
autonomic nervous system, 108, 174, 176, 274
Avalokitesvara, 80, 151, 157
avatāra, 152, 243, 283
Averroes (Muslim mystic), 177
ayurvedic, 103, 105
azimat (also jimat, gangkal, pengaruh/pangaruh, pelian), 58, 237
Babb, L.A. xvii, 261
Bahai, 209
Bartlett, H.H., 190
Basham, A.L., 159
belian (weretiger), 79
belief, xv, xvii, 102, 103, 274, 298
Bellah, R.N., 295
Belo, J., 228
Benjamin, G., 264
beta-endorphin, 59
bhajan (devotional song), 55, 68, 131, 243
bhikṣu (monk), 160, 243
bhikṣunī (nun), 160, 243
bhuta (ghost), 75
Bible, 178, 277
Big Dipper (Ursa Major), 40, 79, 85, 146-148
biofeedback, xviii

331

Index

Blacker, C., 56, 68, 154
bodhisattva, 75, 76, 80, 146, 157, 159, 162, 205, 210, 243, 267, 276
Bogoras, W., 4
bomoh, xxii, 6, 34, 35, 40-42, 44, 53, 55, 72, 73, 90, 95-98, 104-106, 113-115, 186-198, 226, 227, 237, 240, 265
Bon (early Tibetan religion), 12
Bourguignon, E., xxiii, 228, 261
Brahmā, 75, 160, 199, 201, 216, 221, 227, 243, 267, 283
brahmin, 7, 16, 34, 38, 40, 53, 75, 129, 130, 180, 198, 199, 243, 260, 263, 283
Brandon, S.G.F., 255, 256
bridge (p'ing an chiao), 154, 155, 243
Buddha, 11, 37, 38, 57, 75, 76, 79, 89, 104, 110, 134, 136, 139, 151, 159-162, 199, 206-208, 210, 215-217, 221, 222, 243-246, 259, 263, 266, 267, 275, 276, 283
Buddhism, xix, xx, 6, 8, 34, 75, 76, 94, 95, 135, 136, 152, 159, 161, 170, 206, 209, 210, 212, 244, 264, 266, 267, 269, 275
Buddhist, xxiii, 3, 15, 16, 19, 22, 33, 34, 36, 37, 40, 55-57, 73-76, 89, 91, 104, 106-108, 110, 125, 133, 135, 136, 146, 150, 151, 158, 160-162, 198, 201, 204, 206, 208, 210, 214, 216, 222-224, 227, 234, 245, 259, 263, 267, 276, 298, 302
Caraka Samhita, 103
Cardena, E., 67
caste, 263, 283
catharsis, 93, 185, 276

Catholic(ism), 72, 179, 281
chai koo (vegetarian nun), 156
Chao Phi Saen Saeb, 221-224
charisma, 36, 130, 276
charms, 48, 57, 58, 69, 72, 105, 135, 263; see also amulets
Chen, P., 21
ch'i (life force), 154, 281, 291
chianh sin (inviting the spirits), 69
Christ, 178, 210, 261; see also Jesus Christ
Christian, 33, 76, 89, 108, 135, 280, 282, 288, 291
Christianity, xix, 8, 22, 89, 152, 170, 209, 277
Chulalongkorn (King Rama V), 76, 201, 227, 259
Chun-ti, 150, 231, 266
Claus, P., 75
Cohen, A., 58
Comber, L., 52, 78, 80, 146, 149, 150, 263, 264
Communism, 210
Communist, 214
communitas (Turner), xxiii, 99, 104, 127, 131, 134, 179, 266, 277, 296
Confucian(ism), 10, 55, 152, 158, 160, 162, 165, 170, 277, 278
Confucius, 161
coping mechanisms, 110
cosmic, 11
Cuisinier, J., xix
Czaplicka, M.A., 4
Dacher, E.S., 230
dalang (shadow puppet player), 189, 191
Danaraj, A.G.S., 40, 237, 264

dato, 238
Davidson, W.D., xxiii
De Groot, J.J.M., 6, 9, 35, 43, 53, 55, 68, 70, 164-166, 168
De Zoete, B. and W. Spiess, 182, 184
Delaney, W.P., 37, 45, 70, 72, 220, 228
Demetrio, F., S.J., 93
deva(ta), 75; deva raja, 9
Devereux, G., xx, xxiv, 4
dharma (Sanskrit), dhamma (Pāli), 37, 75, 107, 158-161, 205, 207, 217, 221, 222, 243, 269, 283
dhoti (loin cloth), 53, 130, 199, 243
Dickes, R.S., xxiii
DID (dissociative identity disorder), 289
dissociation, 62-64, 67, 175, 176, 262, 279
dissociative, 292
divination, 9, 168, 279, 297
Divine, 35, 41, 48, 72, 91, 99, 102, 103, 105-107, 180, 227, 295, 296, 301, 302
Divine Sages, 203, 204, 208, 210; see also Pu Sawan
DNA, 109
Dore, H., 43, 57, 72, 79, 80, 148, 149, 253, 263, 264, 266
Douglas, M., 228
Doyle, Sir A.C., 174
dragon throne, 69, 128; see also lung wei
dukkha (suffering), 217
Durand, M., 5, 36
Durkheim, E., xviii
Durrenberger, E.P., 226
East India Company, 18
Eberhard, W., 7, 78, 166, 264, 266, 267

ecstasy, 63-65, 185, 280
ecstatic, 5, 39, 178
eggs, 134
ego, 280
Eighteen Lohans, see lohans
Eister, A.W., xxiii
elementary forms of the religious life, xviii, 9, 11-13, 230
Eliade, M., xviii, xix, xxiii, 4, 5, 8, 186, 191, 220, 226, 302
Elliott, A.J.A., xix, 3, 36, 47, 49, 53, 54, 56, 112, 263
entourage, 28, 46, 99, 109, 126-128, 130, 135
Evans-Wentz, W.Y., 51
evocation, 189
exorcism, 31, 38, 40, 41, 50, 64, 65, 105, 128, 140, 191, 211, 281
exorcist, 204, 297
faith, xv, 105, 229, 282
fasting, 8
feng-shen yen-i (Metamorphoses of the Gods), 231, 266
filial piety, 158, 160
fire walking (Timiti), xvii, 3, 7, 62, 64, 163, 257
Fischer, R.W., 58, 228, 295
Four Noble Truths, 217, 267, 275
Fox-Taylor, 174
Frank, J.D., 46, 51, 104, 228
Frankl., V.E., 10, 101, 294
Freed, St.A, and Ruth S. 285
Freud(ian), S., 96, 191, 271, 291, 293
Frigerio, A. 66, 67
fu, 54, 57, 231; see also, amulets; fu-chi (support a winnowing basket) 168, 232; fu-luan (support a phoe-

nix), 168 232; fu-luh (magic script), 57, 232
Furst, P.T., 295
Gak Teh Ia, 232
Gandhi, M., 210
Gaṇeśa, 130, 243, 257, 283
Geertz, C., 11, 12
ghost, xxiv, 145, 282, 292; see also kuei
Gimlette, J.D., xix, 40, 189, 237
glossolalia, xvi, 34, 63, 64, 68, 178-182, 226, 282
Grube, W., 264
guru, 190, 243
hadith (sayings of the prophet), 238, 264
haji (one who has made a pilgrimage to Mecca), 183, 238
Halifax, J., 71, 140
Hallowell, A.I., 228
hallucination, 62, 64, 65, 282
Hamer, J. and I. Hamer, 228
Hansen, V., 77
han-tsin (nominal adoption), 72; see also luk liang
hantu (spirit), 74, 238
Hanuman (monkey god), 6, 75, 120, 243, 258
Harada, J., 149, 152, 162, 163, 267
Harding, M.E., 273
Hariti, 80
Hart, D., 177
Hartog, Y., xx, 40, 41, 237
Hastings, J., 272
HDB (Housing and Development Board), 21, 53, 54, 112, 188, 263
Heinze, R.-I., 6, 12, 37, 41, 42, 61, 67, 76, 94, 99, 200, 207, 263, 265, 267, 273, 277, 287, 292, 296
Hilgard, E.R., 175-177
hilltribe, 120, 225
Hīnayāna, 159, 275
Hinderling, P., 39, 265
Hindu, 19, 74, 75, 91, 94, 107, 108, 134, 146, 201, 222, 227, 239, 240, 243, 246, 257, 258, 261, 267, 268, 275, 283
Hinduism, xix, 8, 22, 34, 76, 89, 152, 283
Hitchcock, J.T., 65
holistic, 106
Holy Arctic Canon, 170, 171
Holy Communion, 57
Holy Ghost, xvi, 180
Holy Mary, 89
Holy Spirit, xvi, 179, 180, 291
Honeger, B., 164, 175, 177
Howells, W., 4
Hsuan-tsang, 6, 79, 232, 234
hun shen (cloud soul), 232
Huang-ti (Yellow Emperor), 232
hypnosis, 63, 67, 176, 185, 284, 301
hypnotism, 290
hypothalamus, 301
hysteria, 4, 64, 96, 106, 181-182, 265, 285, 290, 301
I-Ching, 148, 232
id, 285, 292
imam (leader of a Muslim community), 17, 73, 238
indeterminacy, xxi
Indra, 160, 207
initiation, 43, 44
incantation, 196, 238
inferior temporal lobe, 176

Irwin, J.A., 76
Islam, xix, 8, 16, 19, 22, 95, 152, 170, 209, 241, 286-287, 302
Islamic, 214, 264
Jade Emperor, 80, 89, 149, 251
James, W., 93, 94, 100, 108
jampi (spell), 187, 238; see also, mantra
jamu (traditional medicine), 106
Janet, P., 175
Jesus Christ, 4, 209, 215, 261; see also Christ
Jilek, W., 59, 60, 61
jina (conqueror), 160, 243
jinn (spirit), 73, 239, 264
Jivaka (Buddha's physician), 104
Jones, R., 66
Jordan, D.K., 44, 109
joss paper, 126, 140, 145, 155; see also amulets
joss (incense) sticks, 126, 143, 155, 157
Judaism, 267
Jung, C.G., 71, 182, 272, 273, 294, 295
Kakar, S., 5, 61, 264
Kālī, Mahākālī, 37, 75, 129, 130, 244, 283
kalpa (a day of Brahmā, 4,320 earthly years), 159, 243
Kam T'ien Siong Te, 89, 125, 128. 232, 252, 253
karma (Sanskrit), kamma (Pāli), 34, 39, 74, 94, 95, 107, 220, 243, 267, 283, 287
karuna (compassion), 216
Kau Wong Yeh, 79, 151, 232; see also Nine Imperial Gods
kavaca, 58, 239; see also amulets
kavadi, 7, 25, 56, 63, 243, 261

Keng Yeon Taoist Association, 172
Kennedy, J., 228
Keyes, Ch.F., 111
khon song (spirit medium), xxii, 39, 55, 199, 247
khryang raeng, 38, 57, 247; see also amulets
Khun Suchart, 204-206, 209-215
Khun Vichit Sae Tia, 211, 212
khwan (vital essence), 200, 223, 247, 281
ki (writing stick), 165, 166, 232
kiao (divining block), 55
Kiev, A., xxiii
ki-tong (divining youth), 36
Kildahl, J., 178, 180-182, 289
Kleeman, T.F., 77
Kleinman, A., xx, 41, 104, 265, 266
Kok, L.P., 265, 285
kong t'ung (youth into which a spirit descends), 36
Koran (Qur'an), 40, 53, 58, 73, 91, 184, 237, 241, 263, 264, 277, 286
Krippner, S., 58, 176, 177, 228
Kris, E., 5
Krishna, 134, 222, 257, 283
Kroeber, A., 4, 13
krut (Garuda), 76
Kṣitigarbha, 159, 235, 267
Kuang Kong/Kuan Teh/Kwan-yu, 77, 156, 172, 233, 251, 252, 253
Kuan Yin (Kuanin), 54, 79, 80, 82, 89, 125, 127, 134, 143, 150, 151, 156, 157, 159, 162, 233, 252, 253
kuay oon (removing bad luck), 41, 46, 72, 233
Kuda Kepang, 62, 87, 88, 182-186, 226

Index

kuei, 65, 165, 233; see also ghost
Laderman, C., xix, xxiii, 191, 192
Lambert, G. W., 177
Lao-tzu, 161, 300
Laurentin, R., 179
lemon, 188, 195
len dong (Vietnamese spirit medium), 5
Lessa, W.A. and E. Vogt, xxiii, 7, 296
Levi-Strauss, C., 5
Lewis, I.M., 36, 39, 65, 228, 265
lime, 131, 190
liminal(ity), xxiii, 127, 266, 287, 296
lineage, 217, 218, 221
Litvag, I., 174, 175, 177, 268
Liu-pei, 77, 233
Living Buddha, 44, 81
lohans, eighteen, 136, 253, 266
loh-tang (medium), 36
Lommel, A., 4, 93
lotus chair, 54
Lotus Sūtra, 80
Luang Po (Pu) Tuad, 199, 200, 201, 204, 205, 207, 210-212, 215
Luang Vichit Vadakaran, 206
Ludwig, A.M., 228, 271
luk liang (children adopted by a spirit for protection), 224; see also, han-tsing
Luman-al-Hakim, 104
lung wei (dragon throne), 54, 233
ma khi (horse of spirit, medium), xxii, 5, 39, 221, 247
magic, 9, 41, 102, 187, 191, 288, 297
magical flight, 5, 6, 61, 62, 65, 67, 68
Mahāyāna, xix, 16, 75, 134, 146, 158, 159, 243, 275

main puteri, 113, 114, 189, 191, 226, 239
Maitreya, 160, 210, 253, 267
Manjusri, 80, 160
Manson, J., 264
mantra (magical words; Malay, menteras), 184, 185, 223, 224, 244
margosa (nim, pomegranate), 53
Marīcī (Goddess of Dawn), 150, 266
mass hysteria, 96, 134
Maudsley, Dr., 110
Mecca, 238, 255, 264, 286
Mencius, 57
Merdeka (Malay, Independence Day), 20
Messing, S., 228
Metamorphoses of the Gods, 79, 264; see also feng-shen yen-i
metta (loving kindness), 216
miang (fermented tea leaves), 219, 247
miao (temple for public worship), 233
Miao-shen, 80, 233
millenary movements, 111
Miller, C.J., 98, 103
mindok, 191, 240
Mischel, F. and F.M. Mischel, 228
Moggallana (Pāli), Maudgalyayana (Sanskrit), 76, 204, 221, 222
mokṣa (release), 244, 283
monkey god, 6, 251; see also Hanuman
mortification, 3, 56
MPD (multiple personality disorder), 289
mu bei (divining blocks), 30, 52, 54, 233
mudita (altruistic joy), 216
mudrā, 148, 244

Muehl, A., 176
mufti, 34, 73
Muhammad, 73, 241, 255, 262, 286
muh-yu (wooden fish, skull-shaped block), 55, 233
muni (Sanskrit: sage), 74, 244
Murgam, 38, 75, 129, 130, 134, 222, 243-245, 257, 258, 261, 283
Murphy, G., 177
Muslim, 16, 17, 20, 33, 34, 40, 42, 56, 73, 91, 108, 111, 180, 182-184, 186, 188, 191, 226, 238, 239, 241, 242, 253, 255, 256, 262, 286, 289, 297
Mustapha, S.H., 40, 237
Myers, J.T., 175
mysticism, 290
mystics, xviii, xix
myth, 290
mythology, 13, 290
nag(a) (mystical serpent), 76, 160, 223, 244, 269
nam mon (blessed water), 38, 247
NDE (near-death experience), 62
Neher, A.A., 60
Nei Ching (Book for Internal Diseases), 104
nidāna (cause, underlying factor), 159, 267
nim (pomegranate), 53
Nine Imperial Gods, 6, 79, 82, 146, 148-163, 235, 253, 266; see also Kau Wong Yeh
nirvāṇa (Sanskrit), nibbana (Pāli), 75, 245
Nor Cha Sam T'ai Tze (The Third Prince), 79, 234, 252
Novena Church, 89

Nyce, R., 49
OBE (out of body experience), 61, 62, 64
Olson, J.L. and M. Cramer, 71
omniscience. 72
ong (sacred), 37, 247
Ornstein, R., 180, 228
Osman, M.T., 93
ouija board, 268
Our Lady of Lourdes, xvi, 33, 134, 179, 180
Overmyer, D.L., 9, 10, 164, 165, 167, 168, 170, 172
Pa kua (Eight Trigrams), 54, 234
Pang, D., 148
paññā (wisdom), 205
paraphernalia, 53, 91, 111
pareitta, 263 ; see also mantra
Patanjali, 75, 283, 302
pathological, 185, 294
pathology, xviii, 291
pawang, 183-185, 240
Peace Pagoda, 207, 208, 215
peach, 79; peach tree,; peach garden, 77
pelesit (familiar), 240
Pelletier, K.R., 295
Pen T'sao (Book on Herbs), 104
Pentecostal(ism), 178, 180, 291
peta (hungry ghost), 221
Peters, L., xix
phanung (piece of cloth, wrapped around the hips like a skirt), 218, 247
phoenix (luan), 168
Phra Narai, 42, 76, 118, 215, 217
Phra Sri Ariya Maitreya, 205

Phrom Mali, 36, 116, 117, 201, 202
p'ing an ch'iao (wooden bridge), 56
pitr (ancestor spirit), 75
planchette, 165
p'o ching (embryonic essence), 149
pollution, 4, 70
pomegranate (nim, margosa), 53
Pope Paul VI, 179, 205
possession, xvii, 5, 35, 37-39, 40, 61, 62, 64-71, 74, 75, 96, 146, 168, 180, 200, 202, 203, 205, 211, 216, 218, 219, 221, 222, 262, 292, 297, 298; horse possession, 68, 182; tiger possession, 67, 68, 115
Potter, J., 228
Prabhavananda, S. and Ch. Isherwood, xviii, 75, 89, 283, 302
prasad (food offerings, taken home and eaten to ingest the Divine), 72, 131, 245
Pratyeka Buddha, 159
precepts (rules of discipline), 267, 292
prick ball, 56; see also teng k'au,
Prince, M., 175, 176
Prince, R., xxiii, 60, 228
psychiatrist(s), xviii, 59, 97, 102, 109, 144, 176
psychoneuroimmunology, 228, 229
psychopath(ology), 4, 294
psychopomp (soul guide), 5, 294
psychosis, 4, 294
psychotic, 58
Pu Sawan (Divine Sages), 111, 117, 118, 203, 204, 209-214
pūjā (worship) 129; puṣpa pūjā (flower offerings), 130, 245
puranas, xx, 283

purification, 93
Quah, St., 105
Qur'an, see Koran
raksa (to cure), 219
Rāma, 6, 75, 129, 227, 243, 245, 246, 283
Rama V, 17, 260; see also Chulalongkorn
Ram Kamhaeng, 17
Rashomon effect, xxii, xxiv
Ravana, 6
rebab (spike fiddle), 189, 191, 241
Red Swastika Society, 43, 86, 168
revelation, 42
Rg Veda, 74, 283
rian (to study), 119
rites of passage, 47, 98, 154, 296
ritual, xix, 9, 41, 48, 49, 89, 90, 99, 148, 161, 168, 180, 186, 219, 223, 227, 229, 245, 263, 278, 292, 296
Rituale Romanum, 281
Rizvi, S.A.A., 264
Robinet, I., 147
Rouget, G., 65
sacrifice, 10, 97, 99, 185
sacrificial, 292
Sakyamuni (Shin-chia-mo-ni-fo), 89, 234
samādhi (highest concentration), 205, 216
San Francisco Examiner, 38
sandbox writing, 168
Sangha, xx, 37, 206, 207, 222
Saso, M.R., 147, 148
Schafer, E.H., 147-149, 161, 162, 266
Schipper, K.M., 266
schizophrenic(s), 4, 99, 181, 294

schizophrenia, 296
secret societies,
self-healing powers, 59, 93
Shaw, W., 263
shen (god, spirit), 9, 65, 165, 234
Shen Nung, 104
Shi'ites, 241, 261
Shirokogoroff, S.M., 4
Si-yiu-ki (A Record of Travels in the West), 234
Sikh, 19, 129, 205, 208, 209
Sikhism, 22
sīla (discipline), 205
Sills, D.L., 23
Silverman, J., xviii, 4
sinseh (Chinese healer), 105, 241
Sion Lim Temple, 133
siu-to (stomacher, apron), 53, 234
Sita, 6, 243, 245
Śiva, 37, 38, 75, 238, 243, 244, 245, 257, 258, 268, 283
Smith, A., 278
Somdetch Phra Phutajan Brahma Rangsi (Toh), 204, 207, 209
sonic driving, see auditory driving
Soothill, L.W. and L. Houdous, 267
spike ball, 32
spike chair, 26; see also teng-kio
spirit, bhuta, hantu, jinn, kuei, pelesit, peta, pitr, shen,
spirit medium, see bomoh, khon song, ki-tong, kong t'ung, loh-tang, tang-ki
spirit tiger, 6, 73, 195, 196, 238; see also belian
spiritual, xvi, 5, 7, 9, 37, 43, 71, 73, 74, 95, 98, 99, 101, 108, 110, 111, 138, 205, 226, 227, 229, 234, 290, 297
Spiro, M.E., xix, xxiii, 11, 12, 221, 263, 265
Sri Mariamman Temple, xvii, 25, 26, 261
stomacher, 68; see also siu-to
stūpa (dome-shaped mound), 206
Sun-heu-tze (monkey god), 79, 235, 251
Sunna (body of traditions), 241, 262
Sunni (belief that Muhammad's successor should be elected), 73, 241
Sunn'ite, 242, 262, 286
Supreme Patriarch Luang Pu Tuad, 204 205 207, 210, 212
Susruta Samhita, 103
sūtra (Sanskrit), sutta (Pāli), 75, 245, 263, 276, 302
swami, xxii, 44, 245
Swedenborg, E., 174
symbol(ism), 11, 71, 162, 297, 298
syncretism, 111, 163, 229, 291, 299
syncretistic, 163
Tai Chi Chuan, 156, 235
Tambiah, S.J., xix, 38, 58, 73, 263
t'ang (house altar, shrine), 235, 263
tang-ki (spirit medium), xxii, 36, 43, 235
Tantrayana, xix, 276
tantric, 80, 244
Tao Maha Brahma Jina Panara, 204, 211
Taoism, 22, 33, 76, 95, 150, 152, 162, 167, 170, 299, 300
Taoist, 6, 19, 33, 34, 40, 44, 49, 55, 80, 85, 89, 91, 107, 108, 125, 133, 141, 146-148, 150-152, 156, 158-161, 167, 180, 226, 227, 266, 300

Index

taqdir (Allah's will), 107
Tart, Ch., xxiii, 228, 271
tatoo, 58
teng k'au (prick ball), 56, 235
teng-kio (spike chair), 56, 235
Thaipusam, 3, 25, 35, 258, 261
tham khwan, 201, 249
Thematic Apperception Test (TAT), xxiii
therapeutic, 112
Theravāda, xix, 9, 16, 91, 134, 156, 157, 217, 243, 263, 267, 275, 292
Theravadin (follower of the only extant early Buddhist school), 75, 264
Thomas, M.L., 17
Three Kingdoms (220-280 A.D.), 6, 44-45, 77, 125
Three Worlds, 75
Tibetan Book of the Dead, 51
T'ien Hou (Queen of Heaven), 77, 80, 150, 236
Tillich, P., xv, 101, 102, 299
Timiti (walking on a bed of flowers) see fire walking, xvii, 3, 25, 26, 35, 257, 261
to kio (sword chair), 235
Toa Peh Kong, 78, 235, 251, 253
Totemism, 301
Torrey, E.F., 103, 229
Tou Mu (Goddess of the North Star), 79, 149, 150, 152, 154, 163, 235
trance, xv, 33, 35, 48, 54, 55, 58, 59, 62, 67-71, 88, 89, 130, 183, 184, 187, 200, 223, 297, 301
transcendent(al), 9, 67
transference, 301
transmigration, 34, 94

Triple Gem, 222
Turner, V., xxiii, 99, 104, 127, 179, 229, 277, 296
Turton, V., 219, 221
tying wrists, 266
tz'u (shrine, sanctuary), 235
Tzu-ku, 164, 165
upanisads, 283
upāsaka (layman), 245
upāsikā (laywoman), 245
upekkha (equanimity), 216
upaya (useful means), 38, 73
Ursus Mayor, 266; see also Big Dipper
Vajrapani, 80
Vajrayana, xix, 276
Van Gennep, A., 98, 154, 229, 287, 296
Vedas, xx, 74, 277, 283
vel (Murgam's spear), 75, 130, 245
vibhuti (cow dung ash), 53, 130, 131, 245
Vinaya (227 rules of discipline for Theravāda monks), 263
vision, 42, 64, 301; vision quest, 197
Viṣṇu, 34, 38, 75, 76, 217, 245, 246, 267, 283
wai khru (pay respect to one's teachers), 218, 250, 259
Waldron, Ch., 175
Wallace, A.P.C., 59
Wallnofer, 273, 274, 281, 300
Walpurgis Night, 186
Walters, V.J. and W.G. Walters, 59
Wan Hooi Poh, 69, 70, 165
wan phra (Buddhist Sunday, celebrated at the half phases of the moon), 36, 201, 250
wang (king), 236

Wat Tham Krabod, 106, 116
Watts, A.W., xv
Wavell, St., A. Butt and N. Epton, xxiii, 301
Weber, M., 9, 12, 90, 95, 99, 100, 107, 108, 272, 273, 278
Webster's Third New Dictionary of the English Language, xvi, 178
Wee, V., xix
weretiger, 241; see belian
Winstedt, R.O., xix, 264
Winthrop, R.H., 179
winyan (soul), 216
Wolf, A.P., 76
Wong, C.S., 80
World Red Swastika Society, 166-168, 170, 268; see also Red Swastika Society
Worth, P., 174, 175
Wright, Th., 176

wu (shaman), 9, 10, 236
yak(sa) (Sanskrit), (Pāli) yakka (giant nature spirit), 160, 221, 246, 250
Yama (Lord of Death), 76, 252
yang (light, bright, positive, male principle), 236, 300
Yang, C.K., 7, 47, 90, 165
Yellow Emperor, 104, see also Huang-ti
Yellow Turbans, 77
yin (dark, negative, female principle), 203, 236, 300
yoga, 286, 302
yogi(n), 25, 75
Yu the Great, 148, 236
Zainul-Abidin Bin Ahman, 262
Zinberg, 59
Zoroastrianism, 302
Zoroastric, 288
Zuehlsdorf, V., 39, 219, 220

Thong, Denny, **A PSYCHIATRIST IN PARADISE- Treating Mental Illness in Bali**

A Psychiatrist in Paradise tells the story of a most remarkable attempt by an Indonesian doctor trained in Western medicine, and in charge of a Western-style hospital in Bali, in Indonesia, to use traditional healing practices in the treatment of mental illness. Bali, idealized by many as the archetypal island paradise, has its fair share of mental illness and, within its traditional culture, has developed ways of dealing with such illness that are significantly different from those traditionally espoused by Western medicine but which are now beginning to gain support in the West.

For nearly two decades Dr. Denny Thong strove to integrate modern (Western) health care systems with Balinese customs, decentralizing treatment to the villages, reorganizing the hospital to become a focal point of the community and, most controversially, utilizing the services of traditional healers. Dr. Thong closely studied the ways in which the traditional healers worked, and his survey of the healers and his descriptions and analyses of their procedures add immeasurably to our knowledge of the subject.

(Bangkok 1993) ISBN 974-8495-77-9
216 pp., 150 x 210 mm